Sexual Dysfunction: A New Era

Editors

ALAN W. SHINDEL
TOM F. LUE

UROLOGIC CLINICS OF NORTH AMERICA

www.urologic.theclinics.com

Consulting Editor
KEVIN R. LOUGHLIN

November 2021 • Volume 48 • Number 4

ELSEVIER

1600 John F. Kennedy Boulevard • Suite 1800 • Philadelphia, Pennsylvania, 19103-2899

http://www.theclinics.com

UROLOGIC CLINICS OF NORTH AMERICA Volume 48, Number 4
November 2021 ISSN 0094-0143, ISBN-13: 978-0-323-79829-7

Editor: Kerry Holland
Developmental Editor: Diana Ang

Urologic Clinics of North America (ISSN 0094-0143) is published quarterly by Elsevier Inc., 360 Park Avenue South, New York, NY 10010-1710. Months of issue are February, May, August, and November. Business and Editorial Offices: 1600 John F. Kennedy Blvd., Suite 1800, Philadelphia, PA 19103-2899. Periodicals postage paid at New York, NY and additional mailing offices. Subscription prices are $395.00 per year (US individuals), $1033.00 per year (US institutions), $100.00 per year (US students and residents), $450.00 per year (Canadian individuals), $1059.00 per year (Canadian institutions), $100.00 per year (Canadian students/residents), $520.00 per year (foreign individuals), $1059.00 per year (foreign institutions), and $240.00 per year (foreign students/residents). Foreign air speed delivery is included in all *Clinics* subscription prices. All prices are subject to change without notice. **POSTMASTER:** Send address changes to *Urologic Clinics of North America*, Elsevier Health Sciences Division, Subscription Customer Service, 3251 Riverport Lane, Maryland Heights, MO 63043. **Customer Service: 1-800-654-2452 (US). From outside the United States, call 1-314-447-8871. Fax: 1-314-447-8029. E-mail: JournalsCustomerServiceusa@elsevier.com (for print support)** and **JournalsOnlineSupport-usa@elsevier.com (for online support)**.

Reprints. For copies of 100 or more, of articles in this publication, please contact the Commercial Reprints Department, Elsevier Inc., 360 Park Avenue South, New York, New York 10010-1710. Tel.: 212-633-3874; Fax: 212-633-3820; E-mail: reprints@elsevier.com.

Urologic Clinics of North America is covered in MEDLINE/PubMed (*Index Medicus*), *Excerpta Medica, Current Contents/Clinical Medicine, Science Citation Index,* and *ISI/BIOMED.*

Contributors

CONSULTING EDITOR

KEVIN R. LOUGHLIN, MD, MBA
Emeritus Professor of Surgery (Urology),
Harvard Medical School, Visiting Scientist,
Vascular Biology Research Program at Boston
Children's Hospital, Boston, Massachusetts,
USA

EDITORS

ALAN W. SHINDEL, MD, MAS
Professor, Department of Urology, University
of California San Francisco, San Francisco,
California, USA

TOM F. LUE, MD, ScD (Hon), FACS
Professor of Urology, Emil Tanagho Endowed
Chair in Clinical Urology, Department of
Urology, University of California San Francisco,
San Francisco, California, USA

AUTHORS

MARY KATHRYN ABEL, AB
UCSF School of Medicine, San Francisco,
California, USA

BRYCE BAIRD, MD
Mayo Clinic Florida Urology Department,
Jacksonville, Florida, USA

NIMA BARADARAN, MD
Department of Urology, University of California
San Francisco, San Francisco, California, USA

SHARON L. BOBER, PhD
Director, Sexual Health Program, Department
of Psycho-oncology and Palliative Care, Dana-
Farber Cancer Institute, Associate Professor,
Department of Psychiatry, Harvard Medical
School, Boston, Massachusetts, USA

BENJAMIN N. BREYER, MD
Department of Urology, University of California
San Francisco, San Francisco, California, USA

GREGORY A. BRODERICK, MD
Mayo Clinic Florida Urology Department,
Jacksonville, Florida, USA

ARTHUR L. BURNETT, MD, MBA, FACS
James Buchanan Brady Urological Institute,
Johns Hopkins School of Medicine, Baltimore,
Maryland, USA

KRISTINA BUSCAINO, DO
Clinical Fellow, Sexual Medicine, Department
of Urology, Morsani College of Medicine,
University of South Florida, Tampa, Florida,
USA

RAFAEL CARRION, MD
Chairman, Department of Urology, Morsani
College of Medicine, University of South
Florida, Tampa, Florida, USA

KITTIPAT CHAROENKWAN, MD, MSc
Department of Obstetrics and Gynecology,
Faculty of Medicine, Chiang Mai University,
Chiang Mai, Thailand

BARBARA M. CHUBAK, MD
Assistant Professor, Department of Urology,
Icahn School of Medicine at Mount Sinai, New
York, New York, USA

CARLOS DELGADO, BS
Technologico de Monterrey, School of
Medicine and Health Science, Monterrey,
Nuevo León, Mexico

CHRISTIAN ERICSON, MD
Mayo Clinic Florida Urology Department,
Jacksonville, Florida, USA

RAUL E. FERNANDEZ-CRESPO, MD
Clinical Fellow, Sexual Medicine, Department
of Urology, Morsani College of Medicine,
University of South Florida, Tampa, Florida,
USA

MINDY GOLDMAN, MD
Department of Obstetrics, Gynecology, and
Reproductive Sciences, University of California
San Francisco, San Francisco, California, USA

MARTIN S. GROSS, MD
Assistant Professor, Section of Urology,
Dartmouth-Hitchcock Medical Center,
Dartmouth Geisel School of Medicine,
Lebanon, New Hampshire, USA

TOM F. LUE, MD, ScD (Hon), FACS
Professor of Urology, Emil Tanagho Endowed
Chair in Clinical Urology, Department of
Urology, University of California San Francisco,
San Francisco, California, USA

SUSAN M. MacDONALD, MD
Division of Urology, Penn State Health Milton
S. Hershey Medical Center, Hershey,
Pennsylvania, USA

NATNITA MATTAWANON, MD, MSc
Department of Obstetrics and Gynecology,
Faculty of Medicine, Chiang Mai University,
Chiang Mai, Thailand

ETHAN L. MATZ, MD
Department of Urology, Wake Forest School of
Medicine, Winston-Salem, North Carolina,
USA

**JOHN P. MULHALL, MD, MSc, FECSM,
FACS**
Director, Male Sexual and Reproductive
Medicine Program, Department of Urology,
Memorial Sloan Kettering Cancer Center, New
York, New York, USA

RICARDO MUNARRIZ, MD
Associate Professor, Department of Urology,
Boston University School of Medicine, Boston,
Massachusetts, USA

**JUNO OBEDIN-MALIVER, MD, MPH, MAS,
FACOG**
Assistant Professor, Department of Obstetrics
and Gynecology, Stanford University, Palo
Alto, California, USA

JESSE ORY, MD
Department of Urology, Miller School of
Medicine, University of Miami, Miami, Florida,
USA

RAGHAV PAI, BS
Department of Urology, Miller School of
Medicine, University of Miami, Miami, Florida,
USA

RANJITH RAMASAMY, MD
Department of Urology, Miller School of
Medicine, University of Miami, Miami, Florida,
USA

DAVID L. ROWLAND, PhD
Senior Research Professor, Department of
Psychology, Valparaiso University, Valparaiso,
Indiana, USA

RACHEL RUBIN, MD
IntimMedicine Specialists, Washington, DC,
USA

CAROLYN A. SALTER, MD
Fellow, Male Sexual and Reproductive
Medicine Program, Department of Urology,
Memorial Sloan Kettering Cancer Center, New
York, New York, USA

ALAN W. SHINDEL, MD, MAS
Professor, Department of Urology, University
of California San Francisco, San Francisco,
California, USA

ALEXANDRA SIEGAL, MD
Resident, Department of Urology, Icahn School
of Medicine at Mount Sinai, New York, New
York, USA

ALLEN SIMMS, MD
Department of Urology, University of California
San Francisco, San Francisco, California, USA

BRETT A. STARK, MD, MPH
Resident Physician, Department of Obstetrics, Gynecology, and Reproductive Sciences, University of California San Francisco, California, USA

VIN TANGPRICHA, MD, PhD
Division of Endocrinology, Metabolism and Lipids, Department of Medicine, Emory University School of Medicine, Atlanta, Georgia, USA; Atlanta VA Medical Center, Decatur, Georgia, USA

RYAN P. TERLECKI, MD
Department of Urology, Wake Forest School of Medicine, Winston-Salem, North Carolina, USA

NANNAN THIRUMAVALAVAN, MD
Assistant Professor, Urology Institute, University Hospitals Cleveland Medical Center, Case Western Reserve University School of Medicine, Cleveland, Ohio, USA

MARIA ULOKO, MD
San Diego Sexual Medicine, San Diego, California, USA

DANIELA WITTMANN, PhD, MSW
Associate Professor, Department of Urology, Adjunct Associate Professor, School of Social Work, University of Michigan, Ann Arbor, Michigan, USA

Contents

Foreword: Sexual Dysfunction: Continuing the Pursuit of a Horizontal Desire　　　xiii

Kevin R. Loughlin

Preface: Managing Sexual Dysfunction in 2021 and Beyond　　　xv

Alan W. Shindel and Tom F. Lue

Incorporating the Principles of Sex Therapy into Urologic Care　　　425

Daniela Wittmann and Sharon L. Bober

> Urologic conditions and their treatments can have a significant impact on patients' sexual functioning and sexual health. Although urologists address sexual dysfunction within their scope of practice, sexual health conversations occur rarely and focus narrowly on physiologic sexual function. The sex therapy perspective considers biologic, psychological, relationship, and cultural aspects of sexuality. We propose that urologists benefit from taking this perspective when performing sexual health assessment. Urologists are not required to provide sex therapy but can optimize their patient's sexual well-being by taking a holistic perspective on sex and offering informational resources and referral to colleagues with complementary sexual health expertise.

Sexual Dysfunction in Transgender People: A Systematic Review　　　437

Natnita Mattawanon, Kittipat Charoenkwan, and Vin Tangpricha

> Transgender people may choose to affirm their gender identity with gender-affirming hormone therapy (GAHT) and/or gender-affirming surgery (GAS). The effects of GAHT and GAS on sexual health in transgender people have not been well elucidated. This systematic review aimed to appraise the current scientific literature regarding sexual desire, arousal, orgasm, pain, and satisfaction in transmen and transwomen before, during, and after gender transition. Overall, sexual dysfunction is common in both transmen and transwomen. GAHT and GAS may help to improve sexual satisfaction. More studies that focus on sexual health in the transgender population are urgently needed.

Sexual Wellness in Cisgender Lesbian, Gay, and Bisexual People　　　461

Brett A. Stark, Juno Obedin-Maliver, and Alan W. Shindel

> Cisgender sexual minority persons have sexual wellness needs that go well beyond disease prevention. Despite historical asymmetries in research and clinical attention to sexual wellness in cisgender lesbian, gay, and bisexual persons, a growing body of evidence exists on how to optimally care for these populations. Additional research and development is warranted.

Pharmaceutical and Energy-Based Management of Sexual Problems in Women   473

Alexandra Siegal and Barbara M. Chubak

> This article summarizes and critiques the evidence for use of available pharmaco-
> therapies (vasoactive, psychoactive, and hormonal medications) and energy-
> based therapies (laser, radiofrequency, shockwave, and neurostimulation) for treat-
> ment of female sexual dysfunction. The enthusiasm with which energy-based treat-
> ments for sexual dysfunction have been adopted is disproportionate to the amount
> of data currently available to support their clinical use. Pharmacotherapy for female
> sexual dysfunction has considerably more research evidence to justify its use. Pa-
> tients must be empowered to make an informed, autonomous determination as to
> whether the risk/reward ratio favors the use of pharmacotherapy, energy-based
> therapy, or some other treatment intervention.

Managing Female Sexual Pain   487

Maria Uloko and Rachel Rubin

> Female sexual pain disorder or genito-pelvic pain/penetration disorder (GPPPD),
> previously known as dyspareunia, is defined as persistent or recurrent symptoms
> with one or more of the following for at least 6 months: marked vulvovaginal or pelvic
> pain during penetrative intercourse or penetration attempts, marked fear or anxiety
> about vulvovaginal or pelvic pain in anticipation of, during, or as a result of penetra-
> tion, and marked tensing or tightening of the pelvic floor muscles during attempted
> vaginal penetration. In this review, we discuss etiology, diagnosis, and treatment for
> common disorders that cause GPPD.

Oncology Survivorship and Sexual Wellness for Women   499

Mindy Goldman and Mary Kathryn Abel

> Sexual dysfunction is extremely common in cancer survivors. Cancer survivors are
> living longer, and survivorship issues like sexual functioning are now a part of routine
> cancer care. Oncology providers need to be as comfortable assessing and address-
> ing these issues as they would any other aspect relating to cancer care. Providers
> should know how to perform an evaluation for sexual dysfunction, understand basic
> treatment options, and have appropriate referrals available to ensure that the pa-
> tient's needs are met. This review provides an overview of sexual dysfunction per-
> taining to women who are survivors of cancer and articulates areas needing
> further research.

Physiology of Erection and Pathophysiology of Erectile Dysfunction   513

Susan M. MacDonald and Arthur L. Burnett

> The science of penile erection, including recent advances in its molecular physiology
> and neuroanatomic pathways, is described. The pathophysiology of erectile
> dysfunction is presented, acknowledging associated disease states, and accord-
> ingly follows a practical classification scheme: vasculogenic, neurogenic, endocrine,
> and psychogenic.

Optimizing Outcomes in Penile Implant Surgery   527

Raul E. Fernandez-Crespo, Kristina Buscaino, and Rafael Carrion

 Video content accompanies this article at http://www.urologic.theclinics.com.

Since their initial release in the 1970s, modern penile prostheses have been subjected to continuous improvement with respect to both device engineering and surgical technique. Proper implantation begins with appropriate patient selection and counseling; these are essential elements to optimize results and set expectations postoperatively. An evidence-based protocol for the prevention of infections is essential. A pain management protocol should be initiated even before surgery. Strict adherence to recommended intraoperative techniques minimizes the risk complications; when complications occur, a step-by-step process for management improves odds of resolution. Safe techniques to increase the perceived or actual penile length postimplant can markedly improve patient satisfaction. Postoperatively, the surgeon and the patient should follow strict evidence-based instructions to optimize the overall outcomes of penile prosthesis surgery.

Is There a Role for Vascular Surgery in the Contemporary Management of Erectile Dysfunction?   543

Ricardo Munarriz, Nannan Thirumavalavan, and Martin S. Gross

Erectile dysfunction management is intended to restore capacity for penile erection. Although effective, none of the currently available treatments approved by the US Food and Drug Administration reverse erectile dysfunction pathophysiology. Penile arterial bypass surgery is intended to restore erectile function without the need for the chronic use of vasoactive medications or penile prosthesis placement. In select cases, venous ligation surgery may be beneficial, but this approach is not supported by the most recent guidelines on erectile dysfunction management. The lack of high-quality research surrounding penile vascular surgery has limited its use.

Penile Fractures: Evaluation and Management   557

Allen Simms, Nima Baradaran, Tom F. Lue, and Benjamin N. Breyer

Penile fracture is a urologic injury with an etiology that varies based on the cultural milieu. Diagnosis can be made based on history and physical examination alone. Patients should be evaluated with RUG or cystoscopy when urethral injury is suspected. Ultrasound or MRI is a helpful adjunct when the diagnosis is unclear, and can assist in identifying the location of the rupture. Surgical management is favored over conservative measures to improve outcomes. Delayed surgical repair may not be inferior to immediate intervention.

Management of Priapism: 2021 Update   565

Christian Ericson, Bryce Baird, and Gregory A. Broderick

Priapism is defined as a persistent penile erection lasting more than 4 hours. Priapism is a rare condition but when present it requires prompt evaluation and definitive diagnosis. Priapism has 2 pathophysiologic subtypes: ischemic and nonischemic. Ischemic priapism accounts for a majority of cases reported. Ischemic priapism is a urologic emergency and requires intervention to alleviate pain and prevent irreversible damage to erectile tissues. This article highlights current guidelines and the contemporary literature on priapism.

A Conceptual Approach to Understanding and Managing Men's Orgasmic Difficulties   577

David L. Rowland

Premature ejaculation (PE) and delayed/inhibited ejaculation (DE) are 2 ejaculatory problems that may negatively affect the sexual relationship and cause distress. Although no specific cause explains these problems when they have been lifelong conditions, understanding both biological and psychological factors may be relevant to treatment choices, with options ranging from pharmacologic to psychobehavioral. Integrating treatment modalities may lead to better outcomes but may also require greater psychological and resource investment from the patient or couple.

Oncosexology: Sexual Issues in the Male Cancer Survivor   591

Carolyn A. Salter and John P. Mulhall

Oncosexology is a multidisciplinary field composed of physicians, nurses, psychologists, and other health care professionals focusing on sexual issues in patients with cancer. Although any cancer diagnosis or treatment can be associated with sexual dysfunction, pelvic malignancies (such as prostate, bladder, or colorectal cancer) have the highest rates of sexual dysfunction in men. This includes erectile dysfunction, testosterone deficiency, ejaculatory dysfunction, orgasmic dysfunction, sexual incontinence, and penile shortening. Testicular cancer and hematologic malignancies also have a significant impact on patients' sexual function. Health care providers should address sexual dysfunction with their patients, including any adverse effects of potential treatment options.

Energy-Based Therapies for Erectile Dysfunction: Current and Future Directions   603

Raghav Pai, Jesse Ory, Carlos Delgado, and Ranjith Ramasamy

Energy-based therapies are novel treatments for erectile dysfunction that are thought to work by stimulation of tissue vasodilation, neoangiogenesis, and so forth. Low-intensity extracorporeal shock wave therapy (Li-ESWT) is the energy-based therapy with the most robust evidence basis demonstrating efficacy and safety. Among this evidence, randomized controlled trials (RCTs) evaluating Li-ESWT have largely been focused on responders to phosphodiesterase-5 inhibitors. Many of these RCTs have limitations including short follow-up durations, inconsistent protocols, and small sample sizes. Until more diverse patient populations are studied and these limitations are addressed, the use of Li-ESWT should remain limited to IRB-approved clinical research trials.

Stem Cell and Gene-Based Therapy for Erectile Dysfunction: Current Status and Future Needs   611

Ethan L. Matz and Ryan P. Terlecki

Erectile dysfunction affects an increasing number of men. The mainstays of management include oral medications, local erectogenic agents, and surgical placement of prosthetic devices. Newer technologies such as stem cell and gene therapy have been investigated as a means to restore spontaneous erectile capacity. Mesenchymal stem cells are thought to produce a local immunomodulatory and pro-repair milieu at the area of injury or needed repair. Gene therapy involves targeting the erectogenic pathway to augment factors involved in producing a natural erection. Such therapies are considered experimental and should be used in the setting of a clinical trial with appropriate oversight.

UROLOGIC CLINICS OF NORTH AMERICA

FORTHCOMING ISSUES

February 2022
Minimally Invasive Urology: Past, Present, and Future
John Denstedt, *Editor*

May 2022
Urologic Pharmacology
Craig Comiter, *Editor*

August 2022
Urologic Reconstructive Surgery
Jill Buckley, *Editor*

RECENT ISSUES

August 2021
Prostate Cancer Genetics: Changing the Paradigm of Care
Leonard G. Gomella and Veda N. Giri, *Editors*

May 2021
The Changing Landscape of Urologic Practice
Deepak A. Kapoor, *Editor*

February 2021
Robotic Urology: The Next Frontier
Jim C. Hu and Jonathan E. Shoag, *Editors*

SERIES OF RELATED INTEREST
Surgical Clinics of North America
https://www.surgical.theclinics.com/

Foreword

Sexual Dysfunction: Continuing the Pursuit of a Horizontal Desire

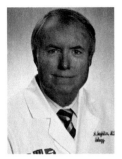

Kevin R. Loughlin, MD, MBA
Consulting Editor

"Dancing is a perpendicular expression of a horizontal desire." This quote has been attributed to the playwright George Bernard Shaw.[1] Since the dawn of time, humanity has been obsessed with sexual function and dysfunction. After all, besides other issues, it is the way we perpetuate our species.

Doctors Shindel and Lue have produced a truly landmark work in this issue of *Urologic Clinics of North America*. It is notable, that, for years, this area of medicine was often referred to as male sexual dysfunction, a rather myopic and gender-biased view of the topic. This issue provides an overview of the issues involved in both male and female dysfunction as well as issues involved in lesbian/gay/bisexual/transgender (LGBT) patients. The topics covered are both current and forward looking.

The interest in sexual function can be traced to the beginnings of recorded history. Reports have been found in Egyptian tombs, on Greek paintings, and in the *Old Testament*.[2] In the modern era, the Massachusetts Male Aging Study revealed that in otherwise healthy men, aged 40 to 70 years, 52% reported erectile dysfunction.[3]

The ancient Greeks and Romans wore talismans of rooster and goat genitals, and in the thirteenth century, the friar Albertus Magnus advocated ingesting roasted wolf penis as remedies for sexual dysfunction.[4] By the eighteenth century,

Doctor Samuel Solomon created a balm composed of cardamon, brandy, and cantharides that was applied to the testicles in a cold-water bath.[4] This was intended to prevent a man's desire to masturbate, which was thought to decrease his semen reserves and therefore contribute to sexual dysfunction.

By the nineteenth century, the role of testosterone in male sexual function was beginning to become appreciated. The French physician, Charles Edward Brown-Sequard, began injecting himself with testicular extracts from dogs and guinea pigs.[5] This progressed to the Russian surgeon, Serge Voronoff, who performed testicular graft transplants from apes into human testes.[6] These attempts were all unsuccessful in increasing testosterone levels, but they provided an underpinning for further research. In 1935, Adolph Butenandt was able to synthetize testosterone from cholesterol, which resulted in his sharing the Nobel Prize with Leopold Ruzica in 1939.[7]

In 1998, the Food and Drug Administration approved the first oral treatment for erectile dysfunction, sildenafil.[7] This ushered in a series of new oral, injectable, intraurethral, and topical treatments for erectile dysfunction over the next two decades.

Parallel to these medical treatments for male sexual dysfunction were surgical treatments as well. In 1936, Nicolas Borgoras fashioned the first

Urol Clin N Am 48 (2021) xiii–xiv
https://doi.org/10.1016/j.ucl.2021.07.005
0094-0143/21/© 2021 Published by Elsevier Inc.

penile implant using rib cartilage and bone. In the 1950s, Willard Goodwin and William Scott used acrylic rods to treat impotence.[8] In 1973, Brantley Scott implanted the first three-piece implantable penile prosthesis, which introduced a new era of surgery.[9]

Doctors Shindel and Lue have produced a unique work that both captures the present and provides a glimpse of the future. Sexual Dysfunction: A New Era encompasses not just therapies for the traditional view of male sexual dysfunction but also significantly expands the discussion to include female sexual dysfunction and dysfunction in those with alternative lifestyles as well. They include discussions of sexual wellness and pain in women as well as sexual wellness in the LGBT community. It is truly a state-of-the-art issue. The horizontal desire continues unabated throughout humanity.

Kevin R. Loughlin, MD, MBA
Vascular Biology Research Program at
Boston Children's Hospital
300 Longwood Avenue
Boston, MA 02115, USA

E-mail address:
kloughlin@partners.org

REFERENCES

1. Dancing is a perpendicular passion of a horizontal desire. Quote Investigator. Available at: https://quoteinvestigator.com/2016/09/11/dancing. Accessed July 3, 2021.
2. Carson CC. History of urologic prosthesis. In: CC Carson, editor. Urologic prosthesis: the complete practical guide to devices, their implantation and patient follow up. Tatawa, NJ: Humana Press; 2002. p. 1–7.
3. O'Donnell AB, Araujo AB, McKinlay JB. The health of normally aging men: the Massachusetts Male Aging Study (1987-2004). Exp Gerontol 2004;39:975–84.
4. McLaren A. Impotence: a cultural history. Chicago: University of Chicago Press; 2007.
5. Brown-Sequard EC. The effects produced on man by subcutaneous injections of liquid from the testicles of mammals. Lancet 1889;134:105–7.
6. Voronoff S. Rejuvenation by grafting. London: Allen and Unwin; 1925.
7. Payne R. Erectile dysfunction: a historical review. In: Whitelaw WA, editor. Proceedings of the 13th Annual History of Medicine Days. Calgary, Alberta, Canada: Faculty of Medicine, University of Calgary; p. 365–377.
8. Goodwin WE, Scott WW. Phalloplasty. J Urol 1952;68:903–8.
9. Scott FB, Bradley WE, Timm GW. Management of erectile impotence: use of implantable inflatable prosthesis. Urology 1973;2(1):80–2.

Preface

Managing Sexual Dysfunction in 2021 and Beyond

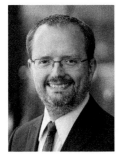

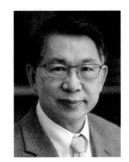

Alan W. Shindel, MD, MAS   Tom F. Lue, MD, ScD (Hon), FACS

Editors

The tumultuous events of 2020 have challenged our health care system. In the face of such upheaval and challenge, should we as health care providers be concerned with issues of sexual wellness and satisfaction? Aren't there bigger problems to address?

The editors and authors of this current issue of *Urologic Clinics of North America* reply emphatically that sexual wellness matters. Sexuality is a uniquely human phenomenon; sexual reproduction is present in many species, but the meaning we assign to it is part of what makes us different from other living things. Because sex is so human, it plays an essential role in human well-being. Hence, the value we add to our patients lives by helping them achieve sexual wellness is substantial and important.

The biomedical approach to sexual wellness was pioneered by Masters and Johnson a little over 60 years ago. It was about 50 years ago that modern penile prostheses first became available. Approximately 40 years ago, nonsurgical management of erectile dysfunction (ED) came of age with the development of the intracavernosal injection of vasodilators, which were followed by intraurethral vasodilators and vacuum erection devices. The nitric oxide pathway that regulates genital vasodilation was elucidated approximately 30 years ago, leading to release of phosphodiesterase type 5 inhibitors as the first highly efficacious oral therapy for ED about 20 years ago. After decades of progress in the management of ED, the first oral pharmacotherapy for female sexual dysfunction was submitted for regulatory approval 10 years ago.

So, what is next? In this issue, expert clinicians and researchers on the cutting edge articulate their visions for the current state-of-the-art and what is next in management of sexual dysfunction.

We consider "Principles of Sex Therapy that Clinicians can Incorporate into Their Care of Patients" (Wittman, Bober) in the first article. Psychology and emotion cannot be extricated from sexuality; no matter the specifics of one's practice, an ability to understand what sex and sexual dysfunction mean to a patient is critical. We devote the articles "Sexual Wellness in Transgender Persons" (Mattawanon, Charoenkwan, Tangpricha) and "Sexual Wellness in Gay, Lesbian, and Bisexual Patients" (Stark, Obedin-Maliver, Shindel) to the care of lesbian/gay/bisexual/transgender (LGBT) persons. LGBT communities have been marginalized and neglected for many years, so improvement in our ability to care for these and other sexual minority groups is a priority.

We next consider the sexual wellness needs of women, another group that has been historically overlooked in the sexual medicine literature. Novel medical and procedural interventions have revolutionized our ability to care for women with sexual concerns and are considered in "Pharmaceutical and Energy-Based Management of Sexual Problems in Women" (Siegal, Chubak). Women experiencing sexual issues need no longer be told that sexual problems are "all in your head"; a

Urol Clin N Am 48 (2021) xv–xvi

https://doi.org/10.1016/j.ucl.2021.07.004

0094-0143/21/© 2021 Published by Elsevier Inc.

multidisciplinary biopsychosocial approach to women's sexual wellness is now possible. Sexual pain is a common issue in women of all sexual orientations and is considered in "Managing Female Sexual Pain" (Uloko, Rubin). We conclude our section on female sexual wellness with consideration of the special needs of women who have survived cancer in "Oncology Survivorship and Sexual Wellness for Women" (Goldman, Abel).

An update on our contemporary understanding of penile erection is included in "Physiology of Erection and Pathophysiology of Erectile Dysfunction" (MacDonald, Burnett). Optimization of penile injection therapy and penile prosthesis surgery is considered in "Optimizing Outcomes in Penile Implant Surgery" (Fernandez-Crespo, Buscaino, Carrion). These highly effective therapies have been available for decades, but many patients remain hesitant to consider them. "Is There a Role for Vascular Surgery in the Contemporary Management of Erectile Dysfunction?" (Munarriz, Thirumavalavan, Martin) is devoted to consideration of the role for vascular surgery in management of ED in 2021. Consideration of the two most common forms of "penile emergency" follows with updates on contemporary management of penile fracture in "Penile Fractures: Evaluation and Management" (Simms, Baradaran, Lue, Breyer) and priapism in "Management of Priapism: 2021 Update" (Ericson, Baird, Broderick). "A Conceptual Approach to Understanding and Managing Men's Orgasmic Difficulties" (Rowland) provides principles and advice germane to the assessment and management of male ejaculation/orgasm difficulties, a poorly understood and vexing set of problems. We conclude this section with the article, "Oncosexology: Sexual Issues in the Male Cancer Survivor" (Salter, Muhall), wherein we consider the needs of men who are survivors of cancer.

Energy transfer ("Energy-Based Therapies for Erectile Dysfunction: Current and Future Directions" [Pai, Ory, Delgado, Ramasamy]) and stem/gene therapy ("Stem Cell and Gene-Based Therapy for Erectile Dysfunction: Current Status and Future Needs" [Matz, Terlecki]) have the potential to restore erectile capacity without the need for "on-demand" therapies nor invasive procedures. Whether these technologies will find a place in the armamentarium of the sexual medicine remains ambiguous, but the current state-of-the-art is discussed herein.

We are hopeful you will find these articles of value in your care of patients.

Alan W. Shindel, MD, MAS
Department of Urology
University of California, San Francisco
400 Parnassus Avenue, Suite A-610
San Francisco, CA 94143-0739, USA

Tom F. Lue, MD, ScD (Hon), FACS
Department of Urology
University of California, San Francisco
400 Parnassus Avenue, Suite A-610
San Francisco, CA 94143-0739, USA

E-mail addresses:
alan.shindel@Ucsf.edu (A.W. Shindel)
tom.lue@ucsf.edu (T.F. Lue)

Incorporating the Principles of Sex Therapy into Urologic Care

Daniela Wittmann, PhD, MSW[a],*, Sharon L. Bober, PhD[b,c]

KEYWORDS

- Sex therapy • Urologic conditions • Biopsychosocial sexuality • Culture

KEY POINTS

- Most urologic conditions, such as lower urinary tract symptoms, neurogenic bladder, and urologic cancers, are associated with sexual dysfunction.
- The impact of urologic conditions on sexual function has implication for the patient, the partner, and for their relationship.
- The patient's sexual orientation, religion, and cultural background are integral to the patient's sexual experience.
- A screening sexual health assessment can help orient the patient to relevant sexual health specialists and resources.
- Sexuality is a biopsychosocial experience. Including the partner in the assessment and asking about unique needs related to sexual orientation, religion, or culture makes the patient feel seen and heard, and facilitates a more complete and effective evaluation of sexual issues.
- The availability of sexual health resources, such as informational brochures and links to educational and support programs, goes a long way to meeting patient informational needs.
- Providing patients with referral to a sexual health specialist can optimize patients' sexual well-being in the context of urologic conditions.

INTRODUCTION

Although sexual dysfunction is one of the most prevalent consequences of many urologic conditions, it is notable that counseling about sexual health is not routinely incorporated into care for most urology patients.[1,2] In a recent study of practice patterns regarding sexual health counseling among urologic oncologists, 75% of clinicians reported that they did not routinely discuss sexual function with their patients.[2] This is consistent with several previous studies showing that sexual health is typically not addressed by physicians.[3] In addition, the lack of attention to sexual health may reflect specific gender disparities. Urology providers are significantly less likely to counsel female patients undergoing radical cystectomy about various domains of sexual function compared with male cystectomy patients.[2] Studies of urology patients confirm this gap in care. Survivors of urologic cancers report significant unmet needs regarding information and support related to sexual function.[4]

Despite the clear gap in physician-patient communication about sexual health, almost all urologists believe sexual health counseling falls within their scope of practice and urologists and urology residents report a need for more training

[a] Department of Urology, School of Social Work, University of Michigan, 2800 Plymouth Road, Building 16, Room 110E, Ann Arbor, MI 49108-2800, USA; [b] Sexual Health Program, Department of Psycho-oncology and Palliative Care, Dana-Farber Cancer Institute, 450 Brookline Avenue, SW320, Boston, MA 02215, USA; [c] Department of Psychiatry, Harvard Medical School, Boston, MA, USA
* Corresponding author.
E-mail address: dwittman@med.umich.edu
Twitter: @DrWittmann (D.W.); @drsharonbober (S.L.B.)

Urol Clin N Am 48 (2021) 425–436
https://doi.org/10.1016/j.ucl.2021.06.003
0094-0143/21/© 2021 Elsevier Inc. All rights reserved.

in how to address this topic.[2,5–7] Clinical guidelines including those from the American Urologic Association, the American Cancer Society, and the American Society for Clinical Oncology state that clinicians should address sexual health, including counseling patients regarding the impact of treatment on sexual function and sexual rehabilitation.[8–10] It is therefore imperative to begin addressing specific barriers, such as providers' lack of knowledge about sexual health, their lack of communication training, and lack of awareness of resources and intervention strategies. A roadmap for urologists would incorporate inquiry and intervention about sexual health into routine clinical practice. In this article, we offer the principles of sex therapy, including a biopsychosocial understanding of sexuality, the need for sexual health assessment, and the value of multidisciplinary care as a framework for integrating sexual health as a routine aspect of urologic care.

SEXUAL HEALTH: A BIOPSYCHOSOCIAL MODEL

The World Health Organization states that sexual health is not merely the absence of disease, dysfunction, or infirmity, but rather a state of physical, emotional, mental, and social well-being in relation to sexuality that must be respected and protected.[11] This broad definition of sexual health is consistent with a biopsychosocial understanding of sexuality, which directs the clinician to consider the biologic/physiologic, psychological, and social/interpersonal elements of a presenting dysfunction.[12] It positions the experience of sexual heath and sexual function at the intersection of physiologic, psychological, and sociocultural factors.

When assessing a patient with a sexual concern the clinician must undertake not only a physical review of systems but also consider an individual's lived experiences; this should include assessment of past and present history of sexual trauma, depression, anxiety, or other psychological distress that may be contributing to their current experience of sexual dysfunction. Individual experiences also vary with regard to perceived body image, perceived attractiveness, and sexual self-efficacy. For example, when an ostomy patient is struggling with feeling damaged, uncomfortable, or ashamed, it is insufficient to assess only the mechanical aspects of sexual function, such as capacity to get an erection or the ability to reach orgasm.

This model underscores the necessity of assessing the interpersonal sexual context, including the romantic relationship, and the partner's experience. It has been demonstrated that the partner's sexual function is directly impacted by the patient's experience and that partners have a direct impact on one another.[13] For example, partners of patients with prostate cancer often report more distress than patients themselves and prostate cancer treatment has been shown to have a profound impact on the partner as an individual and the couple as a unit.[14] Single, older patients, and/or patients with disability may experience apprehension and concerns related to dating and sexuality; these concerns, whereas distressing, are commonly overlooked because assumptions are made that older, single, widowed, disabled, or divorced individuals may not be sexually active.[15]

Clinicians must also be aware of the influence of the broader sociocultural context on sexual health when attempting to inquire about and treat sexual dysfunction. Culture influences many aspects of sexual functioning, including what is acceptable sexual activity, how patients express symptoms, and how likely they are to feel distress and engage in help-seeking. It is therefore particularly important for urologists to provide culturally competent health care. Culturally competent health care is defined as adapting care to the cultural needs of individuals, providing equitable care, and having empathy for the individual.[16] Specific examples include accommodating, wherever feasible, a patient's preferences regarding the gender or other factors of their health care provider and inquiring about religious factors that may place restrictions on potentially therapeutic interventions that may involve practices, such as guided masturbation or extravaginal ejaculation.[17]

THE IMPACT OF UROLOGIC CONDITIONS ON SEXUALITY

Given the close proximity of organs and neurovascular systems in the pelvis, it is only natural to deduce that dysfunction in any part of this carefully organized functional system will affect others. Nearly every condition that involves the lower urinary tract affects sexuality, as do most urologic cancers and nonurologic lesions that impact on lower urinary tract function (eg spinal cord injury, neurodegenerative disease). Physical discomfort or pain that accompanies these conditions can lead to anxiety, depression, and loss of desire to be sexually engaged. The physical discomfort and anxiety about pain may lead the patient to increase tension in pelvic muscles, leading to high-tone pelvic floor dysfunction. Observing and interacting with the unhappy patient who is uncomfortable or in pain can become a source of uncertainty and psychological distress in the partner who, at some point, recognizes that his or her sex life has been altered. This cascade of effects underlies the complexity of sexual problems in patients with urologic conditions that are addressed in sex therapy, but should also be a part of the urologist's conceptual template.

LOWER URINARY TRACT SYMPTOMS

A large swath of urologic patients suffers from lower urinary tract symptoms (LUTS). LUTS are characterized by urinary urgency, frequency, nocturia, postvoid dribbling, and incontinence. In a global study of LUTS, Irwin and colleagues[18] found that 45% of the worldwide population were affected by at least one LUTS problem and predicted increasing prevalence of LUTS because of increasing population growth and overall aging of the worldwide general population. In an earlier population-based study reported on a European and Canadian sample, of the surveyed 19,165 participants, symptoms of LUTS were reported by 62.5% of men and 66.5% women.[19] LUTS are associated with several urologic conditions. Sexual desire, sexual function, and the ability to enjoy sexual activity may be impacted by LUTS, which can therefore negatively affect the sexual relationship.

Benign prostatic hyperplasia (BPH) is a common condition that occurs in aging men. According to Egan,[20] a review of the epidemiology of BPH and LUTS estimated that approximately 50% to 70% of men older than 50 experience BPH and LUTS, as do approximately 80% of men older than 70. Sexual function was evaluated by Rosen and colleagues[21] on a sample of 12,815 European men with BPH and LUTS. According to their study findings, 49% of the men reported erectile dysfunction (ED). Bother with ED increased with increased LUTS symptoms. The authors also report reduced ejaculation in 46% of men and no ejaculation in 5% of men. Ejaculation problems also increased with age and severity of LUTS symptoms. Sexual dysfunctions were shown to be independently related to age and LUTS severity and not related to comorbidities.[21] Leong and colleagues,[22] in a summary of surgical treatments to relieve the symptoms of LUTS, recognize that LUTS have a potential to induce ED and ejaculatory problems. He points to the more recent, minimally invasive treatments, such as UroLift, Rezum, and Aquablation, as having a better chance of preserving sexual function.[22] Medical treatments for BPH can compromise sexual function. Roehrborn and colleagues[23] assessed, in a randomized controlled trial of 389 men with BPH, the effect of combined tamsulosin and dutasteride treatment of erectile function and ejaculation. They found that there was a significant diminution of ejaculation and satisfaction, whereas erectile function was not affected.[23] The relationship between treatment with finasteride and men with ED has been noted in some studies but has not been fully demonstrated in randomized controlled trials.[24]

Incontinence or urine leakage is an aspect of other conditions, but as a singular phenomenon may simply appear and increase as a condition of the aging body. A study of community-dwelling men and women aged 50 to 90 (n= 391 women and 141 men) in the English Longitudinal Study of Aging (ELSA) reported the presence of urinary incontinence in 20% of women and 6.9% of men in the last 12 months.[25] In women, incontinence was associated with lower ability to become aroused and lower frequency of sexual activity. In men, incontinence was additionally associated with erectile and orgasmic difficulties. In a study comparing 66 couples coping with incontinence in the female partner and 95 control subjects who were younger, the patients and the male partners reported more sexual dysfunction than control subjects. The patients reported poorer sexual function, more sexual dissatisfaction, and avoidance, whereas the partners reported more sexual dissatisfaction, more ED, and less frequent sexual activity.[26] Similar findings were reported by Stadnicka and colleagues[27] who assessed women after labor and delivery. Of the 193 women participating, 16.6% had symptoms of stress incontinence and a significantly lower satisfaction with sex life, compared with women who did not have those symptoms.[27] These studies that originate in different parts of the world document a pervasive concern about sexual health that is, to date, largely not addressed in clinical care or research.

The impact of overactive bladder (OAB), a condition that includes urinary urgency, frequency, and incontinence, on sexual function has been described in men and women. According to Milsom and colleagues[28] who reported on a sample of 16,776 participants in six European countries, 42% of men and 58% of women endorsed LUTS symptoms associated with OAB. Irwin and colleagues[29] compared 502 male patients with OAB with 502 control subjects and found a higher level of ED in men with OAB (25.2% vs 15.6%; $P \leq .05$). Similarly, in a sample of 458 of Korean women, 19.9% of the participants reported that OAB symptoms affected their sexual life as compared with only 3.5% of participants without OAB ($P \leq .001$). Their emotional health was also affected: 22.7% reported anxiety and 39.3% reported depression, compared with 9.7% of participants in the control group who reported anxiety and 22.9% who reported depression. Only a small proportion (19.7%) of the participants with OAB reported that they had spoken to their health care provider about their urinary symptoms, although 50% were open to it.[30] Given the earlier noted lack of discussion of sexual concerns in urology practice, it is likely that most patients with OAB did not discuss their sexual concerns either as a part of their care, and that the lack of these discussions may be common worldwide.

Some urologic conditions, such as interstitial cystitis and prostatitis, include the experience of pelvic pain and pelvic floor dysfunction in men and women. Pelvic pain and pelvic floor dysfunction may be associated with sexual pain in women and some men, with ejaculation being the pain syndrome most common in men with these conditions.[31] The pathophysiology of both of these conditions remains elusive, but both are considered to be complex and influential factors in sexual dysfunctions.[15]

Interstitial cystitis, a noninfectious condition, is characterized by urinary urgency and frequency, nocturia, and pain with intercourse for women. A physical examination during which there is a mild pressure on the urethra can help recognize bladder pain and distinguish interstitial cystitis from dyspareunia that is gynecologically driven.[32] However, women with interstitial cystitis may also suffer from vaginal dryness, particularly if they are postmenopausal.[33] According to a review by Tonyali and Yilmaz,[34] more than 50% of women with interstitial cystitis report sexual dysfunctions in several studies. Gupta and colleagues[35] describe the complex nature of the condition, recognizing that pelvic floor issues and sexual health should be addressed in clinical care.

Chronic pelvic pain syndrome (formerly known as chronic prostatitis) is a common condition in men and is often associated with significant sexual dysfunction. Urinary urgency and frequency are presenting problems, but pelvic and testicular pain and pain with ejaculation can also be a part of the symptom complex. In two reviews, Muller and Mulhall[36] and Sadeghi-Nejad and Seftel[37] singled out chronic prostatitis and chronic pelvic pain syndrome as conditions that have been reported to result in significant sexual difficulties, including low libido, ED, and pain with ejaculation. Men with chronic prostatitis/chronic pelvic pain syndrome can present with low libido, premature ejaculation, ED, and pain with ejaculation. All lead to a decrease in quality of life. Cohen and colleagues[38] argue that pain with ejaculation may be caused by pelvic floor dysfunction and, in a review, propose pelvic floor rehabilitation as a methodology for alleviating it.

The need for sexual health care in neurogenic conditions, such as spinal cord injury, spina bifida, Parkinson disease, and multiple sclerosis, is gaining attention as sexual dysfunction in these conditions is increasingly documented. As with the other urologic conditions, there is a tendency to focus on physiologic function. However, attending to the whole person has been advocated more recently.[15,39–41] The patients' challenges have also been made evident recently. Streur and colleagues[15] describe the frustrations of women with spina bifida with not getting education about the impact of their condition on sexual function and ability to bear children, with being seen as asexual and therefore not provided with appropriate sexual and reproductive care support, and with having to navigate sexual relationships and health care "flying blind." Elliott[42] has written about sexual issues in spinal cord injury for many years, recognizing that clinicians are often poorly educated about the complex nature of sexual dysfunctions of patients with injured spines. Strategies are promoted that can leverage medications, devices, pelvic floor physical therapy as rehabilitation resources, include partners in the enterprise, and even reimagine sexual stimulation and arousal using human capacity for neuroplasticity.[42]

The impact of genitourologic cancers and their treatments on sexuality is probably the most studied area among urologic conditions. Surgical and radiation treatments for prostate and muscle-invasive bladder cancer in men result in ED and changes in orgasm; hormonal therapy for prostate cancer also diminishes libido, because of the loss of testosterone.[43–47] Patients and partners report significant distress and disruption of their relationships.[48–50] Women with muscle-invasive bladder cancer often undergo resection of the anterior vaginal wall, which may make vaginal intercourse painful or even impossible. Oophorectomy for ovarian or other gynecologic cancers can induce surgical menopause, which is often associated with low or no libido, vaginal dryness, and consequent dyspareunia.[51] Men and women with non-muscle invasive bladder cancer report disrupted and potentially diminished sexual activity during and after treatments, and fear of transmitting their disease to their partners through sexual intercourse.[52] Penile cancer may require partial or total penectomy, leading to partial or complete loss of capacity to have penetrative intercourse. Orchiectomy for testicular cancer may compromise testosterone production and can exert a negative psychological impact on the generally young men who must be treated with this surgery. Sexual health of patients with cancer has been, at least conceptually, recognized as an important aspect of cancer survivorship. Interventions have been developed and tested in prostate cancer.[53] Models exist that not only describe the experience of sexual recovery, but also provide guidance for sexual rehabilitation. These models emphasize the need to prepare patients and partners for the side effects of treatment and rehabilitation and the emotional impacts that these side effects bring to them. Patients and partners must be prepared for feelings of grief about the loss of sexual function and of the template for sexual interaction that they had developed in their relationship over time; the experience of frustration and failure as they learn to use sexual aids; for the need to be patient, use humor, and be optimistic about their ability to use their emotional strengths to move into a new sexual paradigm that accommodates these changes. The ability to work through this process has been known to bring couples closer together with a feeling of greater emotional intimacy and, in some cases, improved mutuality in their sex lives.[54,55]

SEXUAL HEALTH ASSESSMENT: PRINCIPLES OF SEX THERAPY

Sexual health assessment encompasses all domains of sexuality: the patient's biologic function, psychological experience, and the interaction of the couple in a cultural context. Comprehensive assessment can potentially uncover the origin of the dysfunction and reveal how the problem impacts other domains of function, which in turn informs the approach to treatment. Although busy clinicians often do not have the time or clinical capacity to undertake time-intensive sexual health assessment with all patients, an overview of the core domains of assessment is provided to demonstrate the key elements of evaluation that can optimally guide intervention. Thorough evaluation is often conducted in the context of multidisciplinary collaboration.

Sexual dysfunction has been defined by Vroege and colleagues[56] as "the various ways in which an individual is unable to participate in a sexual relationship as he or she would wish," including lack or loss of sexual desire, sexual aversion disorder, failure of genital response (eg, ED, rapid or dry ejaculation, poor vaginal lubrication), orgasmic dysfunction, nonorganic vaginismus, nonorganic dyspareunia, and excessive sexual drive." It is also important to add that this definition should include inability to engage in sexually stimulating oneself to one's satisfaction because not everyone is in a relationship.

Physiologic function domain assessment includes questions about desire, arousal, erectile function for men and lubrication and/or pain with intercourse for women, orgasmic capacity, and satisfaction. In urologic conditions, men's and women's pelvic pain must also be assessed to facilitate differential diagnosis. The history of the complaint and its pervasiveness must be elicited to understand whether it is lifelong or is triggered by events, whether it is situational or occurring in all circumstances. The Diagnostic and Statistical Manual of Mental Disorders, 5th edition emphasizes the importance of distress in conducting a functional evaluation. Functional variants, such as low desire/hypoactive sexual desire disorder and early ejaculation, were considered de facto dysfunctions in the past. In contemporary thinking these conditions are now considered true dysfunctions only if they cause bother within the person or within a couple.[57,58]

Psychological domain assessment focuses on the patient's feelings, beliefs, and cognitions about his/her dysfunction and on the patient's overall feeling of confidence as a sexual partner. Sexual dysfunction can trigger psychological distress in a person who had been sexually confident previously. A person who struggles with perceived lack of attractiveness or worries about feeling skilled as a sexual partner may face further deficit in sexual efficacy because of stress. Often there is a reciprocal influence of psychological and physiologic factors that need to be taken into consideration in the course of assessment and treatment.

Relationship domain evaluation comprises enquiring about the index patient's partner (or partners), including assessment of overall relationship quality, partner interest in sex, and the partner's own experience of sexual problems/difficulties that were preexisting or have developed since onset of the patient's sexual dysfunction.

Cultural and religious investigation explores the patient's beliefs and practices with respect to sexual expression, taboos, and interdictions that may be germane to sexual issues or their treatment.

Sexual history is an aspect of sexual health assessment that provides an opportunity to learn about the early influences on a patient's attitudes to sexuality, early experiences that were positive or negative, and experience of sexual relationships throughout puberty and adult life. This history includes inquiry about sexual abuse and trauma.

Personal history assessment helps identify any important life events that may have been influential, such as losses, experience of success and failure, and overall social integration. A personal history is a window into the patient's capacity for attachment, self-observation, reality testing and ability to flexibly adapt to challenges, and optimism versus pessimism. Potentially relevant issues also include history of medical illness, mental illness, substance abuse, physical abuse, and comorbidities.

BIOPSYCHOSOCIAL CASE CONCEPTUALIZATION AND TREATMENT RECOMMENDATIONS

Organizing sexual health assessment findings into a formulation that incorporates all dimensions of sexuality allows for a thoughtful approach to sexual rehabilitation. It begins with recognizing the biologic and physiologic realities, such as dysfunction based on hormone insufficiency or the impact of injury, a chronic condition, and/or medical treatments. The patient's psychological response reveals his/her strengths and vulnerabilities. Particular areas of import include ability to realistically appraise the situation, express and cope with feelings (eg, grief, loss), and engage internally and with others in the process of recovery. Historical events become relevant when assessing psychological coping. The availability and quality of a relationship either enhances or challenges the patient's coping, and cultural and religious factors influence the psychological and relationship resources and options for rehabilitation.

Conceptualization of the assessment findings can assist with making decisions about treatment recommendations. The decision making process is illustrated in **Fig. 1**.

TREATMENT OPTIONS

Sex therapy is typically tailored to the patient or the couple, based on the biopsychosocial assessment. Treatment is often an iterative process in the sense that there is an ongoing assessment of the patient's needs, based on newly uncovered information and progress. This means that a patient may begin in individual sex therapy, but later transition to a couple-based therapy or vice versa. Various techniques may become more relevant as treatment evolves (**Table 1**). It is not unusual that feelings of loss and grief are initially dominant as the patient (and partner) come to terms with changes that have resulted in sexual dysfunction. Patients and partners may have to accept that they may never return to baseline sexual function. As patients begin to accept the part that physiology plays in their sexual experience, they may begin to work on physical and psychological strategies for coping with sexual dysfunction and modifying couple sexual interactions. One example is use of sensate focus, a structured set of intentional touching exercises that reduce performance anxiety, and increase communication and nonjudging awareness of sensation. Psychological issues, such as depression, anxiety, and relationship dysfunction, complicate work on sexual recovery and are best addressed concurrently.

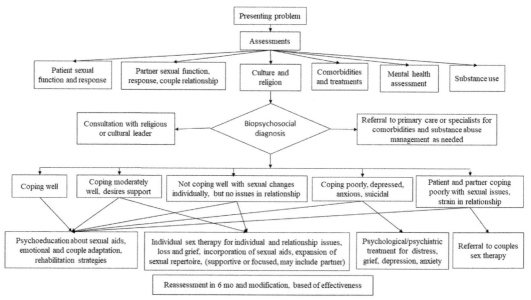

Fig. 1. Sex therapy treatment recommendations. (*Adapted from* Wittmann. Psychological treatment of individual sexual dysfunction. In Watson M and Kissane D (Eds), Sexual Health Fertility and Relationships in Cancer Care, 2020, Oxford University Press, New York).

Table 1
Sex therapy interventions to address sexual dysfunction

Intervention	Format	Desired Outcome
Psychoeducation review: sexual side effects, emotional and relationship impacts, rehabilitation options. Outline realistic expectations.	Individual patient, patient and partner or group setting for patients and partners.	Actionable sexual recovery plan, increased patient (and partner) competence and self-efficacy.
Sex therapy/counseling: coping with grief about sexual losses, addressing barriers to recovery, using strength-based approach to improve communication, and relationship engagement.	Individual patient, patient and partner.	Increased cognitive flexibility and coping skills to address sexual losses. Use of sexual aids as needed, increased engagement or re-engagement in sexual relationship. Improved communication.
Mindfulness meditation to increase sexual arousal.	Individual patient or group setting.	Increased nonjudging awareness of cognition and sensation. Use of curiosity for addressing negative thought interference.
Sensate focus exercise to re-engage comfortably in sensual and sexual activity.	Preferably as a couple, but can be used as self-exploration.	Discovery of sensual and sexual body foci, capacity to overcome embarrassment, anxiety, and enhanced focus on pleasure.
Expansion of sexual repertoire.	Individual patient may invite partner.	Increased awareness of sexual pleasure for the individual and in the relationship.
Couple's therapy.	Patient and partner.	Resolution of long-term issues, improved communication, and sexual dynamics.

Adapted from Wittmann. Psychological treatment of individual sexual dysfunction. In Watson M and Kissane D (Eds), Sexual Health Fertility and Relationships in Cancer Care, 2020, Oxford University Press, New York.

Collaboration with specialists in mental health, physical therapy, urology, gynecology, medical oncology, and radiation oncology may be needed for the patient with a sexual health problem related to urologic conditions to achieve his/her treatment goals (**Table 2**).

CLINICAL GUIDANCE FOR UROLOGISTS: ASK THE QUESTION

Most urologists and urology residents receive little to no training about how to initiate communication about sexual health. Often providers worry about opening a "Pandora's Box" (eg, the patient may ask questions that are too complicated or difficult to address within the scope of a busy clinical practice) if they start to inquire. It is our strong belief that it is incumbent on clinicians to incorporate inquiry about sexual health into a routine review of systems. It is critical that clinicians are equipped with tools and resources, so they can offer treatment of sexual problems directly and/or provide appropriate educational materials or referrals to appropriate sexual health experts for further treatment as needed.

Recent empirical research regarding enhancement of clinician communication about sexual health points to two key points: the need to improve clinicians' perceived confidence around sexual health communication, and the need to promote clinicians' beliefs that communication about sexual health will result in positive outcomes for their patients.[59] It is critical for urology providers to have the skills to initiate conversation about sexual health and the confidence that sexual health discussions can lead to positive outcomes for their patients.

Clinicians are more motivated to inquire about sexual health if they know how to ask and they are more likely to offer consultation if they know what to offer patients with regard to concrete referrals and resources. Two recent initiatives from different consensus groups offer useful tools to address these needs. The International Society

Table 2
Collateral medical interventions

Collateral Intervention	Format	Aim
Pelvic floor physical therapy	Individual patient	Improved strength and function of pelvic floor, increased capacity to relax and stretch pelvic floor muscles, decreased pain
Sexual medicine/urology evaluation	Individual patient, male partner	Evaluation to identify and treat symptoms including low testosterone, erectile dysfunction, genitourinary dysfunction
Gynecologic evaluation	Individual female partner	Conduct comprehensive physical examination to identify normal and abnormal findings and determine relationship to presenting sexual problems
Endocrine consultation	Individual patient	Evaluation to identify and treat endocrine abnormality, such as pituitary or thyroid disorder
Psychiatric consultation	Individual patient	Evaluation and medical management of mental health disorder including major depression and anxiety
General medicine consultation	Individual patient	Evaluation and treatment of comorbidities effecting sexual function, such as diabetes, cardiac disease, asthma, and substance abuse
Menopause consultation	Individual female partner	Evaluation and treatment of menopausal symptoms including hot flashes, sleep disruption, and estrogen deprivation

for the Study of Women's Sexual Health recently outlined a four-step process of care model for the identification of women's sexual concerns.[60] Steps include eliciting the patient's story, naming/reframing the sexual problem, empathic witnessing, and assessment and treatment. Consistent with this approach, we recommend initiating assessment by offering a ubiquity statement that assures the patient that sexual concerns are common and acknowledges that sexual concerns can be addressed. Such a statement also delivers an implicit message that sexual health is an aspect of care that is worthy of attention.

The International Consultation in Sexual Medicine-5 stepwise diagnostic and treatment algorithm identifies three basic principles including: (1) adoption of a patient-centered framework, (2) application of evidence-based medicine in diagnostic and treatment planning, and (3) use of a unified management approach in evaluating and treating sexual problems.[61] We agree that systematic use of a universal clinical checklist promotes uniformity of assessment and evaluation and suggest that the Brief Sexual Symptoms Checklists for Men and Women offer clinicians a useful tool for clinical evaluation (**Table 3**). Finally, it is imperative that clinicians build a referral network to call on and have access to basic educational resources that can be given to patients when a patient endorses a problem.

Table 3
Brief sexual health assessment

Brief Sexual Symptom Checklist for Men (BSSC-M)	Brief Sexual Symptom Checklist for Women (BSSC-W)
Please answer the following questions about your overall sexual function 1. Are you satisfied with your sexual function? ☐ Yes ☐ No If No, please continue. 2. How long have you been dissatisfied with your sexual function? 3a. The problem(s) with your sexual function is: (mark one or more) ☐ 1 Problem with little or no interest in sex ☐ 2 Problem with erection ☐ 3 Problem ejaculating too early during sexual activity ☐ 4 Problem taking too long, or not being able to ejaculate or have orgasm ☐ 5 Problem with pain during sex ☐ Problem with penile curvature during erection ☐ Other: 3b. Which problem is most bothersome (circle) 1 2 3 4 5 4. Would you like to talk about it with your doctor? ☐ Yes ☐ No	Please answer the following questions about your overall sexual function 1. Are you satisfied with your sexual function? ☐ Yes ☐ No If No, please continue. 2. How long have you been dissatisfied with your sexual function? 3a. The problem(s) with your sexual function is: (mark one or more) ☐ 1 Problem with little or no interest in sex ☐ 2 Problem with decreased genital sensation (feeling) ☐ 3 Problem with decreased vaginal lubrication (dryness) ☐ 4 Problem reaching orgasm ☐ 4 Problem with pain during sex ☐ 5 Other: 3b. Which problem is most bothersome (circle) 1 2 3 4 5 4. Would you like to talk about it with your doctor? ☐ Yes ☐ No

Adapted from Bober SL, Reese JB, Barbera L, et al. How to ask and what to do: a guide for clinical inquiry and intervention regarding female sexual health after cancer. Current Opinion in Supportive and Palliative Care, 2015; 10(1):44-54.

Clinicians will be more motivated to address this problem and start a conversation if they have a roadmap for clinical inquiry and resources to refer to as needed.

TAKE HOME POINTS

- Educating patients about the sexual impacts of their conditions and subsequent treatment is a good opening for normalizing patients' sexual concerns and making the topic open for discussion.
- It is important that clinicians ask about sexual health concerns when patients with urologic problems present for care, regardless of the condition, and assess how important and distressing identified sexual issues are to the patient. The four-question Brief Sexual Symptom Checklist screening tool[61] can help signpost the direction of a potential referral for sexual health care.
- A biopsychosocial perspective on sexuality should be a part of a urologist's mental assessment template. This means

recognizing that the patient may have feelings about his or her dysfunction and that including the partner, if one exists, gives room to the patient to fully communicate sexual concerns. Sociocultural factors may play a significant role with regard to a patient's sexual health and need to be considered as part of referral decision making. Most simply, a patient should respectfully be asked about any religious or cultural concerns that should be considered during a conversation about sexual health.

- A urologist should not feel pressured to go beyond his/her scope of practice. To minimize such pressure, it is helpful to establish reliable resources, such as brochures from the Urology Care Foundation or the American Cancer Society, that address specific issues in sexual health or develop brochures on site with the knowledge of the specific practice needs. For patients with cancer, online resources, such as cancersexnetwork.org, Will2Love.com, or SexualRecoveryAfterProstateCancer.org, are helpful. An online program for spinal cord injury patients, developed in Canada (https://scisexualhealth.ca/) provides sexual health information and support. The American Association of Sex Therapy Educators, Counselors and Therapists (aasect.org) helps identify sex therapists in every state in the United States. Sexual health professionals are also found on the Web sites of the Society for Sex Therapy and Research (sstar.org) and Sexual Medicine Society of North America (smsna.org).

- Clinicians who do not feel comfortable addressing sexual issues in their practice can pursue training available in established sexual health training programs, such as the University of Michigan Postgraduate Sexual Health Certificate Program (https://ssw.umich.edu/offices/continuing-education/certificate-courses/sexual-health), which provides targeted education for health care professionals, including physicians, nurses, physical therapists, physicians assistants, and others.

CLINICS CARE POINTS

- Patients frequently report unmet informational needs about the impact of urologic conditions on sexuality.
- A brief sexual health assessment, using a checklist, can facilitate a discussion of sexual health concerns that the patient may not bring up spontaneously. It can help evaluate what type of resources are needed.
- Providing education about the impact of a urologic condition on sexual function and sexual health reduces the stigma of having sexual problems.

DISCLOSURE

Dr. Wittmann is funded by the Movember Foundation to lead the International True North Sexual Recovery in Prostate Cancer Work Group. She is a member of the Board of Directors of the Sexual Medicine Society of North America (this ends in November 2021). She is Associate Editor of the Journal of Sexual Medicine. Dr. Bober is the Chair of the Scientific Network on Female Sexual Health and Cancer.

REFERENCES

1. Paterson C, Jensen BT, Jensen JB, et al. Unmet informational and supportive care needs of patients with muscle invasive bladder cancer: a systematic review of the evidence. Eur J Oncol Nurs 2018;35:92–101.
2. Gupta N, Kucirka LM, Semerjian A, et al. Comparing provider-led sexual health counseling of male and female patients undergoing radical cystectomy. J Sex Med 2020;17(5):949–56.
3. Parish SJ, Clayton AH. Sexual medicine education: review and commentary. J Sex Med 2007;4(2):240–68.
4. Bessa A, Martin R, Häggström C, et al. Unmet needs in sexual health in bladder cancer patients: a systematic review of the evidence. BMC Urol 2020;20(1):64.
5. Schloegl I, Köhn FM, Dinkel A, et al. Education in sexual medicine: a nationwide study among German urologists/andrologists and urology residents. Andrologia 2017;49(2):1–11.
6. Foley S, Wittmann D, Balon R. A multidisciplinary approach to sexual dysfunction in medical education. Acad Psychiatry 2010;34(5):386–9.
7. Krouwel EM, Grondhuis Palacios LA, Putter H, et al. Omissions in urology residency training regarding sexual dysfunction subsequent to prostate cancer treatment: identifying a need. Urology 2016;90:19–25.
8. Chang SS, Bochner BH, Chou R, et al. Treatment of non-metastatic muscle-invasive bladder cancer: AUA/ASCO/ASTRO/SUO guideline. J Urol 2017;198(3):552–9.
9. Skolarus TA, Wolf AM, Erb NL, et al. American Cancer Society prostate cancer survivorship care guidelines. CA Cancer J Clin 2014;64(4):225–49.
10. Carter J, Lacchetti C, Rowland JH. Interventions to address sexual problems in people with cancer: American Society of Clinical Oncology clinical practice guideline adaptation summary. J Oncol Pract 2018;14(3):173–9.
11. WHO SHDS. Defining sexual health: a report of a technical consultation on sexual health. World Health Organization, Sexual Health Document Series; 2002. Available at: https://www.who.int/health-topics/sexual-health#tab=tab_1.
12. Berry MD, Berry PD. Contemporary treatment of sexual dysfunction: reexamining the biopsychosocial model. J Sex Med 2013;1(11):2627–43.
13. Metz M, McCarthy B. The "good-enough sex" model for couple sexual satisfaction. J Sex Relations Ther 2007;351–62.
14. Wittmann D, Northouse L, Foley S, et al. The psychosocial aspects of sexual recovery after prostate cancer treatment. Int J Impot Res 2009;21(2):99–106.
15. Streur CS, Schafer CL, Garcia VP, et al. "If everyone else is having this talk with their doctor, why am I not having this talk with mine?": the experiences of sexuality and sexual health education of young women with spina bifida. J Sex Med 2019;16(6):853–9.

16. Henderson S, Horne M, Hills R, et al. Cultural competence in healthcare in the community: a concept analysis. Health Soc Care Community 2018;26(4):590–603.

17. Atallah S, Johnson-Agbakwu C, Rosenbaum T, et al. Ethical and sociocultural aspects of sexual function and dysfunction in both sexes. J Sex Med 2016; 13(4):591–606.

18. Irwin DE, Kopp Z, Agatep B, et al. Worldwide prevalence estimates of lower urinary tract symptoms, overactive bladder, urinary incontinence and bladder outlet obstruction. BJU Int 2011;108(7):1132–8.

19. Irwin DE, Milsom I, Hunskaar S, et al. Population-based survey of urinary incontinence, overactive bladder, and other lower urinary tract symptoms in five countries: results of the EPIC study. Eur Urol 2006;50(6):1306–14.

20. Egan KB. The epidemiology of benign prostatic hyperplasia associated with lower urinary tract symptoms prevalence and incident rates. Urol Clin North Am 2016;43:289–97.

21. Rosen R, Altwein J, Boyle P, et al. Lower urinary tract symptoms and male sexual dysfunction: the multinational survey of the aging male (MSAM-7). Eur Urol 2003;44:637–49.

22. Leong JY, Patel AS, Ramasamy R. Minimizing sexual dysfunction in BPH surgery. Curr Sex Health Rep 2019;111(3):190–200.

23. Roehrborn CG, Manyak MJ, Palacios-Moreno JM, et al. A prospective randomised placebo-controlled study of the impact of dutasteride/tamsulosin combination therapy on sexual function domains in sexually active men with lower urinary tract symptoms (LUTS) secondary to benign prostatic hyperplasia (BPH). BJU Int 2017;121(4):647–58.

24. Shin YS, Karna KK, Choi BR, et al. Finasteride and erectile dysfunction in patients with benign prostatic hyperplasia or male androgenetic alopecia. World J Mens Health 2018;37(2):157–65.

25. Lee DM, Telley J, Pendleton N. Urinary incontinence and sexual health in a population sample of older people. BJU Int 2017;(122):300–8.

26. Lim R, Liong ML, Leong WS, et al. Effect of stress urinary incontinence on the sexual function of couples and the quality of life of patients. J Urol 2016; 196:153–8.

27. Stadnicka G, Stodolak A, Pilewska-Kozak AB. Stress urinary incontinence after labor and satisfaction with sex life. Ginekologia Polska 2019;90:500–6.

28. Milsom P, Abrams L, Cardozo RG, et al. How widespread are the symptoms of an overactive bladder and how are they managed? A population-based prevalence study. BJU Int 2001;87:760–6.

29. Irwin DE, Milsom I, Reilly K, et al. Overactive bladder is associated with erectile dysfunction and reduced sexual quality of life in men. J Sex Med 2008;5: 2904–10.

30. Yoo ES, Kim BS, Oh SJ, et al. The impact of overactive bladder on health-related quality of life, sexual life and psychological health in Korea. Int Neurourol 2011;15:143–51.

31. Luzzi GA, Law IA. The male sexual pain syndromes. Int J STD AIDS 2006;17(11):720–6.

32. Wittmann D and Clemens JQ. The painful bladder syndrome and other urologic causes of chronic pelvic pain. In Chronic Pelvic Pain, Vercellini P (Ed) Wiley-Blackwell, Oxford, 2011. Ch. 9, pp. 86-97.

33. McLennan MT. Interstitial cystitis: epidemiology, pathophysiology and clinical presentation. Obstet Gynecol Clin North Am 2014;41:385–95.

34. Tonyali S, Yilmaz M. Sexual dysfunction in interstitial cystitis. Curr Urol 2017;11:1–3.

35. Gupta P, Gaines N, Sirls LT, et al. A multidisciplinary approach to the evaluation and management of interstitial cystitis/bladder pain syndrome: an ideal model of care. Transl Androl Urol 2015;4(6):611–9.

36. Muller A, Mulhall JP. Sexual dysfunction in the patient with prostatitis. Curr Urol Rep 2006;7:307–12.

37. Sadeghi-Nejad H, Seftel AD. Sexual dysfunction and prostatitis. Curr Urol Rep 2006;7:479–84.

38. Cohen D, Gonzalez J, Goldstein I. The role of pelvic floor muscles in male sexual dysfunction and pelvic pain. Sex Med Rev 2015;4:53–62.

39. Delaney KE, Donovan J. Multiple sclerosis and sexual dysfunction: a need for further education and interdisciplinary care. NeuroRehabilitation 2017; 41(2):317–29.

40. Stoffel JT, Van der Aa F, Wittmann D, et al. Fertility and sexuality in the spinal cord injury patient. World J Urol 2018;36(10):1577–85.

41. Bhattacharyya KB, Rosa-Grilo M. Sexual dysfunctions in Parkinson's disease. An underrated problem in a much discussed disorder. Int Rev Neurobiol 2017;134:859–76.

42. Elliott S. Sexual Dysfunction and infertility in individuals with spinal cord disorders. In Spinal Cord Medicine 3rd Edition, Kirshblum S & Lin VW (Eds), 2018, Demos Medical Publishing, Springer, New York.

43. Resnick MJ, Koyama T, Fan KH, et al. Long-term functional outcomes after treatment for localized prostate cancer. N Engl J Med 2013;368(5): 436–45.

44. Fode M, Serefoglu EC, Albersen M, et al. Sexuality following radical prostatectomy: is restoration of erectile function enough? Sex Med Rev 2017;5(1):110–9.

45. Incrocci L. Sexual function after external-beam radiotherapy for prostate cancer: what do we know? Crit Rev Oncol Hematol 2006;57(2):165–73.

46. Loi M, Wortel RC, Francolini G, et al. Sexual function in patients treated with stereotactic radiotherapy for prostate cancer: a systematic review of the current evidence. J Sex Med 2019;16(9):1409–20.

47. Gomella LG. Contemporary use of hormonal therapy in prostate cancer: managing complications and

addressing quality-of-life issues. BJU Int 2007; 99(Suppl 1):25–9 [discussion 30].

48. Hedestig O, Sandman PO, Tomic R, et al. Living after radical prostatectomy for localized prostate cancer: a qualitative analysis of patient narratives. Acta Oncol 2005;44(7):679–86.

49. Tanner T, Galbraith M, Hays L. From a woman's perspective: life as a partner of a prostate cancer survivor. J Midwifery Womens Health 2011;56(2): 154–60.

50. Wittmann D, Carolan M, Given B, et al. What couples say about their recovery of sexual intimacy after prostatectomy: toward the development of a conceptual model of couples' sexual recovery after surgery for prostate cancer. J Sex Med 2015;12(2): 494–504.

51. Avulova S. Optimizing women's sexual experience after radical cystectomy. Urol Gold J 2020;151: 138–44.

52. Kowalkowski MA, Chandrashekar A, Amiel GE, et al. Examining sexual dysfunction in non-muscle-invasive bladder cancer: results of cross-sectional mixed-methods research. Sex Med 2014;2(3): 141–51.

53. Wittmann D, Koontz BF. Evidence supporting couple-based interventions for the recovery of sexual intimacy after prostate cancer treatment. Curr Sex Health Rep 2017;9(1):32–41.

54. Walker LM, Wassersug RJ, Robinson JW. Psychosocial perspectives on sexual recovery after prostate cancer treatment. Nat Rev Urol 2015;12(3):167–76.

55. Elliott S, Matthew A. Sexual recovery following prostate cancer: recommendations from 2 established Canadian Sexual Rehabilitation Clinics. Sex Med Rev 2018;6(2):279–94.

56. Vroege JA, Gijs L, Hengeveld MW. Classification of sexual dysfunctions: towards DSM-V and ICD-11. Compr Psychiatry 1998;39(6):333–7.

57. Association AP: Washington, DC. Diagnostic and statistical manual of mental disorders. 5th edition 2013.

58. Parish SJ, Hahn SR. Hypoactive sexual desire disorder: a review of epidemiology, biopsychology, diagnosis and treatment. Sex Med Rev 2016;4(2): 103–20.

59. Reese JB, Lepore SJ, Daly MB, et al. A brief intervention to enhance breast cancer clinicians' communication about sexual health: feasibility, acceptability, and preliminary outcomes. Psychooncology 2019;28(4):872–9.

60. Parish SJ, Hahn SR, Goldstein SW, et al. The international society for the study of women's sexual health process of care for the identification of sexual concerns and problems in women. Mayo Clinic Proc 2019;95:5842–56.

61. Hatzichristou D, Rosen RC, Derogatis LR, et al. Recommendations for the clinical evaluation of men and women with sexual dysfunction. J Sex Med 2010;7(1 Pt 2):337–48.

Sexual Dysfunction in Transgender People
A Systematic Review

Natnita Mattawanon, MD, MSc[a],*, Kittipat Charoenkwan, MD, MSc[a], Vin Tangpricha, MD, PhD[b,c]

KEYWORDS

- Transgender health • Sexual dysfunction • Sexual distress • Transwomen • Transmen
- Transgender

KEY POINTS

- Sexual dysfunction is common in transgender people
- Gender-affirming hormone therapy decreases sexual desire and activity in transwomen but increases sexual desire and activity in transmen
- Gender-affirming surgery helps to improve sexual satisfaction in both transmen and transwomen
- Differences in hormone regimens and surgeries may impact sexual function
- There is a need for validated tools to assess sexual function and satisfaction in the transgender population

INTRODUCTION

There has been increased interest in transgender health over the past decade but less focus on the sexual health of transgender people. The current diagnostic criteria in the DSM 5 categorizes sexual health problems into 4 broad categories for both men and women. Men may experience delayed ejaculation, erectile disorder, male hypoactive sexual desire disorder, and premature ejaculation. Women may be diagnosed with female orgasmic disorder, female sexual interest/arousal disorder, and genito-pelvic pain/penetration disorder.[1]

There are no standard diagnostic criteria specific for sexual dysfunction in the transgender population. Transgender and gender nonbinary people may take gender-affirming hormone therapy (GAHT) or undergo gender-affirming surgery (GAS) procedures to align their gender identity with their appearance.[2,3] A transgender man or transman (TGM) is an individual who was assigned female at birth and has a gender identity of boy/man/male and most often seeks to transition their body and/or gender role to a more masculine body or role. A transgender woman or transwoman (TGW) is an individual who was assigned male at birth and has a gender identity of girl/woman/female and most often seeks to transition their body and/or gender role to a more feminine body or role. GAHT differs for transmen and women, which may alter sexual function differently. GAS for transmen includes chest reconstruction surgery, hysterectomy (with/without oophorectomy), vaginectomy, metoidioplasty, and phalloplasty. For TGW, GAS includes breast augmentation, orchiectomy, penectomy, and a creation of neovagina.[2] These GAS procedures change the genital

Conflict of Interest: The authors have nothing to disclose.
[a] Department of Obstetrics and Gynecology, Faculty of Medicine, Chiang Mai University, 110 Intawaroros road, Chiang Mai 50200, Thailand; [b] Division of Endocrinology, Metabolism and Lipids, Department of Medicine, Emory University School of Medicine, 101 Woodruff Circle NE-WRMB1301, Atlanta, GA 30322, USA; [c] Atlanta VA Medical Center, Decatur, GA, USA
* Corresponding author. Reproductive Medicine Unit, Department of Obstetrics and Gynecology, Faculty of Medicine, Chiang Mai University, 110 Intawaroros Road, Chiang Mai, Thailand, 50200.
E-mail address: Natnita.m@cmu.ac.th

anatomy, sexual response physiology, and psychological response to sexual stimuli that may unavoidably impact the sexual health of transgender people.[4] It is incompletely understood how GAHT and GAS impact the sexual health of transgender populations but the effects are likely highly variable.

Most existing literature on sexual wellness in transgender people is centered around the risk of HIV and/or living with HIV.[5] Research on the impact of GAHT and GAS on sexual wellness in the general transgender population is not well described. The purpose of this systematic review is to assess the currently published scientific literature regarding sexual satisfaction, sexual function, and dysfunction in the transgender population after receipt of GAHT and/or GAS. The review focuses on the 5 main areas in sexual health: desire, arousal, orgasm, pain, and sexual behavior in both transgender men and women.

MATERIALS AND METHODS
Eligibility Criteria

We included studies that reported outcomes on transgender, gender diverse, or gender nonbinary people into this systematic review. Only studies with full text available in English were included. We excluded studies on transgender youth. Our study outcomes of interest were as follows: sexual dysfunction, sexual desire, sexual arousal, pain from sexual intercourse, orgasm, and sexual behavior in the transgender men and women population.

Information Sources

We used the electronic databases Pubmed.gov and www.embase.com. The search included studies published between January 1, 2000 and October 2020. Additional studies were identified from the references of the articles identified during our search strategy.

Search Strategy

The example of the algorithm used for PubMed database searching was: ((("Transgender Persons"[MeSH Terms] OR "Transgender women"[All Fields] OR "Trans men"[All Fields] OR "Transmen"[All Fields] OR "Trans women"[All Fields] OR "transwomen"[All Fields] OR "Transgender men"[All Fields]) OR ("gender nonbinary")) OR ("gender non-binary")) AND ("Libido"[MeSH Terms] OR "sexual dysfunction, physiological"[MeSH Terms] OR "sexual dysfunctions, psychological"[MeSH Terms] OR "sexual behavior"[MeSH Terms]). Only studies in humans that had an available full manuscript published in English after the year 2000 were included. This filter was applied: Case Reports, Clinical Study, Clinical Trial, Clinical Trial Protocol, Clinical Trial, Phase I, Clinical Trial, Phase II, Clinical Trial, Phase III, Clinical Trial, Phase IV, Comparative Study, Controlled Clinical Trial, Multicenter Study, Observational Study, Pragmatic Clinical Trial, Preprint, Randomized Controlled Trial, Validation Study, Humans.

Study Selection

Two researchers reviewed the title and abstracts from the two databases for the first round of review of the studies. Any disagreement regarding the eligibility of the study was reviewed, discussed, and a second vote was held on whether to include or exclude. If the disagreement remained, a third author was consulted to break the tie. Duplicate studies, studies that did not include our study outcomes of interest, or studies that did not have full electronic manuscripts available were excluded. On the second round of review, each potentially eligible manuscript underwent a full review to exclude additional studies that were irrelevant or failed to measure the study outcomes of our research questions. Finally, the references of the included studies were reviewed to identify additional studies that contained our outcomes of interest.

Data Collection Process

Data obtained from all studies were collected and stored on a spreadsheet that included the authors' name, year of publication, title of the manuscript, number of the participants, study design, intervention, measurement tools, key findings, and the study outcomes of interest (Supplement Tables 1 and 2).

Risk of Bias in Individual Studies

As there are so few studies on our outcomes of interest, we included a variety of different study designs. This included prospective cohort studies, retrospective cohort studies, case-control studies, case reports, or case series. No randomized controlled trials were found in our search strategy.

Summary Measures

We collected data on outcomes before and after GAHT and/or GAS. The data were primarily descriptive in nature. We summarized data as percentages or by qualitative terms.

RESULTS
Study Selection

Our initial search strategy identified 340 studies of which 25 studies were duplicates. Another 262 studies were excluded by the review of title and abstract. We then excluded an additional 36 studies based on full-text review leaving 17 studies that met our inclusion and exclusion criteria. The review of the references of these 17 studies identified another 27 more studies. A total of 44 studies were included in this review (**Fig. 1**).

TRANSMEN
Sexual Desire in Transmen

We identified 8 studies that focused on sexual desire in 1034 TGM[6–13] (**Table 1**). The majority of these studies primarily focused on the effects of GAHT and GAS on sexual desire. There was only a study by Kerckhof and colleagues[6] that assessed sexual desire before GAHT and GAS. The prevalence of low sexual desire and sexual aversion among 170 TGM in this study were 42.9% and 28.6%, respectively. After transition, Wierckx and colleagues[12] reported the prevalence of hypoactive sexual desire disorder (HSDD) according to DSM-IV TR diagnostic criteria to be 5% in a group of 138 TGM receiving GAHT with the majority (85%) of these subjects having completed GAS.

Testosterone therapy, the major form of GAHT in TGM, was associated with increased sexual desire. Six studies that included 843 TGM with GAHT reported an increase in sexual desire after GAHT.[7–12] A study in 53 TGM found that 60% of the participants reported an increase in sexual desire,[11] and the other 5 studies reported a significantly higher mean score for sexual desire after GAHT based on various types of questionnaires.[7–10,12] The desire tended to increase within months of starting GAHT[7,8,12] and remained increased by 1 year.[10] A long-term study by Defreyne and colleagues[7] found that sexual desire that involved a partner (dyadic sexual desire) returned to baseline levels after a 3-year of GAHT. Route of testosterone administration did not influence sexual desire.[12] However, the level of serum testosterone had a positive correlation with a frequency of sexual activity in a cohort of 50 TGM.[10] Elevated sexual desire can be problematic in some individuals. Wierckx and colleagues[12] reported that 3.6% of TGM on GAHT experienced distress from a sexual desire that was elevated.

Few studies reported on the impact of GAS on sexual desire with inconsistent results. A study by van de Grift and colleagues[13] in a cohort of 21 TGM after GAS found a decrease in sexual desire. The mean age of the participants was 40.1 years with a mean follow-up period of 31.4 months. In contrast, a study from Wierckx and colleagues[8] in 2011 reported an increase in sexual desire using the sexual desire inventory score after GAS in 72.7% of participants. Wierckx and colleagues later reported, in 2014, no change in sexual desire after GAS in a group of 138 TGM. They also found that phalloplasty or erectile prosthesis also did not

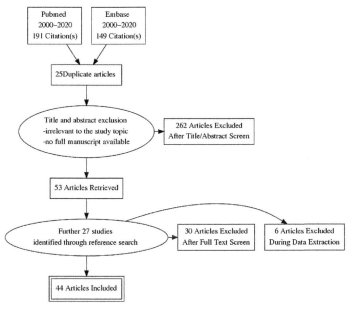

Fig. 1. Flow chart of data selection. Further search on the references of all studies identifies 27 more studies to include in this meta-analysis.

Table 1
Studies in transmen examining sexual desire

Authors, Year	Number of Participants	Study Design	Measurement	Main Findings
Impact of GAHT on sexual desire				
Costantino et al,[10] 2013	50	Prospective cohort study	Sexual desire during the first 12 mo of GAHT	Increased
Defreyne et al,[7] 2020	364	Prospective cohort study	Sexual desire during the first 3 y of GAHT	Increased (transient)
van Dijk et al,[9] 2019	193	Prospective cohort study	Sexual desire after GAHT	Increased (transient)
Wierckx et al,[8] 2011	45	Cross-sectional study	Sexual desire after GAHT	Increased
Wierckx et al,[11] 2014	53	Prospective cohort study	Sexual desire during the first 12 mo of GAHT	Increased
Wierckx et al,[12] 2014	138	Cross-sectional study	Sexual desire after GAHT	Increased (transient)
Impact of GAS on sexual desire				
Defreyne et al,[7] 2020	364	Prospective cohort study	Sexual desire and GAS	Similar
Kerckhof et al,[5] 2019	170	Cross-sectional study	Prevalence of low sexual desire and sexual aversion after GAS	Decreased
van de Grift et al,[13] 2017	21	Retrospective cohort study	Sexual desire after GAS	Decreased
Wierckx et al,[12] 2014	138	Cross-sectional study	Sexual desire after GAS	Similar
Wierckx et al,[8] 2011	45	Cross-sectional study	Sexual desire after GAS	Increased

affect sexual desire.[12] Another recent study by Defreyne and colleagues[7] in 364 TGM also found no correlation between mastectomy or phalloplasty and sexual desire. Finally, Kerckhof and colleagues[6] found that GAS decreased the prevalence of low sexual desire and sexual aversion, but there were no effects on the prevalence of people who had elevated sexual desire.

Sexual Arousal in Transmen

There were 4 studies examining sexual arousal in a total of 451 TGM[6,10,14,15] (**Table 2**). All studies found a positive correlation between GAHT and sexual arousal, whereas GAS had mixed effects on sexual arousal. A cross-sectional study in 141 TGM mostly (91%) naïve to GAHT by Ristori and colleagues[14] found that body dissatisfaction correlated with sexual dysfunction and led to difficulties in sexual arousal. Later, these investigators found that initiation of GAHT had a positive effect on sexual arousal.[14] Wierckx and colleagues (2011)[15] reported that 65% of 49 TGM were easier to be sexually aroused after GAHT/GAS than

before GAHT. Another prospective cohort study by Costantino and colleagues in 50 TGM also found an increase in sexual arousal after 12 months of GAHT.[10]

Effects of GAS on sexual arousal in TGM have mixed results. Studies by Wierckx and colleagues in 49 TGM[15] and Kerckhof and colleagues in 211 TGM[6] found a positive effect of GAS on sexual arousal. GAS was associated with a lower prevalence of arousal dysfunction. The prevalence of arousal dysfunction in Kerckhof and colleagues study decreased from 28.6% in prior to GAHT/GAS group to 9.7% in postmastectomy and hysterectomy group, and 5.4% in TGM after phalloplasty; however, the rates were not statistically different.[6] In contrast, Costantino and colleagues[10] found that the frequency of sexual arousal after GAS was less than those before GAS in 50 TGM. The insertion of an erectile prosthesis did not alter sexual arousal in 46 TGM postphalloplasty in Wierckx and colleagues study.[15] Data regarding sexual arousal after GAS in TGM are inconsistent to make a firm conclusion about the impact of GAS on sexual arousal.

Table 2
Studies in transmen examining sexual arousal

Authors, Year	Number of Participants	Study Design	Measurement	Main Findings
Costantino et al,[10] 2013	50	Prospective cohort study	Sexual arousal after GAHT	Increased
Ristori et al,[14] 2020	141	Cross-sectional study (n = 141) and prospective cohort study (n = 36)	Sexual dysfunction and sexual arousal Sexual arousal after GAHT	Sexual dysfunction was negatively associated with sexual arousal Improved
Wierckx et al,[15] 2011	49	Cross-sectional study	Sexual arousal after GAHT	Increased (much faster)
Costantino et al,[10] 2013	50	Prospective cohort study	Sexual arousal after GAS	Decreased
Kerckhof et al,[6] 2019	211	Cross-sectional study	Sexual arousal after GAS	Increased
Wierckx et al,[15] 2011	49	Cross-sectional study	Sexual arousal after GAS	Increased

Orgasm in Transmen

There were 7 studies that assessed orgasm in a total of 531 TGM[6,10,15–19] (**Table 3**). Orgasm at the baseline before GAS and GAHT was explored in 2 studies. The first study in a cohort of 163 TGM by Cerwenka and colleagues found that 36.8% of the participants always felt pleasant with orgasm, whereas 4.9% never found orgasm pleasant.[16] Another study by Kerckhof and colleagues found that 42.9% of 211 TGM had orgasmic difficulties that impacted daily life.[6]

The effect of GAHT on orgasm was assessed in only one study with 50 participants by Costantino and colleagues[10] They found no impact of GAHT on orgasmic function and serum testosterone levels did not correlate with an ability of orgasm.[10] The effect of GAS assessed in 6 studies with a total of 368 TGM found mixed results.[6,10,15,17–19] The prevalence of orgasmic dysfunction was significantly less in individuals receiving GAS compared with those not receiving GAS.[6] However, a study by De Cuypere and colleagues in 23 TGM found an increase in the ability to attain orgasm during sexual intercourse from 45.5% before GAS to 77.8% after GAS.[17] The ability to orgasm by masturbation was reported to be in the range of 65.1% to 92% of the participants after GAS.[15,17–19] Phalloplasty also had a positive effect on orgasm with 2 reports that included 67 TGM with neophallus showing that orgasm was more intense and more powerful.[15,17] Erectile prosthesis did not impact orgasm according to a study by Wierckx and colleagues in a group of 46 TGM with neophallus.[15] Yet, the time duration to

achieve orgasm did not change after GAS.[18] A study in 50 TGM by Costantino and colleagues found no effect of GAS on orgasm.[10] Apart from GAHT/GAS, a good relationship had a positive impact on the sexual pleasure and frequency of orgasm.[15]

Sexual Pain in Transmen

There were only 2 studies that provided information on this topic. Kerckhof and colleagues reported that 12% of the 211 subjects experienced pain, which led to sexual dysfunction.[6] This pain was not influenced by receipt of GAS.[6] The other study by De Cuypere and colleagues reported pain related to erectile prosthesis. They found that 63.5% of 12 participants with an erectile prosthesis experienced pain.[17]

Sexual Behavior and Sexual Activity in Transmen

Masturbation and sexual activity

There were 3 studies that explored the frequency of sexual activity and/or masturbation in TGM before GAHT/GAS. Cerwenka and colleagues found that 59% of 172 TGM before GAHT/GAS practiced masturbation.[16] Nikkelen & Kreukels[20] found that 87% of 251 TGM practiced masturbation once a month to once a week and the mean frequency of sexual intercourse was less than once a month. And Wierckx and colleagues (2011)[15] reported that 35.4% of 49 TGM masturbated daily to weekly (**Table 4**).

The effects of GAHT on the frequency of masturbation were assessed in only 1 study by Costantino

Table 3
Studies in transmen examining orgasm

Authors, Year	Number of Participants	Study Design	Measurement	Main Findings
Cerwenka et al,[16] 2014	163	Cross sectional study	Orgasmic quality before GAHT/GAS	36.8% had a pleasant orgasm 4.9% never found orgasm pleasant
Impact of GAHT on orgasm				
Costantino et al,[10] 2013	50	Prospective cohort study	Orgasm score before and after GAHT (both by masturbation and sexual activity)	Similar
Impact of GAS on orgasm				
Costantino et al,[10] 2013	50	Prospective cohort study	Orgasm score before and after GAS (by masturbation and sexual intercourse)	Similar
De Cuypere et al,[17] 2005	23	Retrospective cohort study	Frequency of orgasm by sexual activity after GAS	Increased
Garcia et al,[18] 2014	19		Frequency of orgasm by masturbation after GAS	Increased
	23		Change in quality of orgasm after GAS	More powerful and shorter
	25	Cross sectional study	Time to orgasm after phalloplasty	Equal time to orgasm
			Ability to attain orgasm with direct stimulation	92%
			The ability to achieve orgasm with and without penile prosthesis	Similar
Kerckhof et al,[6] 2019	211	Cross sectional study	Orgasmic dysfunction after genital surgery	Decreased
Smith et al,[19] 2001	16	Prospective cohort study	Participants that able to reach orgasm by direct stimulation after genital surgery	68.75% able to reach orgasm regularly
Wierckx et al,[15] 2011	43	Cross-sectional study	Percentage of transmen reaching orgasm by masturbation after GAS	74.4%
	28		Percentage of transmen reaching orgasm by sexual activity after GAS	57.2%
	43		Change in quality of orgasm after GAS	Higher intensity of orgasm

Table 4
Studies in transmen examining sexual activity

Authors, Year	Number of Participants	Study Design	Measurement Tools	Main Findings
Cerwenka et al,[16] 2014	172	Cross sectional study	Ratio of transmen practicing masturbation before GAHT and GAS	59%
Costantino et al,[10] 2013	50	Prospective cohort study	Frequency of masturbation after GAHT	Increased
			Frequency of masturbation after GAS	Increased in 10% of participants Decreased in 24% of participants
			Frequency of sexual intercourse after GAS	No changes
De Cuypere et al,[17] 2005	23	Retrospective cohort study	Frequency of masturbation after GAS (phalloplasty)	Increased
Nikkelen & Kreukels,[20] 2018	251	Cross sectional study	Frequency of masturbation and sexual activity after GAHT and GAS	Increased
Smith et al,[19] 2001	13	Prospective cohort study	Frequency of masturbation after GAS	Increased or no changes
van de Grift et al,[13] 2017	21	Retrospective cohort study	Frequency of masturbation after GAS	Increased
Wierckx et al,[8] 2011	40	Cross sectional study	Percentage of participants who masturbate daily to weekly after GAS	60%
Wierckx et al,[15] 2011	49	Cross sectional study	Percentage of participants who masturbate daily to weekly after GAS	Increased
	27		Frequency of sexual activity with partner after GAS	29.6% Several times/week 48.1% 1–2 times/mo 22.2% Never

and colleagues,[10] which reported a higher frequency of masturbation in 28% of the participants after GAHT. Testosterone level was positively correlated with the frequency of masturbation but not sexual intercourse.[8,10]

Five studies in a total of 357 participants reported a positive effect of GAS on masturbation or sexual activity.[13,15,17,19,20] The frequency of masturbation and sexual intercourse increased after GAS.[13,15,17,19,20] In contrast, a study by Costantino and colleagues found a decrease in the frequency of masturbation in 24% of the 50 participants with no change in sexual activity[10]

Sexual behavior
The use of genitals was examined in 4 publications.[13,15,16,18] Approximately, 50% of 172 TGM before GAHT/GAS used their genitals for sexual activity.[16] After GAHT, only 11% of 44 participants reported having vaginal penetration during sexual intercourse.[15] After phalloplasty, 92% of 25 TGM used their neophallus during masturbation[18] and 78% of 21 TGM used their neophallus for sexual intercourse[13]

The sexual orientation after GAS was reported in Wierckx and colleagues study. Among 50 TGM, 85.7% was gynephilic and 10.2% was

Table 5
Studies in transmen examining sexual behavior

Authors, Year	Number of Participants	Study Design	Measurement Tools	Main Findings
Cerwenka et al,[16] 2014	172	Cross sectional study	Genital involvement in sexual activity before GAHT and GAS	50%
Garcia et al,[18] 2014	25	Cross sectional study	Genital involvement after GAS	92% masturbated with phallus
van de Grift et al,[13] 2017	21	Retrospective cohort study	Genital involvement during sexual intercourse after GAS	Increased genital involvement during sexual intercourse
Wierckx et al,[15] 2011	49	Cross sectional study	Genital involvement during sexual intercourse after GAHT	Less vaginal involvement Similar clitoral involvement
Costantino et al,[10] 2013	50	Prospective cohort study	Change of sexual orientation after GAHT/GAS	Similar to baseline before treatment (98% heterosexual)
Fein et al,[21] 2015	59	Cross sectional study	Change in sexual preference during or after GAHT/GAS	22% of TGM changed sexual preference
Wierckx et al,[15] 2011	50	Cross sectional study	Sexual orientation after GAS	85.7% gynephilic 10.2% androphilic 4.1% bisexual

androphilic.[15] Some TGM reported changes in sexual orientation after GAHT/GAS. Fein and colleagues reported that 22% of 59 TGM changed their sexual orientation after GAHT/GAS.[21] Another study in 50 TGM found no effect of GAHT/GAS on the change in sexual orientation[10] (**Table 5**).

Sexual satisfaction in transmen

The definition of satisfaction is inconsistent among studies. The prevalence of sexual dysfunction before GAS ranged between 32.6% and 53% using the Transmasculine Sexual Functioning Index (TM-SFI) and the WHOQOL, respectively.[22,23] It was reported that TGM with sexual distress were more likely to have a low sexual satisfaction.[14]

Regarding the impact of GAHT/GAS on sexual satisfaction, there were 6 studies in 392 TGM reported an improvement after GAHT/GAS.[8,14,15,17,19,24] A prospective study in 36 TGM found an improvement in sexual distress after GAHT during a 2-year follow-up.[14] The prevalence of people reporting "satisfied" or "very satisfied" after GAS was 64% to 76.2%.[8,15,17,19] A single-center study in 246 participants found that Sex/Dating Life improved significantly after GAS.[24]

There were 3 studies with a total of 305 TGM reported no effects of GAHT/GAS on sexual satisfaction.[13,20,25] Sexual satisfaction appeared to differ depending on the type of GAS. A report in 21 TGM found that TGM with metoidioplasty had a higher sexual satisfaction score on a 5-point Likert scale compared with TGM with phalloplasty.[13] Erectile prosthesis did not correlate to sexual satisfaction in 49 TGM from 2 studies[15,17] (**Table 6**).

Body satisfaction played an important role and positively correlated to all indicators of sexual behavior and feeling.[20] Apart from sexual function, GAS was also associated with improved body image.[13,19,25,26] Therefore, studies report a high rate of sexual satisfaction after GAS despite the presence of surgical complications. Very few TGM were reported to regret undergoing GAS.[13,18,24]

TRANSWOMEN
Sexual Desire in Transwomen

There were 12 studies in a total of 1475 participants that assessed sexual desire in TGW (**Table 7**). These studies were conducted in

Table 6
Studies in transmen examining sexual satisfaction and pain

Authors, Year	Number of Participants	Study Design	Measurement Tools	Main Findings
Sexual satisfaction				
Bartolucci et al,[23] 2015	36 TGM 67 TGW	Cross sectional study	Prevalence of dissatisfaction in sex life in transmen before genital surgery (WHOQOL)	53%
Nikkelen & Kreukels,[20] 2018	251	Cross sectional study	Sexual satisfaction in participants with and without a transition process	Similar
			Sexual esteem	Sexual esteem related to a fulfilled treatment
Reisner et al,[22] 2020	150	Retrospective cohort study	Prevalence of sexual dysfunction in mixed GAHT/GAS status transmen	32.6%[a]
Ristori et al,[14] 2020	141	Cross sectional study	Sexual distress and sexual satisfaction	Sexual distress was negatively associated with sexual satisfaction
	36	Prospective cohort study	Sexual distress after GAHT	Decreased
Sexual satisfaction after GAS				
De Cuypere et al,[17] 2005	21	Retrospective cohort study	Sex life after GAS	Improved in 75%
			Sexual satisfaction after GAS	Satisfied in 76.2%
			Sexual satisfaction with partner after GAS	Improved
McNichols et al,[24] 2020	246	Retrospective cohort study	Sexual satisfaction after GAS	Improved
Smith et al,[19] 2001	16	Prospective cohort study	Ratio of participants that satisfy in their sex life after GAS	70%
	20		Satisfaction with body image after GAS	Increased 80% were satisfied or very satisfied after GAS
van de Grift et al,[13] 2017	21	Retrospective cohort study	Sexual satisfaction after GAS	Similar to before GAS Metoidioplasty had higher sexual satisfaction than phalloplasty
Wierckx et al,[15] 2011	28	Cross sectional study	Overall sexual satisfaction (sexual activity with partner) after GAS	64.2% were satisfy or very satisfy
			Sexual satisfaction after erection prosthesis	No changes
Wierckx et al,[8] 2011	45	Cross sectional study	Sexual satisfaction with partner using sexual desire inventory after GAS	64% satisfied

(*continued on next page*)

Table 6 (continued)				
Authors, Year	Number of Study ParticipantsDesign		Measurement Tools	Main Findings
Sexual pain				
De Cuypere et al,[17] 2005	23	Retrospective cohort study	Sexual pain after erectile prosthesis	63.5% experienced pain
Kerckhof et al,[6] 2019	211	Cross sectional study	Pain dysfunction during sexual intercourse in mixed GAHT/GAS status transmen	12%

[a] TM-SFI: Transmasculine Sexual Functioning Index.

Belgium, The Netherlands, Germany, Norway, Italy, United States, and Canada. Estrogen and antiandrogen therapy resulted in a reduction in sexual desire in many studies. The prevalence of self-reported low sexual desire ranged from 32.7% to 73%[6,12] and the prevalence of HSDD was 22.1% in a cohort of 214 TGW after GAHT/GAS.[12] Although the decreased sexual desire after GAHT was common, most TGW did not found low sexual desire distressing.[12] The impact on sexual desire did not appear to differ based on specific hormonal regimen.[7,12] However, the duration of GAHT impacted sexual desire level. A prospective study in 53 TGW found a significant decrease in sexual desire throughout the first year of the treatment.[11] In contrast, recent studies found that the reduction in sexual desire was transient. A study by van Dijk and colleagues[9] in 205 TGW found a decrease in sexual desire during the first year with a nadir point at the 3rd month before returning to baseline at 12 months of estrogen. A study by Defreyne and colleagues in 401 TGW found a decrease in sexual desire during the 1st year of GAHT.[7] By the 3rd year, solitary sexual desire returned to baseline level, but sexual desire with a partner was still higher than the baseline level.[7]

Regarding the impact of GAS on sexual desire, the prevalence of HSDD in TGW after genital surgery ranged between 18.3% and 33.9%.[6,27,28] Many studies found a positive effect of GAS on sexual desire. A study in 307 TGW by Kerckhof and colleagues found a significantly lower prevalence of low sexual desire in TGW after GAS than before GAS at 18.3% and 32.7%, respectively.[6] A study by Wierckx and colleagues in 138 TGW with neovagina also reported a significant increase in self-reported spontaneous sexual desire compared with those before genital surgery.[12]

Three studies with a total of 130 TGW reported an increase in the FSFI (The Female Sexual Function Index) subscale for sexual desire after GAS.[29–32] On the contrary, Wierckx and colleagues found that 69.7% of 214 TGW reported a decrease in sexual desire after GAS.[12] And a study by van der Sluis and colleagues reported comparable sexual desire scores (FSFI) in 24 TGW underwent intestinal vaginoplasty technique.[33] Type of GAS had different effects on sexual desire. A study in 401 TGW found that orchiectomy decreased sexual desire but vaginoplasty and breast augmentation did not affect sexual desire.[7] Being sexually active related to higher sexual desire scores.[30,32] To compare with cisgender women, 4 studies that include 145 TGW reported a lower sexual desire score in nonclinical TGW with neovagina than cisgender women without sexual problem using FSFI score[30–32] or the Brief Index of Sexual Functioning for Women (BISF-W) score.[34]

Sexual Arousal in Transwomen

Difficulties in sexual arousal were assessed in 8 studies among 599 TGW[6,17,30–35] (Table 8). GAHT demonstrated no impact on arousal difficulties in a study by Kerckhof and colleagues.[6] The prevalence of arousal difficulties in 29 TGW without GAHT and 71 TGW with GAHT was 33.3% and 32.6%, respectively, with no statistical difference. Only 20% of this population considered low arousal as a problem.[6]

The ability to be sexually aroused after genital surgery was explored. Hess and colleagues reported that 71.5% of 91 TGW with neovagina were able to get "aroused easily."[35] There were 4 studies using the Short Questionnaire for Self-Evaluation of Vaginoplasty (SQSV) to evaluate

Table 7
Studies in transwomen examining sexual desire

Study	Number of Participants	Study Design	Measurement	Findings
Impact of GAHT on sexual desire				
Defreyne et al,[7] 2020	401	Prospective cohort study	Total and dyadic sexual desire after GAHT	Transient decrease after the initiation of GAHT. Increase after 3 y after GAHT
			Solitary sexual desire after GAHT	Transient decrease
Kerckhof et al,[6] 2019	307	Cross-sectional study	Prevalence of low sexual desire after GAHT	32.7%
			Prevalence of sexual aversion after GAHT	20%
van Dijk et al,[9] 2019	205	Prospective cohort study	Sexual desire after GAHT	Transient decrease after the initiation of GAHT
Wierckx et al,[11] 2014	53	Prospective cohort study	Sexual desire after GAHT	Decreased
Wierckx et al,[12] 2014	214	Cross-sectional study	Prevalence of low or no sexual desire after GAHT	73%
			Prevalence of HSDD[a] after GAHT	22.1%
			Sexual desire after GAHT after GAHT	Decreased
Impact of GAS on sexual desire				
Elaut et al,[27] 2008	62	Case-control study	Prevalence of HSDD after GAS (control is reproductive age women)	33.9% Similar to control
			Level of sexual desire [b] after GAS	Similar to control
			Sexual desire and androgen level	No significant correlation
Kerckhof et al,[6] 2019	307	Cross-sectional study	Prevalence of low sexual desire after GAS	Decreased
			Prevalence of sexual aversion after GAS	9.1%
Kronawitter et al,[28] 2019	64	Prospective pilot study	Prevalence of HSDD in TGW with GAHT and GAS	28.%
Wierckx et al,[12] 2014	214	Cross-sectional study	Sexual desire after GAS (vaginoplasty)	Increased
Bouman et al,[32] 2016	31	Cross-sectional study	Desire (FSFI score)[c] after GAS	Lower desire score
Buncamper et al,[30] 2015	49	Retrospective cohort study	Desire (FSFI score)[c] after GAS	Lower desire score
van der Sluis et al,[33] 2016	24	Cross-sectional study	Desire (FSFI score)[c] after GAS	Lower desire score
Weyers et al,[31] 2009	50	Retrospective cohort study	Desire (FSFI score)[c] after GAS	Lower desire score
Brotto et al,[34] 2005	15	Cross-sectional study	Desire (BISF-W[d]) after GAS	Lower than control

[a] Sexual Function Health Council's consensus definition.
[b] Sexual desire inventory score.
[c] FSFI: The Female Sexual Function Index (FSFI), control is cis-women without sexual problems.
[d] BISF-W: brief index of sexual functioning for women, control is cis-women experiencing sexual arousal difficulties.

Table 8
Studies in transwomen examining sexual arousal

Study	Number of Participants	Study Design	Measurement	Findings
Impact of GAHT on sexual arousal				
Kerckhof et al,[6] 2019	307	Cross-sectional study	Sexual arousal after GAHT	Similar to before GAHT
Impact of GAS on sexual arousal				
De Cuypere et al,[17] 2005	32	Retrospective cohort study	Sexual arousal after GAS	More often
Kerckhof et al,[6] 2019	307	Cross-sectional study	Sexual arousal after GAS	Improved
Hess et al,[35] 2018	91	Retrospective cohort study	Percentage of participants that get arouse easily after GAS	71.5% of the participant
Bouman et al,[32] 2016	31	Cross-sectional study	Ability to be sexually aroused[a] after GAS	100%
			Sexual arousal (FSFI score)[b] after GAS	Lower arousal score
			Lubrication (FSFI score)[b] after GAS	Lower lubrication score
Buncamper et al,[30] 2015	49	Retrospective cohort study	Ability to be sexually aroused[a] after GAS	89.8%
			Sexual arousal (FSFI score)[b] after GAS	Lower arousal score
			Lubrication (FSFI score)[b] after GAS	Lower lubrication score
van der Sluis et al,[33] 2016	24	Cross-sectional study	Ability to be sexually aroused[a] after GAS	100%
			Sexual arousal (FSFI score)[b] after GAS	Lower arousal score
			Lubrication (FSFI score)[b] after GAS	Lower lubrication score
Weyers et al,[31] 2009	50	Retrospective cohort study	Sexual arousal (FSFI score)[b] after GAS	Lower arousal score
			Lubrication (FSFI score)[b] after GAS	Lower lubrication score
Brotto et al,[34] 2005	15	Cross-sectional study	Arousal (BISF-W[c]) after GAS	Lower arousal score
Lawrence et al,[36] 2006	232	Prospective cohort study	Lubrication after GAS	Low satisfaction with vaginal lubrication
Zavlin et al,[37] 2018	39	Prospective cohort study	Lubrication after GAS	Medium level of satisfaction

[a] SQSV: Short Questionnaire for Self-Evaluation of vaginoplasty.
[b] FSFI: The Female Sexual Function Index (FSFI), control is cis-women without sexual problems.
[c] BISF-W: brief index of sexual functioning for women, control is cis-women experiencing sexual arousal difficulties.

outcomes after vaginoplasty.[30–33] Among a total cohort of 154 TGW with neovagina, 89.8% to 100% of them reported being able to be sexually aroused after GAS.[30–33] However, the sexual arousal subscale of FSFI was lower than nonclinical cisgender women.[30–33] Brotto and colleagues found an average level of mental and physical sexual arousal scores in 15 TGW with GAS as measured by Detailed Assessment of Sexual Arousal scale.[34]

GAS demonstrated a positive impact on sexual arousal in 2 studies.[6,17] A study in 307 TGW found that the proportion of participants with sexual arousal problems decreased from 33.3% in

Table 9
Studies in transwomen examining orgasm

Study	Number of Participants	Study Design	Measurement	Findings
Cerwenka et al,[16] 2014	208	Cross-sectional study	Orgasmic quality before GAHT and GAS	18.3% never found orgasm pleasant
Kerckhof et al,[6] 2019	29	Cross-sectional study	Prevalence of orgasmic dysfunction before GAHT and GAS	46.7%
Impact of GAHT on orgasm				
Kerckhof et al, 2019[6]	71	Cross-sectional study	Orgasmic dysfunction after GAHT	29.2%
Impact of GAS on orgasm				
Kerckhof et al,[6] 2019	207	Cross-sectional study	Orgasmic dysfunction after GAS	28.8%
Zavlin et al,[37] 2018	40	Prospective cohort study	Orgasmic satisfaction after GAS	High
De Cuypere et al,[17] 2005	32	Retrospective cohort study	Frequency of orgasm by sexual intercourse after GAS	Increased
			Always able to achieve orgasm by masturbation (N = 23)	65.2%
			Quality of orgasm after GAS	More intense, smoother, and longer
Selvaggi et al,[39] 2007	30	Retrospective cohort study	Orgasm after GAS	85% able to orgasm 18% unable to orgasm
			Pleasure of orgasm after GAS	Improved
Hess et al,[35] 2018	91	Retrospective cohort study	Frequency of orgasm after GAS n = 78	52.6% less frequently 26.9% more frequently
			Orgasm quality after GAS n = 77	More intense 55.8% Less intense 23.4%
Lawrence et al,[36] 2006	232	Prospective cohort study	Frequency of orgasm after GAS	More than half or almost always in 48%
Bouman et al,[32] 2016	31	Cross-sectional study	Ability to orgasm[a] after GAS	84%
			Orgasm FSFI score[b] after GAS	Lower orgasmic score
			Orgasmic quality after GAS	Equal sensation in 62.5%

(continued on next page)

Table 9
(continued)

Study	Number of Participants	Study Design	Measurement	Findings
Buncamper et al,[30] 2015	49	Retrospective cohort study	Ability to orgasm[a] after GAS (n = 41)	83.7%
			Orgasmic score (FSFI)[a] after GAS	Lower orgasmic score
			Orgasmic quality after GAS	46.9% More sensation, 28.6% Less sensation
van der Sluis et al,[33] 2016	24	Cross-sectional study	Ability to orgasm[a] after GAS	100%
			Orgasm FSFI score[b] after GAS	Lower orgasmic score
Weyers et al,[31] 2009	50	Retrospective cohort study	Orgasm FSFI score[b] after GAS	Lower orgasmic score
Brotto et al,[34] 2005	15	Cross-sectional study	Ability to orgasm after GAS	40%
LeBreton et al,[42] 2017	25	Prospective cohort study	Ability to orgasm after GAS	80%
			Frequency of orgasm by masturbation after GAS	Similar
			Frequency of orgasm by sexual intercourse after GAS	Similar
Perovic et al,[40] 2000	89	Cross-sectional study	Ability to orgasm after GAS	82%
Raigosa et al,[43] 2015	60	Retrospective cohort study	Ability to orgasm after GAS	100%
Soli et al,[47] 2008	15	Prognosis (outcomes research)	Ability to orgasm after GAS	46.6%
Smith et al,[19] 2001	16	Prospective cohort study (TGW + TGM)	Ability to reach orgasm regularly after GAS	68.75%
Lawrence et al (2005)[38]	227	Retrospective cohort study	Ability to orgasm Pleasure of the orgasm (n=218)	85% Better than before GAS
Amend et al,[45] 2013	24	Retrospective cohort study	Ability to orgasm by clitoris stimulation after GAS	96%
Goddard et al,[46] 2007	64	Prognosis (outcomes research)	Ability to orgasm by clitoris stimulation after GAS	48%
Krege et al,[44] 2001	31	Prospective cohort study	Ability to orgasm by clitoris stimulation after GAS	87%
Wagner et al,[41] 2010	50	Prospective cohort study	Ability to orgasm by clitoris stimulation after GAS	70%

[a] SQSV: Short Questionnaire for Self-Evaluation of vaginoplasty.
[b] FSFI: The Female Sexual Function Index (FSFI), control is cis-women without sexual problems.

TGW without GAHT/GAS to 15.9% in post-GAS group.[6] The other study in 32 TGW reported that the percentage of TGW who were able to get sexually aroused "often" or "very often" increased from 17.2% to 46.9% after GAS.[17] Being sexually active significantly improves sexual arousal.[30,32] Sensitivity of neoclitoris was also associated with more sexual arousal in TGW after vaginoplasty.[35]

Another marker of sexual arousal is vaginal lubrication. In TGW, vaginal lubrication may not occur depending on the type of vaginoplasty performed. Many studies reported a dissatisfaction of vaginal lubrication after GAS.[36,37] Not surprisingly, TGW had lower lubrication scores by FSFI compared with cisgender women in 4 studies.[30–33] The reference FSFI subscore for vaginal lubrication from cisgender women was 5.7 ± 1.0[29] compared with the scores ranging 2.39 ± 2.29 to 2.8 ± 2.4 in TGW with penile inversion vaginoplasties and 4.0 ± 2.6 in TGW with intestinal neovagina.[30–33] The prevalence of TGW that experienced vaginal fluid during sexual arousal was 64.3%[17] and during orgasm was 55% to 76%.[17,38]

Orgasm in Transwomen

There were 22 studies in a total of 1483 TGW, that studied orgasm in TGW[6,16,17,19,30–47] (**Table 9**). Without GAHT/GAS, Kerckhof and colleagues[6] reported that the prevalence of orgasmic dysfunction was 46.7% among 29 participants. This prevalence decreased to 29.2% in a group of 71 TGW with GAHT.[6] Ejaculation was considered a negative experience in 12% of the subjects in this study.[6] Another study by Cerwenka and colleagues reported that 18.3% of 208 TGW before GAHT/GAS never found orgasm a pleasant feeling.[16]

The ability to attain orgasm after genital surgery was explored in 13 studies, which included 1175 TGW.[30,32–34,39–47] The percentage of participants who were able to orgasm after GAS ranged from 40% to 100%.[30,32–34,39–47] It was found that masturbation or direct neoclitoral stimulation had a higher orgasm rate than sexual intercourse.[35] The frequency of orgasm was also reported in some studies. A study by Lawrence and colleagues (2006) reported that 48% of the 232 participants able to attain orgasm in "more than half of the time" or "almost always."[36] De Cuypere and colleagues[17] reported that 65.2% of 32 participants could always orgasm by masturbation. A study by Smith and colleagues in a mixed TGM and TGW population found that 68.75% can reach orgasm regularly.[19] The FSFI subscore for orgasm after vaginoplasty was assessed in 4 studies that included 154 TGW.

The overall orgasmic score ranges from 2.82 ± 2.29 to 4.0 ± 2.2,[30–33] which were lower than cisgender women without sexual problems (5.1 ± 1.1).[29,30] TGW with neovagina who were sexually active had a higher score than sexually inactive TGW.[30,32]

The effect of GAS on orgasm in TGW is inconclusive. De Cuypere and colleagues[17] reported an increase in the frequency of orgasm by sexual activity after GAS. However, a study by Hess and colleagues[35] found that 52.6% of a group of 91 participants experience orgasms less frequently after GAS and only 20.5% of the participants reported more frequent orgasms.[35] And Kerckhof and colleagues[6] found a comparable prevalence of orgasmic dysfunction in participants before and after GAS. The effect of GAS on the quality of orgasm was evaluated in 5 studies that included 421 participants. In 4 of the 5 studies, orgasms improved after GAS. A study by Lawrence and colleagues (2005)[38] found that 51% of the 218 participants found more pleasurable orgasms after GAS. Orgasms were reported to be more sensitive,[30] intense,[17,35] smoother, and longer after GAS.[17] However, Bouman and colleagues[32] found that 62.5% of 31 TGW in their study reported no changes in their orgasmic feeling after GAS. Duration since the surgery demonstrated no correlation to intensity of orgasm in a study of 91 TGW with neovagina.[35] However, Lawrence and colleagues (2006) found that the frequency of orgasm inversely correlated with duration since surgery.[36]

Sexual Pain in Transwomen

There were 11 studies in a total of 990 TGW that included sexual pain as a study outcome[6,30–34,36,37,41,44,46] (**Table 10**). Kerckhof and colleagues reported that 24% of 307 TGW had sexual pain that led to sexual dysfunction, which was significantly higher in TGW with neovagina compared with TGW without a neovagina.[6] The rate of pain on penetration of the neovagina ranged from 4.76% to 11.11% based on 3 studies in 300 TGW.[36,41,44] Painful or uncomfortable sensation at the neoclitoris was found in 2.2% of 183 TGW in a study by Goddard and colleagues.[46] Regarding pain score, Brotto and colleagues found very low mean pain score (1/10) during the insertion of a probe to test sensation of the neovagina.[34] Zavlin and colleagues reported a mean sexual pain score 2.33/10 for a masturbation/intercourse after GAS, which was not considered to impact sexual functioning in most of the 39 subjects.[37] The pain/comfort FSFI score demonstrated a significantly lower comfort level in TGW compared with cisgender women without sexual problem (at

Table 10
Studies in transwomen on sexual pain

Study	Number of Participants	Study Design	Measurement	Findings
Kerckhof et al,[6] 2019	307	Cross-sectional study	Pain during sexual activity	24% reported pain that resulting in sexual dysfunction
Post-vaginoplasty				
Goddard et al,[46] 2007	183	Prognosis (outcomes research)	Pain or uncomfort of clitoral sensation	2.2%
Krege et al,[44] 2001	18	Prospective cohort study	Pain during penetration of neovagina	11.11%
Lawrence et al,[36] 2006	232	Prospective cohort study	Pain during penetration of neovagina	8.65%
Wagner et al,[41] 2010	42	Prospective cohort study	Pain during penetration of neovagina	4.76%
Brotto et al,[34] 2005	15	Cross-sectional study	Pain score[a]	1/10
Zavlin et al,[37] 2018	39	Prospective cohort study	Pain score	2.33/10
Bouman et al,[32] 2016	31	Cross-sectional study	Pain (FSFI score)[b] after GAS	Lower comfort score
Buncamper et al,[30] 2015	49	Retrospective cohort study	Pain (FSFI score)[b] after GAS	Lower comfort score
van der Sluis et al,[33] 2016	24	Cross-sectional study	Pain (FSFI score)[b] after GAS	Lower comfort score
Weyers et al,[31] 2009	50	Retrospective cohort study	Pain (FSFI score)[b] after GAS	Lower comfort score

[a] Pain during vaginal probe insertion.
[b] FSFI: The Female Sexual Function Index (FSFI), control is cis-women without sexual problems.

2.2 ± 2.7 and 5.7 ± 0.8, respectively).[29,30] This lower comfort level was found in both penile-skin neovagina[30,31] and intestinal neovagina.[32,33] Bouman and colleagues reported a significantly more sexual comfort in the sexually active TGW group than the sexually inactive TGW group.[32]

Sexual Behavior and Sexual Activity in Transwomen

Masturbation and sexual activity

Before GAHT/GAS, Cerwenka and colleagues reported that, in 208 TGW, 72.4% practiced masturbation, 79.7% had sexual activity with a partner, and 60.4% involved their penis in the activity.[16]

After GAS, the frequency of masturbation decreased in 3 studies that included 357 TGW.[19,20,42] LeBreton and colleagues also found a reduction in the frequency of sexual fantasy after GAS.[42] De Cuypere and colleagues, however, found no change in frequency of masturbation after GAS in 32 TGW.[17]

Regarding the frequency of sexual activity after GAS, 7 studies that included 319 TGW reported that 36.7% to 89% of TGW after vaginoplasty had sexual activity.[30,32,33,40,41,43,44] Having regular or frequent sexual intercourse was reported in 33% to 89% of 124 participants.[32,33,43,45] Neovaginal involvement in sexual activity was found in 52% to 89%.[32,33,37] In contrast, Hess and colleagues reported that 56.3% of 91 TGW were sexually inactive after GAS.[35] Time interval between surgery and frequency of sexual activity were not correlated.[35]

The effect of GAS on sexual activity was evaluated by Zavlin and colleagues in 39 TGW. The prevalence of people with regular vaginal receptive intercourse significantly increased from 17.5% to 57.5% after GAS.[37] LeBreton and colleagues and Lobato and colleagues also found an increase in the frequency of vaginal receptive intercourse or sexual activity after GAS.[42,48] Cardoso da Silva and colleagues evaluated sexual activity by WHOQOL and found an improvement in

Table 11
Studies in transwomen examining sexual activity

Study	Number of Participants	Study Design	Measurement	Findings
Before transition				
Cerwenka et al,[16] 2014	208	Cross-sectional study	Genital involvement in sexual activity Practice masturbation	60.4% 72.4%
Impact of GAS on sexual activity				
Cardoso da Silva et al,[49] 2016	47	Prospective cohort study	Sexual activity after GAS (WHOQOL-100)	Improved
Zavlin et al,[37] 2018	39	Prospective cohort study	Sexual activity after GAS	Increased
De Cuypere et al,[17] 2005	32	Retrospective cohort study	Frequency of masturbation after GAS	Similar Frequency
LeBreton et al,[42] 2017	25	Prospective cohort study	Frequency of masturbation after GAS	Decreased
			Frequency of vaginal receptive intercourse after GAS	Increased
			Frequency of sexual fantasy after GAS	Decreased
Nikkelen and Kreukels[20] 2018	325	Cross-sectional study	Frequency of masturbation after GAS	Less frequent
			Frequency of sexual activity after GAS	Similar Frequency
Smith et al,[19] 2001	7	Prospective cohort study	Frequency of masturbation after GAS	Decreased
Lobato et al,[48] 2006	18	Prospective cohort study	Frequency of sexual activity after GAS	More frequent
Amend et al,[45] 2013	24	Retrospective cohort study	Sexual activity after GAS	33% have regular intercourse
Buncamper et al,[30] 2015	49	Retrospective cohort study	Sexual activity after GAS	36.7% sexually active
Bouman et al,[32] 2016	31	Cross-sectional study	Sexual activity after GAS	69% sexually active 52% intercourse with neovagina 43.5% have regular intercourse
Hess et al,[35] 2018	91	Retrospective cohort study	Sexual activity after GAS	56.3% sexually inactive
Krege et al,[44] 2001	31	Prospective cohort study	Sexual activity after GAS	58% sexually active
Perovic et al,[40] 2000	89	Cross-sectional study	Sexual activity after GAS	79% sexually active
Raigosa et al,[43] 2015	60	Retrospective cohort study	Sexual activity after GAS	86% sexually active
van der Sluis et al,[33] 2016	9	Cross-sectional study	Sexual activity after GAS	89% have regular intercourse
Wagner et al,[41] 2010	50	Prospective cohort study	Sexual activity after GAS	84% sexually active

Table 12
Studies in transwomen examining sexual satisfaction

Study	Number of Participants	Study Design	Measurement	Findings
Before GAS				
Bartolucc et al,[23] 2015	67	Cross sectional study 36 TGM 67 TGW	Sexual satisfaction after GAHT (WHOQOL)[a]	22% very dissatisfied 31% poor/ Dissatisfied
Cerwenka et al,[16] 2014	208	Cross sectional study	Perception of penile sensation before transition	45.1% reported unpleasurable sensations
Ristori et al,[14] 2020	36	Prospective cohort study	Sexual distress after GAHT	Decreased
Impact of GAS on sexual satisfaction				
De Cuypere et al,[17] 2005	29	Retrospective cohort study	Sexual satisfaction after GAS	Improved
			Sexual satisfaction with partner after GAS (n = 32)	Similar
Elaut et al,[27] 2008	62	Case-control study	Sexual satisfaction after GAS compared to reproductive cis-women	Less than control group
Lawrence et al,[36] 2006	232	Prospective cohort study	Level of sexual satisfaction after GAS	Good
Zavlin et al,[37] 2018	40	Prospective cohort study	Level of sexual satisfaction after GAS (n = 40)	Good
			Satisfaction with intercourse (n = 23)	Improved
Hess et al,[35] 2018	91	Retrospective cohort study	Ratio of participants that reported satisfaction their sex life	35.2% always pleasurable 14.8% never felt pleasure
Özkan et al,[50] 2018	9	Cross sectional study	Ratio of participants that reported satisfaction in their sex life	88.89%
Smith et al,[19] 2001	10	Prospective cohort study TGW + TGM	Ratio of participants that reported satisfaction their sex life	70%
Bouman et al,[32] 2016	31	Cross sectional study	Sexual satisfaction (FSFI score)[b] after GAS	Lower satisfaction score
			Total FSFI score[b] after GAS	Lower than cut-off point
			Genital Self-Image Scale[c] after GAS	20.0 ± 4.5
			Prevalence of sexual	31%

(continued on next page)

Table 12
(continued)

Study	Number of Participants	Study Design	Measurement	Findings
			dysfunction after GAS	
Buncamper et al,[30] 2015	49	Retrospective cohort study	Sexual satisfaction (FSFI score)[b] after GAS	Lower satisfaction score
			Total FSFI score[b] after GAS	Lower than cut-off point
			Genital Self-Image Scale[c] after GAS	22.6 ± 4.1[c]
			Prevalence of sexual dysfunction after GAS	67%
van der Sluis et al,[33] 2016	24	Cross sectional study	Sexual satisfaction (FSFI score)[b] after GAS	Lower satisfaction score
			Total FSFI score[b] after GAS	Lower than cut-off point
			Genital Self-Image Scale[c] after GAS	21.5
			Prevalence of sexual dysfunction after GAS	44.4%
Weyers et al,[31] 2009	50	Retrospective cohort study	Sexual satisfaction (FSFI score)[b] after GAS	Lower satisfaction score
			Total FSFI score[b] after GAS	Lower than cut-off point
Lobato et al,[48] 2006	18	Prospective cohort study	Sexual satisfaction after GAS	Improved by 83.3% of patients
LeBreton et al,[42] 2017	25	Prospective cohort study	Sexual satisfaction after GAS	Improved
			Genital sensation after GAS	Satisfied to very satisfied
Amend et al,[45] 2013	24	Retrospective cohort study	Genital sensation after GAS	Good or excellent neoclitoral sensation in 97%
Goddard et al,[46] 2007	64	Prognosis (Outcomes Research)	Genital sensation after GAS	Uncomfortable clitoral sensation in 14%
Soli et al,[47] 2008	15	Cross sectional study	Genital sensation after GAS	Good neoclitoral sensitivity in 100%

[a] WHOQOL: measure for quality of life by world health organization.
[b] FSFI: The Female Sexual Function Index (FSFI), total score cut-off point is 26.55.[51]
[c] FGSIS: The Female Genital Self-Image Scale (FGSIS) mean total score in cis-women is 21.3 ± 5.4.[52]

the frequency of sexual activity after GAS compared with before the surgery in 47 TGW.[49] However, Nikkelen & Kreukels reported a comparable frequency of sexual activity between no treatment group and post-transition group[20] (**Table 11**).

Genital sensation

After GAS, neoclitoral sensation was good in many studies.[35,42,45,47] Neoclitoral sensation was "good" or "excellent" in 97% to 100% of 39 participants in studies by Amend and colleagues and Soli and colleagues[45,47] Neoclitoral sensation was "satisfied" in 73.9% of 119 participants in Hess and colleagues study.[35] LeBreton and colleagues reported a mean score in the range of "satisfied/very satisfied" in 25 participants.[42] However, Goddard and colleagues reported that 14% of 64 participants experienced uncomfortable sensation at neoclitoris.[46]

Sexual satisfaction in transwomen

Perceptions regarding pleasurable genital sensations varied among transgender individuals. A study in 208 TGW before GAHT/GAS by Cerwenka and colleagues found that 45.1% of participants did not perceive penile sensation as a pleasant sensation, whereas 11.6% perceived it as a pleasurable feeling.[16] After GAHT, Bartolucci and colleagues reported that 22% of 67 participants were very dissatisfied and 31% were dissatisfied in their sex life.[23] However, Ristori and colleagues reported that sexual distress correlated to low sexual satisfaction and GAHT helped alleviate sexual distress after 6 months of the treatment in 36 participants.[14]

The effect of GAS on satisfaction with sex life was evaluated in 8 studies[17,19,35–37,42,48,50] (**Table 12**). There was an improvement or positive effect of GAS on satisfaction or happiness in sexual function in 7 studies that included 363 TGW.[17,19,36,37,42,48,50] The largest study by Lawrence and colleagues in 232 TGW with neovagina reported a mean overall happiness with a sexual function score of 7.8/10.[36] However, a study by De Cuypere and colleagues in 29 TGW found a similar level of satisfaction in sexual activity with a partner between before and after GAS.[17] And a study by Hess and colleagues in 91 participants found that 44.3% had a positive satisfaction about their sex life, whereas 14.8% never felt pleasure after GAS.[35]

To compare the level of satisfaction in TGW with neovagina to reproductive age cisgender women, a study of 62 TGW using a 20-item Maudsley Marital Questionnaire reported significantly lower sexual satisfaction compared with cisgender women.[27]

There were 4 studies in a total of 154 TGW using FSFI to evaluate sexual satisfaction.[30–33] All studies reported lower mean score for sexual satisfaction than the mean score in a nonclinical control group of cisgender women.[29] Being sexually active related to a higher score of sexual satisfaction at the mean score of 4.2 ± 1.7 compared with 3.9 ± 1.6 in sexually inactive.[30] The prevalence of sexual dysfunction was 67% of TGW according to FSFI score in Buncamper and colleagues[30] and 31% in Bouman and colleagues.[32] Transgender women reported genital self-image scores comparable to cisgender women[51] in 3 studies that included 104 TGW using the Female Genital Self-Image Scale (FGSIS).[30,32,33]

DISCUSSION

Overall, there were 44 studies included in this review, 20 studies for TGM and 35 for TGW. In TGM, GAHT increased sexual desire and sexual arousal in short-term studies; GAS had mixed results on sexual desire and sexual arousal but was positively associated with more sexual activity and satisfaction from sex. GAHT and GAS did not consistently improve orgasm in TGM. After GAHT/GAS, sexual activity in TGM tended to involve less vaginal stimulation and more use of the clitoris or neophallus. In TGW, GAHT led to a short-term decrease in sexual desire; GAS increased both sexual desire and arousal. The effect of GAHT/GAS on the frequency of orgasm seemed to be mixed but the quality of orgasm was reported to be better after GAS. Pain during vaginal receptive intercourse is not uncommon but the level of pain was often of minimal concern to TGW. After GAS, most TGW involved the neovagina in sexual activity and had more sexual encounters than those TGW who have not yet received GAHT/GAS. In most of the studies, TGW reported that GAS improved their overall sexual satisfaction.

There were limitations of this review and areas of improvement for future research studies on sexual health in TG populations. The biggest limitation was the heterogeneity of the measurement tools of the sexual health outcomes and the differences in GAHT regimens and GAS procedures by both TGW and TGM. Therefore, it is difficult to generalize these findings to the sexual health of all TG people. Some validated tools to capture sexual health outcomes have been used in the cisgender population but these have not been broadly adopted and validated in the TG population.[52] These tools should be modified and adopted for use for TG research. There might be some topics or questions that do not apply to transgender people. For example, the FSFI that was used in many studies involving TGW had a series of questions for vaginal lubrication. This would be only relevant for some but not all genital GAS surgeries.[17,38]

A lack of an appropriate reference group is another limitation of these reported studies. Some of these studies used cisgender controls to interpret the outcomes from transgender people, which may not be appropriate given the outcomes of interest. It may be appropriate to develop reference ranges in various domains in sexual health from a representative population of TG people to better interpret the influence of GAHT/GAS on sexual health outcomes. For example, many studies used the FSFI reference range derived from cisgender women to define sexual dysfunction, which may be inappropriate to apply to TGW and may miscategorize a person's sexual health.[29,53]

Another area that requires further investigation is a better understanding of sexual dysfunction and pleasure in transgender people, which may differ from cisgender people. Sexual perception and satisfaction in transgender people are multidimensional and may be influenced by other factors such as body image, gender dysphoria, and sex hormone levels. Certain sexual activities may be perceived differently among cisgender and transgender people.[4,16] Gender incongruence, particularly before GAHT/GAS, between body and gender identity might be exacerbated by engaging in sexual activity and cause more distress.[16] For instance, TGW with a high level of body dysphoria have significantly lower sexual desire.[7] Many TG people do not seek out sexual activity and are not bothered by absence of sex.[12] An increase in sexual desire (or any sexual health domain) might not be deemed a positive outcome for every transgender people. Although many studies in this review demonstrated an overall improved sexual satisfaction after GAS, it is important to keep in mind that GAHT and GAS alleviate gender dysphoria and improve body esteem, which may be the reasons for the improved sexual satisfaction.

Finally, another major finding of this review is that many studies enrolled very few study participants. The number of participants in these reviewed studies ranged from 9 to 401. There were 26 studies that have less than 50 participants. These smaller studies were likely underpowered to see any significant changes in sexual health outcomes. Furthermore, only 13 studies in this review were prospective in study design, whereas the remaining 31 studies were retrospective or cross-sectional. Selection bias is also a concern of these published studies. The topic of sexual health is difficult to broach in a clinical setting; thus, TG people who were more satisfied may have been more likely to participate in these studies. Moreover, these studies were generally conducted in urban centers in Western countries and thus these results are not generalizable to other parts of the world including Asia, South America, and Africa.

Future Research

Standardized tools to measure all aspects of sexual function for transgender people are urgently needed. Specific criteria for several sexual health outcomes that pertain to the TG population are needed to interpret these study findings. Research in different continents or populations would add more to the understanding of the sexual health of transgender people in non-Western countries.

SUMMARY

There were a limited number of studies on the topic of sexual function and health in transgender people. This review found that TGW tended to have a higher prevalence of sexual dysfunction than TGM. Transition procedures such as GAHT and GAS appear to improve the overall sexual satisfaction in both TGM and TGW. However, the evidence presented in this review come from a wide variety of methodologies, measurement tools, and different hormone and surgeries, which increase the risk of bias and decrease the generalizability of these results. Standardized tools for sexual health outcomes and a normative database specifically for TG people are urgently needed. More research in the sexual health of transgender people should also include gender nonbinary or gender diverse people.

CLINICS CARE POINTS

- Sexuality and sexual function in transgender people are influenced by several factors including hormonal, surgical, physiologic, psychological, and social factors.
- There are no specific criteria or guidelines to assess or diagnose sexual dysfunction in transgender people. However, current criteria for cisgender people may be able to be applied until guidelines specific to transgender people are available.
- Gender-affirming hormone therapy and gender-affirming surgery affect the sexual function of a transgender individual. However, the effects can vary by individual.

- Transgender people may have different goals and expectations for sexual health that may differ from cisgender people.
- Health care providers are encouraged to discuss sexual health and sexual function before, during, and after gender-affirming medical and surgical therapies to provide support that suitable for each individual.

SUPPLEMENTARY DATA

Supplementary data related to this article can be found online at https://doi.org/10.1016/j.ucl.2021.06.004.

REFERENCES

1. American Psychiatric Association. Diagnostic and statistical manual of mental disorders. 5th edition. Arlington: American Psychiatric Association; 2013. p. 451–9.
2. Coleman E, Bockting W, Botzer M, et al. Standards of care for the health of transsexual, transgender, and gender-nonconforming people, version 7. Int J Transgenderism 2012;13(4):165–232.
3. Hembree WC, Cohen-Kettenis PT, Gooren L, et al. Endocrine treatment of gender-dysphoric/gender-incongruent persons: an endocrine society clinical practice guideline. J Clin Endocrinol Metab 2017; 102(11):3869–903.
4. Holmberg M, Arver S, Dhejne C. Supporting sexuality and improving sexual function in transgender persons. Nat Rev Urol 2019;16(2):121–39.
5. Becasen JS, Denard CL, Mullins MM, et al. Estimating the prevalence of HIV and sexual behaviors among the US transgender population: a systematic review and meta-analysis, 2006-2017. Am J Public Health 2019;109(1):e1–8.
6. Kerckhof ME, Kreukels BPC, Nieder TO, et al. Prevalence of sexual dysfunctions in transgender persons: results from the ENIGI follow-up study. J Sex Med 2019;16(12):2018–29.
7. Defreyne J, Elaut E, Kreukels B, et al. Sexual desire changes in transgender individuals upon initiation of hormone treatment: results from the longitudinal european network for the investigation of gender incongruence. J Sex Med 2020;17(4):812–25.
8. Wierckx K, Elaut E, Van Caenegem E, et al. Sexual desire in female-to-male transsexual persons: exploration of the role of testosterone administration. Eur J Endocrinol 2011;165(2):331–7.
9. van Dijk D, Dekker M, Conemans EB, et al. Explorative prospective evaluation of short-term subjective effects of hormonal treatment in trans people-results from the European network for the investigation of gender incongruence. J Sex Med 2019;16(8):1297–309.
10. Costantino A, Cerpolini S, Alvisi S, et al. A prospective study on sexual function and mood in female-to-male transsexuals during testosterone administration and after sex reassignment surgery. J Sex Marital Ther 2013;39(4):321–35.
11. Wierckx K, Van Caenegem E, Schreiner T, et al. Cross-sex hormone therapy in trans persons is safe and effective at short-time follow-up: results from the European network for the investigation of gender incongruence. J Sex Med 2014;11(8): 1999–2011.
12. Wierckx K, Elaut E, Van Hoorde B, et al. Sexual desire in trans persons: associations with sex reassignment treatment. J Sex Med 2014;11(1):107–18.
13. van de Grift TC, Pigot GLS, Boudhan S, et al. A longitudinal study of motivations before and psychosexual outcomes after genital gender-confirming surgery in transmen. J Sex Med 2017; 14(12):1621–8.
14. Ristori J, Cocchetti C, Castellini G, et al. Hormonal treatment effect on sexual distress in transgender persons: 2-year follow-up data. J Sex Med 2020; 17(1):142–51.
15. Wierckx K, Van Caenegem E, Elaut E, et al. Quality of life and sexual health after sex reassignment surgery in transsexual men. J Sex Med 2011;8(12): 3379–88.
16. Cerwenka S, Nieder TO, Cohen-Kettenis P, et al. Sexual behavior of gender-dysphoric individuals before gender-confirming interventions: a European multicenter study. J Sex Marital Ther 2014;40(5): 457–71.
17. De Cuypere G, T'Sjoen G, Beerten R, et al. Sexual and physical health after sex reassignment surgery. Arch Sex Behav 2005;34(6):679–90.
18. Garcia MM, Christopher NA, De Luca F, et al. Overall satisfaction, sexual function, and the durability of neophallus dimensions following staged female to male genital gender confirming surgery: the Institute of Urology, London U.K. experience. Transl Androl Urol 2014;3(2):156–62.
19. Smith YL, van Goozen SH, Cohen-Kettenis PT. Adolescents with gender identity disorder who were accepted or rejected for sex reassignment surgery: a prospective follow-up study. J Am Acad Child Adolesc Psychiatry 2001;40(4):472–81.
20. Nikkelen SWC, Kreukels BPC. Sexual experiences in transgender people: the role of desire for gender-confirming interventions, psychological well-being, and body satisfaction. J sex marital Ther 2018; 44(4):370–81.
21. Fein LA, Salgado CJ, Sputova K, et al. Sexual preferences and partnerships of transgender persons mid- or post-transition. J Homosex 2018;65(5):659–71.
22. Reisner SL, Pletta DR, Potter J, et al. Initial psychometric evaluation of a brief sexual functioning screening

tool for transmasculine adults: transmasculine sexual functioning index. Sex Med 2020;8(3):350–60.

23. Bartolucci C, Gomez-Gil E, Salamero M, et al. Sexual quality of life in gender-dysphoric adults before genital sex reassignment surgery. J Sex Med 2015; 12(1):180–8.

24. McNichols CHL, O'Brien-Coon D, Fischer B. Patient-reported satisfaction and quality of life after trans male gender affirming surgery. Int J Transgender Health 2020;21(4):410–7.

25. van de Grift TC, Kreukels BP, Elfering L, et al. Body image in transmen: multidimensional measurement and the effects of mastectomy. J Sex Med 2016; 13(11):1778–86.

26. Becker I, Auer M, Barkmann C, et al. A cross-sectional multicenter study of multidimensional body image in adolescents and adults with gender dysphoria before and after transition-related medical interventions. Arch Sex Behav 2018;47(8): 2335–47.

27. Elaut E, De Cuypere G, De Sutter P, et al. Hypoactive sexual desire in transsexual women: prevalence and association with testosterone levels. Eur J Endocrinol 2008;158(3):393–9.

28. Kronawitter D, Gooren LJ, Zollver H, et al. Effects of transdermal testosterone or oral dydrogesterone on hypoactive sexual desire disorder in transsexual women: results of a pilot study. Eur J Endocrinol 2009;161(2):363–8.

29. ter Kuile MM, Brauer M, Laan E. The Female Sexual Function Index (FSFI) and the Female Sexual Distress Scale (FSDS): psychometric properties within a Dutch population. J sex marital Ther 2006; 32(4):289–304.

30. Buncamper ME, Honselaar JS, Bouman MB, et al. Aesthetic and functional outcomes of neovaginoplasty using penile skin in male-to-female transsexuals. J Sex Med 2015;12(7):1626–34.

31. Weyers S, Elaut E, De Sutter P, et al. Long-term assessment of the physical, mental, and sexual health among transsexual women. J Sex Med 2009;6(3):752–60.

32. Bouman MB, van der Sluis WB, van Woudenberg Hamstra LE, et al. Patient-reported esthetic and functional outcomes of primary total laparoscopic intestinal vaginoplasty in transgender women with penoscrotal hypoplasia. J Sex Med 2016;13(9):1438–44.

33. van der Sluis WB, Bouman MB, de Boer NK, et al. Long-term follow-up of transgender women after secondary intestinal vaginoplasty. J Sex Med 2016; 13(4):702–10.

34. Brotto LA, Gehring D, Klein C, et al. Psychophysiological and subjective sexual arousal to visual sexual stimuli in new women. J Psychosom Obstet Gynaecol 2005;26(4):237–44.

35. Hess J, Henkel A, Bohr J, et al. Sexuality after male-to-female gender affirmation surgery. Biomed Res Int 2018;2018:9037979.

36. Lawrence AA. Patient-reported complications and functional outcomes of male-to-female sex reassignment surgery. Arch Sex Behav 2006;35(6):717–27.

37. Zavlin D, Schaff J, Lelle JD, et al. Male-to-female sex reassignment surgery using the combined vaginoplasty technique: satisfaction of transgender patients with aesthetic, functional, and sexual outcomes. Aesthet Plast Surg 2018;42(1):178–87.

38. Lawrence AA. Sexuality before and after male-to-female sex reassignment surgery. Arch Sex Behav 2005;34(2):147–66.

39. Selvaggi G, Monstrey S, Ceulemans P, et al. Genital sensitivity after sex reassignment surgery in transsexual patients. Ann Plast Surg 2007;58(4): 427–33.

40. Perovic SV, Stanojevic DS, Djordjevic ML. Vaginoplasty in male transsexuals using penile skin and a urethral flap. BJU Int 2000;86(7):843–50.

41. Wagner S, Greco F, Hoda MR, et al. Male-to-female transsexualism: technique, results and 3-year follow-up in 50 patients. Urol Int 2010;84(3):330–3.

42. LeBreton M, Courtois F, Journel NM, et al. Genital sensory detection thresholds and patient satisfaction with vaginoplasty in male-to-female transgender women. J Sex Med 2017;14(2):274–81.

43. Raigosa M, Avvedimento S, Yoon TS, et al. Male-to-female genital reassignment surgery: a retrospective review of surgical technique and complications in 60 patients. J Sex Med 2015;12(8):1837–45.

44. Krege S, Bex A, Lummen G, et al. Male-to-female transsexualism: a technique, results and long-term follow-up in 66 patients. BJU Int 2001;88(4): 396–402.

45. Amend B, Seibold J, Toomey P, et al. Surgical reconstruction for male-to-female sex reassignment. Eur Urol 2013;64(1):141–9.

46. Goddard JC, Vickery RM, Qureshi A, et al. Feminizing genitoplasty in adult transsexuals: early and long-term surgical results. BJU Int 2007;100(3): 607–13.

47. Soli M, Brunocilla E, Bertaccini A, et al. Male to female gender reassignment: modified surgical technique for creating the neoclitoris and mons veneris. J Sex Med 2008;5(1):210–6.

48. Lobato MI, Koff WJ, Manenti C, et al. Follow-up of sex reassignment surgery in transsexuals: a Brazilian cohort. Arch Sex Behav 2006;35(6):711–5.

49. Cardoso da Silva D, Schwarz K, Fontanari AM, et al. WHOQOL-100 before and after sex reassignment surgery in brazilian male-to-female transsexual individuals. J Sex Med 2016;13(6):988–93.

50. Ozkan O, Ozkan O, Cinpolat A, et al. Vaginal reconstruction with the modified rectosigmoid colon:

surgical technique, long-term results and sexual outcomes. J Plast Surg Hand Surg 2018;52(4):210–6.

51. Herbenick D, Schick V, Reece M, et al. The Female Genital Self-Image Scale (FGSIS): results from a nationally representative probability sample of women in the United States. J Sex Med 2011;8(1):158–66.

52. Vedovo F, Di Blas L, Perin C, et al. Operated male-to-female sexual function index: validity of the first questionnaire developed to assess sexual function after male-to-female gender affirming surgery. J Urol 2020;204(1):115–20.

53. Wiegel M, Meston C, Rosen R. The female sexual function index (FSFI): cross-validation and development of clinical cutoff scores. J Sex Marital Ther 2005;31(1):1–20.

Sexual Wellness in Cisgender Lesbian, Gay, and Bisexual People

Brett A. Stark, MD, MPH[a], Juno Obedin-Maliver, MD, MPH, MAS, FACOG[b],
Alan W. Shindel, MD, MAS[c],*

KEYWORDS

- Lesbian • Gay • Bisexual • Sexual wellness • Sexual dysfunction • Sexuality

KEY POINTS

- Sexual orientation is a fundamental aspect of most people's self-identity. Healthcare outcomes are optimized when patients are able to disclose and discuss their sexual orientation and behavior with their provider without fear of recrimination.
- A habit of non-judgmental inquiry and provision of evidence-based advice (when available) is essential to care of patients who are part of a sexual minority group. Clinical judgement and informed counseling is are required in circumstances where evidence basis is lacking.
- Sexual dysfunction is prevalent in sexual minority women and men. The prevalence and ramifications of sexual concerns tends to be similar to non-sexual minority women and men but subtle differences may exist which influence what constitutes optimal care.
- Treatment options for sexual dysfunction in sexual minority persons should proceed according to standard practice and protocol with shared decision making a key element in all treatment selections.

INTRODUCTION

Sexual attraction to persons of the same gender was until recently considered a mental disorder in most Western nations. "Homosexuality" as an intrinsic disorder was dropped from the third edition of the *Diagnostic and Statistical Manual of Mental Disorders* (DSM-III) in 1973. "Ego-Dystonic homosexuality" (ie, personal distress related to having attraction to same-gender partners) was retained, but was removed from the DSM-III revision (DSM-IIII-R) in 1987. Attraction to same-gender partners is no longer considered a mental disturbance, but rather a variant of normal human sexuality.

Estimates vary, but approximately 4.5% of the US adult population identifies as lesbian, gay, bisexual, transgender, queer (LGBTQ) and/or a sexual/gender minority population.[1,2] Although the last few decades have seen marked increase in societal acceptance and visibility of same-gender sexuality and relationships, bias against cisgender (ie, those individuals whose gender identity aligns with that commonly associated with their sex assigned at birth) sexual minority people continues to be an issue with legal, social, public health, and medical implications.[3] Cisgender sexual minority individuals are less likely to have access to health care and more likely to have some specific health issues when compared with the general population.[4,5] Health and health care disparities are thought to stem in large part from discrimination and stigma and may be mediated on an individual level by minority stress (ie,

a Department of Obstetrics, Gynecology, and Reproductive Sciences, University of California, San Francisco, 490 Illinois Street, 10th Floor, Box 0132, San Francisco, CA 94158, USA; b Department of Obstetrics and Gynecology, Stanford University, 1701 Page Mill Road, Palo Alto, CA 94304, USA; c Department of Urology, University of California, San Francisco, 400 Parnassus Avenue, Suite A-610, San Francisco, CA 94143-0738, USA
* Corresponding author.
E-mail address: alan.shindel@ucsf.edu

Urol Clin N Am 48 (2021) 461–472
https://doi.org/10.1016/j.ucl.2021.06.005
0094-0143/21/© 2021 Elsevier Inc. All rights reserved.

persistent and often ubiquitous interpersonal, intrapersonal, and systemic discrimination against a person from a minority group).[6]

Sexual wellness is defined by the World Health Organization and Pan-American Health Organization as "a state of physical, emotional, mental and social well-being in relation to sexuality; it is not merely the absence of disease, dysfunction or infirmity."[7] Insufficiency and inequity in provision of health care for LGBTQ persons extends to the provision of care for sexual wellness. Biomedical studies of the sexual lives of cisgender sexual minority people have been historically neglected but rose to prominence as a consequence of the human immunodeficiency virus (HIV) epidemic. Attention to the sexual practices of cisgender men who have sex with men (MSM) became an area of particular concern with a focus on HIV risk mitigation, rather than optimizing sexual wellness.[8,9] Data on both sexual wellness and risk mitigation strategies in cisgender women who have sex with women are scant. The dearth of biomedical data on sexual wellness in cisgender women who have sex with women may stem from prejudice, the false assumption that women who have sex with women are not at risk of sexually transmitted infections, a perception that women's sexual wellness is not a biomedical issue, and/or other factors.[10]

In this article, we review current best practices and supporting evidence for treating sexual concerns in cisgender lesbian, gay, and bisexual individuals. We recognize that some cisgender individuals may engage in sexual activity with partners of the same gender and/or have same gender attraction without endorsing a gay, lesbian, or bisexual sexual orientation and or identity. Although discordance between an individual's sexual attraction, behavior, and orientation or identity are well-known and have health implications, the consideration of these unique circumstances is beyond the scope of this review.[11–15]

We also recognize the importance of considering sexual wellness needs of transgender, gender nonbinary, and other gender minority individuals who may endorse a gay, lesbian, or bisexual orientation. The care of transgender and gender nonbinary persons is considered in another article published in this volume. Space limitations also prohibit us from devoting consideration to other sexual minority groups, specifically individuals who (1) identify as asexual, queer, or hold multiple sexual identities, (2) engage in consensual nonmonogamy (eg, polyamory, open relationships), and (3) engage in relationship dynamics that feature consensual power exchange and/or fetishistic activity (eg, bondage/discipline/

sadomasochism [BDSM], "kink"). Interested readers are referred to recent publications on the particular health care needs of these populations.[16–18]

DEFINITIONS

A full discussion of sexuality and gender is beyond the scope of this article. However, some terms are essential to any discussion of sexual wellness. It is important to recognize that sex, sexual orientation, and gender identity are separate constructs. Simplistically, sex assigned at birth is "what body parts was one born with," gender identity is "who one has sex AS," and sexual orientation is "WITH WHOM one has sex." For example, a person who was born with a penis and testicles (male sex assigned at birth) and identifies as a woman (transgender) who is sexually attracted to and engages in sexual behavior with women (lesbian) may conceptualize themselves as a lesbian woman, regardless of their genitalia or external appearance. An individual who was born with a vagina, uterus, and ovaries (female sex assigned at birth) and identifies as a woman (cisgender) and is sexually attracted to women (lesbian) may also conceptualize themselves as a lesbian woman, although their lived experience will likely be quite different from the aforementioned lesbian woman.

CARE OF CISGENDER SEXUAL MINORITY PATIENTS

Fundamentally, the basic physiology of sexual response does not differ between cisgender heterosexual and cisgender sexual minority individuals. Interpersonal dynamics and sexuality-related concerns also tend to be similar between heterosexual and cisgender sexual minority persons.[19] The care of the cisgender sexual minority patients should in most circumstances proceed according to well-established protocols on proper inquiry, evaluation, and treatment of the patient with sexual concerns.[20–29] Although the fundamentals of evaluation and respect for patient autonomy apply, some specific issues merit consideration.

Many cisgender sexual minority patients have experienced bias when seeking health care. This bias may be explicit and intentional (eg, hostile comments, neglect, refusal to provide care) or subtle and potentially unintentional (eg, assumption of heterosexual orientation, failure to use preferred terminology).[3] It is essential that health care providers remain agnostic with respect to a given patient's sexual orientation until the patient themselves discloses.[3] Disclosure of sexual orientation to health care providers is associated with superior clinical outcomes and hence should be deemed an essential element of the history.[30] Providers can help to facilitate this disclosure by avoiding heteronormative assumptions, making clear that the clinical encounter is a "safe space," and tactfully eliciting the patient's gender identity, sexual orientation, and sex assigned at birth.

Health care providers need not be expert on every aspect of cisgender sexual minority sexuality nor familiar with every term. Providers should be willing to ask for clarification of any terms or concepts with which they are not familiar. A habit of "humble inquiry" (an approach that is based on tactful, nonprurient curiosity and interest in the other person) and a willingness to use a patient's preferred terms tends to help put patients at ease.[31]

It is essential that the provider maintain a nonjudgmental attitude. Ultimately, all persons, including health care providers, are entitled to their personal beliefs about the appropriateness of sexual activity between persons of the same gender. Nevertheless, professionalism dictates that the wellness of patients is our priority; we must not allow personal biases or beliefs to interfere with the provision of evidence-based care.[32] This consideration extends to recommendations about risk mitigation strategies, including safer sex practices. For example, the safest form of sexual expression is one that involves no skin-to-skin contact between people (ie, celibacy). Celibacy may entail avoidance of all sexual intimacy, but some self-identified celibate individuals may engage in isolated self-masturbation with or without a partner present, concurrent self-masturbation with a partner, and/or clothed tribadism (ie, genital to genital stimulation without penetration, colloquially known as "dry humping"). A celibate lifestyle is not tolerable to most individuals and hence risk mitigation strategies (eg, barrier protection, routine testing for sexually transmitted infections) are used to decrease (but not eliminate) the odds of unwanted health outcomes. In the context of sexual activity between consenting adults of any sexual orientation or gender identity, the health care provider's obligation is to understand preferred sexual activities and provide evidence-based guidance on risk mitigation so as optimize patient well-being.

SEXUAL MINORITY WOMEN AND SEXUAL DYSFUNCTION

Sexual minority women (SMW) in an umbrella term inclusive but not limited to women who define themselves by sexual identity (eg, lesbian,

bisexual, queer, questioning), behavior (eg, women who have sex with women, women who have sex with men and women), or relationship status (eg, women who are married to or cohabit with other women). It is important to consider all 3 aspects of sexual identity. The gender identity of sexual partners of SMW cannot be ascertained by sexual identity alone, because 77.3% of SMW who identify as lesbian report a cisgender male partner in their lifetime, with 5.7% reporting sexual contact with a cisgender man in the last year.[33] Conversely, many women who identify as heterosexual report a history of sexual contact with another woman.[34] SMW are more likely to endorse frequent masturbation, a higher total number of partners, and greater sexual desire compared with non-SMW. SMW are also more likely to experience an earlier sexual debut with a mean age at sexual debut of 14.4 versus 15.7 years for SMW versus non-SMW, respectively ($P<.001$).[35]

SMW women participate in a variety of sexual activities, including vaginal and anal penetrative sex, orogenital sex (cunnilingus), masturbation, oroanal sex (analingus), and vibrator use.[36] A 2012 study of 3116 (presumably) cisgender lesbian and bisexual women reported that the most commonly cited sexual practices between women in the last year included genital rubbing (99.5%) vaginal fingering (98.2%), cunnilingus (97.6%), vibrator use (59.6%), and nonvibrating dildo use (55.6%).[37] Less commonly used sexual practices included use of a nonvibrating strap-on, vaginal fisting, butt plugs, and anal beads, with 43.5%, 53.5%, 89.5%, and 93.4% of participants stating they had never used these practices, respectively.[37]

Studies on women's sexuality in general have been fraught with limitations and misconceptions; for instance, a 43% prevalence of sexual dysfunction in American women was promulgated for many years based on studies such as that of by Laumann and colleagues,[38] which reported out subject responses to 7 dichotomous questions on specific sexual issues over the past 12 months. This study did not assess chronicity, frequency, or sex-related distress, which are essential elements for the accurate diagnosis of a sexual dysfunction in any person. A 2008 American study that drew distinctions between "sexual problems" (eg, self-perceived low sexual desire or arousal, difficulty reaching orgasm) and sex-related distress confirmed that, although sexual problems were present in 43% of women, sex-related distress was present in 22% and concomitant sexual distress and problem(s) was present in just 12% of women.[39]

It is noteworthy that sexual orientation and partner gender were not explicitly assessed in the aforementioned "nationally representative" study.[39] The prevalence of sexual dysfunction in SMW remains incompletely characterized, although quantitative biomedical data on these populations do exist.[40] Interestingly, the 1999 study by Laumann et al did not report any statistically significant differences in sexual dysfunction between women who had or had not had lifetime sexual contact with another woman.[38] More contemporary data have supported the notion that the prevalence of sexual problems and distress is relatively similar between lesbians and heterosexual women, although bisexual women may be at greater risk of sexual dissatisfaction than either other group.[41] Sexuality factors known to be strongly associated with one another in non-SMW (eg, sexual frequency with orgasm frequency, orgasm frequency with sexual satisfaction, sexual satisfaction with relationship satisfaction) seem to be related to one another in SMW as well.[42,43] The results of individual studies do vary, with some suggesting superior functioning in terms of orgasm and lubrication among lesbian women in comparison with heterosexual women.[44]

Several quantitative metrics have been developed to allow for large-scale and comparative study of sexual function in women. Among these instruments, the Female Sexual Functioning Index (FSFI)[45] is the most widely used and has been validated in multiple populations, including validation studies in lesbian women.[46,47] Some specific modifications made for FSFI versions useable in SMW include replacing the term "penile penetration" with "vaginal penetration."

The FSFI is a brief self-report measure composed of the following subscales: desire, arousal, lubrication, orgasm, satisfaction, and pain.[45] An FSFI total score of 26.55 or less suggests a risk for sexual dysfunction. It is important to remember that FSFI alone cannot diagnose dysfunction because it does not include a distress criterion.[48] The FSFI total score also does not provide specifics on the nature of the sexual concern/problem. The FSFI may also be misinterpreted as a response of "no sexual activity" is typically scored as zero, although it may not reflect a bothersome state of affairs over short periods of time in some SMW couples. To rectify this potential FSFI scoring problem, Meyer-Bahlburg and Dolezal[47] suggest transforming zeros to missing values, whereas Boehmer and colleagues[49] recommended replacing missing values through simple mean imputation. Both of these methods have been used to validate the FSFI in SMW populations. These issues and the generally heteronormative focus on the FSFI

suggest that a novel tool or tools may be useful for more nuanced quantitative studies of sexual wellness in SMW.

"Bed death" is a colloquial term used to describe longitudinal decreases in sexual activity in SMW relationships not necessarily associated with concomitant decline in emotional intimacy.[50,51] In a population-based study by Flynn and colleagues,[44] SMW reported less partnered sexual activity in the past 30 days as compared with heterosexual women (47% vs 56%, respectively) despite reporting similar rates of "single and not dating" relationship status (21% vs 22%, respectively). One semistructured interview of 30 SMW with a partner of more than 6 months reported a majority experienced bed death and felt it was related to decreased sexual initiative and sexual desire.[50] However, Cohen and colleagues[51] argue that the presence of this phenomenon does not always correlate with relationship problems or sexual dysfunction, because SMW who reported they could discuss sexual problems freely with their partners reported greater overall sexual satisfaction despite the presence of bed death. It also remains unclear whether the decrease in sexual frequency in SMW relationships differs substantively from the general trend toward less frequent sexual activity often seen in most long-term relationships.

SMW may experience genitopelvic pain/penetration disorder, regardless of whether or not they engage in vaginal or anal penetrative sex. Blair and colleagues[52] in a cross-sectional convenience study of heterosexual and SMW aged 18 to 45 years reported pain inside the vagina was the most commonly reported location for sexual pain, followed by pain in the pelvic/abdominal pain and/or the vaginal introitus. The prevalence of reported genitopelvic pain/penetration disorder in SMW varies across populations and is estimated to be between 5.9% and 24.2%.[52–55] This prevalence is generally lower than what is reported in studies of non-SMW.[52] However, 1 web-based study demonstrated no significant differences in the percentage of distressing sexual symptoms between lesbian and heterosexual women.[56] Although SMW may experience sex-related genital pain, communication with the partner is associated with the perception of pain having less of an effect on relationship and sexual functioning.[52]

The prevalence of female orgasmic disorder is poorly characterized in SMW. Risk factors for orgasm issues seem to be similar between SMW and non-SMW, with psychosocial and anxiety figuring prominently in orgasmic disorders for both groups.[57] There are mixed data on the impact of anxiety on the ability of SMW to achieve orgasm under stress, with 1 study showing a decreased ability climax, whereas another showed no change, leading the authors to postulate that anxiety for SMW may manifest in ways other than sexual problems[46,57]

SMW may experience unique risk factors that increase their risk for sexual dysfunction. For example, SMW are at higher risk for tobacco or recreational drug use, mental illness including major depressive disease, poor general physical health, and interpersonal violence.[58–61] Mental health disorders and psychological domains have been associated with sexual dysfunction in men and women, although mainly studied in heterosexual populations. Substance abuse and antidepressant medications have long been associated with sexual dysfunctions including inhibited orgasm and diminished sexual desire and excitement.[62,63] Although data assessing the impact of anxiety and depression on SMW sexual health is limited, it is possible that depression and anxiety in SMW are associated with worsening sexual function through negative effects on arousal, orgasm, satisfaction and lubrication.[64]

It is important to consider the role of breast cancer in the sexual health of SMW. Although there is no causal evidence that SMW experience breast cancer at higher rates than non-SMW, there are data to suggest that SMW have more risk factors for breast cancer (lower parity and lactation) and lower rates of mammography screening.[65] One study of SMW diagnosed with breast cancer reported lower rates of sexual desire, a decreased ability to reach orgasm, less sexual frequency, and higher rates of sexual pain.[66]

The American College of Obstetrics and Gynecology and the International Society for the Study of Women's Sexual Health have provided evidence-based guidelines for the management of sexual dysfunction in cisgender women.[20,28,29,67] These guidelines were largely developed through research in heterosexual cisgender women, and the guidelines do not specifically discuss the management of sexual dysfunction in SMW. Given the lack of evidence-based treatment options for SMW, the authors recommend use of these, or similar, guidelines in the management of sexual dysfunction for SMW while calling for studies and guidelines that actively include and center an evidence-based approach for cisgender SMW.

All professional society recommendation on sexual wellness in women advocate discussing sexuality with patients during routine care visits to help identify potential problems early and destigmatize the discussion of sexual function with patients. This screening can be performed using validated questionnaires, such as the previously described FSFI. Once sexual dysfunction is recognized, the initial management should include obtaining a detailed history and performing a physical examination. Depending on the underlying etiology of sexual dysfunction, treatment options may include pelvic floor physical therapy, hormonal and nonhormonal medical management, and lifestyle changes, such as the inclusion of vaginal lubricants. Continuing research is needed to study and classify the differences in sexual function and dysfunction among SMW, and to help identify potentially unique therapeutic interventions that could be useful in this population.

SEXUAL WELLNESS IN SEXUAL MINORITY MEN

Sexual and romantic relationships in sexual minority men (SMM) vary; the interpersonal dynamics and relationship structure of among SMM (including bisexual and gay men) can be as heterogeneous as in any other dyad. Unpartnered bisexual and gay men are often sexually active; the United States National Survey of Sexual Health and Behavior reported that less than 25% of unpartnered gay men had not engaged partnered sexual activity in the past year, compared with more than 75% of unpartnered heterosexual and bisexual men.[68] Consensual nonmonogamy and BDSM are more frequently features of gay male relationships when compared with the general population. Although these practices are more common in LGB couples compared with strictly heterosexual couples, they represent a minority of all gay male relationships.[69,70]

Sexual activity between cisgender SMM may take the form of full body contact, mutual masturbation, oral sex, and anal sex.[68,69,71] Anal sex may involve the insertion of an erect penis into the rectum; other means of sexual expression involving the anus or rectum include oral to anal contact (analingus or "rimming") and fisting (insertion of a finger or hand into the rectum).[72] Oral sex is the most common means used to achieve climax in gay male encounters.[71] Interestingly, approximately one-third of gay men report having had lifetime oral or vaginal sex with a female partner.[68]

Sexual activity involving the anus and rectum is commonly associated with gay men, but these practices are not ubiquitous. Although more than 80% of gay men report a lifetime experience with both receptive and insertive anal sex, a 2011 study (n = 24,787 gay and bisexual men) reported that just 34% and 36% report either insertive or receptive anal sex as part of their most recent sexual encounter.[68,69,71] Among SMM who do engage in anal intercourse, some men prefer being the insertive partner ("top"), the receptive partner ("bottom"), or both ("switch" or "versatile").

Some consideration should be devoted to the importance of ejaculation in SMM. Ejaculation is an essential element of sexual experience for many men (of any sexual orientation), aside from its obvious relevance for procreation and strong association with the pleasurable sensation of orgasm. Studies from Australia and the United States indicated that semen itself is eroticized and/or used as a component of sexual play for approximately 1 out of 6 gay men.[73,74] Ejaculation disorders may be a particular source for concern in SMM, particularly if there is a sense of comparison between men who are both expected to ejaculate during sex.

EPIDEMIOLOGY OF SEXUAL PROBLEMS IN SEXUAL MINORITY MEN

Estimates of the prevalence of sexual problems in SMM is hampered by limited existing data and a lack of fully validated metrics for assessment. Older studies which included nonheterosexual men most often used sexual orientation as an independent variable for use in analyses of the prevalence of sexual problems. Data from these studies tended to indicate that SMM are at increased risk of erectile dysfunction (ED), but have similar or lower risk for premature ejaculation (PE) compared with heterosexual men.[23,75] More recent comparative evidence has suggested that the prevalence of PE may be generally similar between SMM and strictly heterosexual men although variability in data acquisition and metrics used confuse this issue.[76]

Data on Peyronie's disease in SMM are very limited; a single study of 27 gay men with Peyronie's disease reported that disease parameters are generally similar between groups with the exception of MSM presenting more often with noncurvature deformities compared with strictly heterosexual men (11% vs 1%, respectively).[77]

A major limitation of older data is the absence of validated quantitative survey instruments. The International Index of Erectile Function (IIEF) and the Erectile Function subdomain of the IIEF are the most commonly used tools for research on men's erectile response. A version of the IIEF has been validated for use in gay, HIV-positive men (IIEF-MSM). The principal modifications of this instrument include removal of "vaginal penetration" as a metric and inclusion of erection responses during masturbation, oral sex, and anal penetration.[78] Although the instrument has not been validated in non–HIV-positive men, nothing in the instrument itself invokes HIV status and hence this may be a useful tool for the assessment of erectile function in MSM.

The bulk of contemporary studies on sexual problems in men are focused on heterosexual men and frequently invoke "vaginal penetration" as the outcome measure of greatest interest. The varied nature of sexual expression in SMM makes comparison of outcomes challenging. Existing studies do suggest that some of the same variables known to be associated with impairment of sexual wellness in heterosexual men (eg, increasing age, lack of exercise, mental health concerns, interpersonal stressors) are also predictors of sexual problems in MSM.[69,79]

Certain risk factors for sexual dysfunction are more prevalent in SMM. HIV and the medications used to control the condition have been associated with ED.[4,80] Tobacco use is approximately 50% more prevalent in bisexual and gay men compared with heterosexual men.[81] Studies on the particular contribution of tobacco use to the burden of sexual dysfunction in SMM are lacking, but the clear relationship between ED and tobacco makes this a source of concern.[82] Body image also seems to be more frequently a contributing factor to sexual concerns among SMM, particularly with regard to ED and PE[83,84]

The experience of discrimination is also associated with a greater risk of sexual concerns.[83] A study of young bisexual and gay men in Poland, a nation that is not generally accepting of nonheterosexual persons, reported that at least some degree of ED was present in 76% of gay men and 62% of bisexual men. The experience of discrimination and internalized homophobia were associated with worse overall sexual quality of life in this cohort.[79] A study from the United States that focused on young SMM indicated that (after multivariable analysis) there was a weak association between internalized homophobia and decreased overall sexual quality of life, but no significant association between stigma and sexual desire or erectile function.[85] Cultural milieu and overall societal acceptance seem to be play important roles in sexual wellness for SMM.

The largest contemporary report on sexual concerns in MSM enrolled 7001 participants (mean age, 38 years; 81% Caucasian) in an internet-based study.[86] The study used a single item binary response question on the presence of specific sexual problems over the past 12 months. Low sexual desire was the most prevalent concern, with 57% of respondents responding in the affirmative. ED, lack of sexual pleasure, anorgasmia, PE, and pain with sex were reported by 45%,

37%, 36%, 34%, and 14% of men, respectively.[86] The nature of the question makes it impossible to determine if these men were experiencing what would be classified as clinically relevant sexual dysfunctions or as situational or reactive impairments in sexual response.

Another recent study of urinary and sexual wellness in MSM reported out data on 2783 men (mean age, 39 ± 12 years; 85% Caucasian) who participated in an online survey.[69] The IIEF-MSM was administered to participants; participants also completed the Premature Ejaculation Diagnostic Tool, a metric validated (although not specifically in MSM) for assessment and risk stratification regarding bothersome PE.[87]

Validated cut-points for stratification of ED based on the erectile function domain of the IIEF-MSM do not exist; based on existing validation of cut-points for the original IIEF in heterosexual men and a score range of 0 to 30, a score of 10 or less was defined as severe ED, 11 to 15 as moderate ED, and 16 to 24 as mild ED. ED of some severity was present in more than one-half of men over the age of 60; interestingly, approximately 15% of men even in the youngest age cohort (18–29 years) endorsed ED. This estimate is slightly higher than existing estimates from the age-matched general population, although variation in sampling and means of assessment may drive some of these differences.[38] Between 15% and 20% of men in this study had Premature Ejaculation Diagnostic Tool results indicative of possible PE, with the prevalence lower albeit only slightly in older cohorts.

MANAGING SEXUAL PROBLEMS IN SEXUAL MINORITY MEN

A robust body of evidence based-guidance has been promulgated for the management of a variety of sexual problems in men. Specifically, consensus documents from the International Society for Sexual Medicine and the American Urologic Association have provided guidance for practitioners on the evaluation of sexual problems generally and managing specific male sexual problems, including PE, ED, testosterone deficiency, and Peyronie's disease.[21,23,25,26,88] The data from which these evidenced-based recommendations were derived are based heavily on heterosexual populations; nevertheless, there is no reason to conclude that these recommendations are not by and large applicable to SMM.

Briefly, it is recommended that any man with a sexual concern be evaluated with a detailed history.[21] Physical examination and laboratory assessment, particularly assessment of serum testosterone, may be useful based on clinical judgment and risk factors.[23,25,26] Specialized testing may be indicated in select cases.[25,26] Mental health evaluation and encouragement of healthy lifestyle behaviors is oftentimes of great value. ED may be managed with oral phosphodiesterase type 5 inhibitors, intracavernous injection of vasodilators, vacuum tumescence devices, intraurethral prostaglandins suppositories, and/or the placement of penile prostheses.[26] Men with Peyronie's disease may benefit from intratunical injections of clostridial collagenase or surgical correction.[25] There are no therapies approved by the US Food and Drug Administration for PE, but a robust body of evidence supports the use of selective serotonin reuptake inhibitors and/or topical anesthetics for this indication.[23] Although management may follow similar lines for sexual minority (bisexual and gay) and sexual majority (heterosexual/straight) cisgender men, establishing clinician training that frames interventions as being suitable for SMM, continuing to study differences in sexual function and dysfunction by sexual orientation, and finally considering targeted materials and interventions that look at differential outcomes and effects by sexual orientation will move the field forward in ensuring equitable and appropriate health care.

PROSTATE CANCER AND SEXUALITY AMONG SEXUAL MINORITY MEN

Prostate cancer is the most common noncutaneous solid malignancy in North American men and the second leading cause of cancer death.[89] The prevalence of prostate cancer seems to be generally similar in SMM compared with the general cisgender heterosexual population.[90] Gay men are less likely than their heterosexual counterparts to be screened for prostate cancer and hence may present with more advanced disease.[91] Prostate cancer itself tends to be clinically indolent, but may merit treatment depending on issues of longevity and cancer characteristics. All treatments for prostate cancer (prostatectomy, radiotherapy, androgen ablation) carry a high risk of disrupting sexual responses, particularly penile erections and ejaculation.

The prevalence of ED and anejaculation after prostate cancer treatment is well-understood and can affect men of any sexual orientation. Comparative data suggest that SMM who have been treated for prostate cancer tend to experience greater psychological stress and lower health-related quality of life, masculine self-esteem, and treatment satisfaction. Interestingly, despite these findings, SMM treated for prostate cancer reported higher overall ratings of sexual confidence and satisfaction than matched heterosexual men.[92]

The prostate is an erogenous organ for many cisgender SMM, particularly those who engage in anal receptive sex.[93] Loss of this sexual organ may significantly impair sexual enjoyment for these men. Changes in anal sensation and/or the development of bowel issues related to radiotherapy may also be of particular concern to SMM who engage in receptive anal sex[94] SMM may also be more bothered by the loss of ejaculation that accompanies prostate cancer treatment; this greater degree of concern may stem in part from the eroticized role that semen has for some SMM.[93,95,96] SMM may also be particularly impacted by the loss of erectile or ejaculatory function in comparison with their partner(s).[97–100] Like their heterosexual counterparts, the challenges are greater for unpartnered SMM.[93,99]

Heterosexual sexual relationships tend to center on coitus, which requires at least a moderate degree of penile tumescence that can be difficult to attain after prostate cancer treatment. Loss of erectile hardness may be of particular concern for men who engage in anal insertive sex given the high degree of tumescence required for anal penetration[93,100] However, the diversity of SMM sexual expression may facilitate adaptive practices to loss of erectile function from prostate cancer treatment.[101] The loss of once preferred sexual activities (eg, "topping" during anal sex) in the postprostate cancer treatment SMM patient should not, however, be construed as trivial; the goal of therapy should ultimately always be to restoration of sexual activity to pretreatment levels, in as much as this is possible.

FUTURE DIRECTIONS

Research on sexual wellness in cisgender sexual minority populations will be facilitated by the development of new scales and/or the validation of existing scales to quantify relevant domains of sexual response. The National Institutes of Health have designated sexual and gender minority people as a health disparities population for research and this extends to considerations of sexual health and well-being.[102] Such scales will facilitate study of novel therapies. Careful consideration should be given to the variable nature of sexual expression in cisgender sexual minority populations and care taken to be inclusive of this diversity.

Despite positive trends, prejudice against cisgender sexual minority populations at the societal level will most likely persist for the foreseeable future. Health care inequities are thus likely to persist as well. These inequities will continue to exacerbate existing disparities in sexual wellness in cisgender sexual minority individuals; it is hence incumbent on health care providers to emphasize appropriate care for these populations as an element of medical professionalism.

SUMMARY

Cisgender sexual minority persons have sexual wellness needs that go well beyond disease prevention. Despite historical asymmetries research and clinical attention to sexual wellness in cisgender LGB persons, a growing body of evidence exists on how to optimally care for these populations. Additional research and development is warranted.

CLINICS CARE POINTS

- Sexual orientation is a fundamental aspect of most people's self-identity. Health care outcomes are optimized when patients are able to disclose and discuss their sexual orientation and practices with their provider without fear of recrimination.

- A practice of nonjudgmental inquiry and provision of evidence-based advice (when available) is essential to care of patients who are part of a sexual minority group. Clinical judgment and informed counseling is are required in circumstances where an evidence basis is lacking.

- Sexual dysfunction is prevalent in SMW and SMM. The prevalence and ramifications of sexual concerns tends to be similar to non-SMW and non-SMM but subtle differences may exist that influence what constitutes optimal care.

- Treatment options for sexual dysfunction in sexual minority persons should proceed according to standard practice and protocol with shared decision making a key element in all treatment selections.

REFERENCES

1. University of California. Los Angeles School of Law. Williams Institute. LGBT Proportion of Population: United States. LGBT Data & Demographics. 2018. Available at: https://williamsinstitute.law.ucla.edu/visualization/lgbt-stats/?topic=LGBT#density. Accessed August 7, 2020.

2. "Sexual & Gender Minority Research Office." National Institutes of Health, U.S. Department of Health and Human Services. 2020. Available at: dpcpsi.nih.gov/sgmro. Accessed March 10, 2021.

3. Committee on Lesbian, Gay, Bisexual, and Transgender Health Issues and Research Gaps and Opportunities. The health of lesbian, gay, bisexual, and transgender people: Building a foundation for better understanding. Washington, DC: Institute of Medicine; 2011. p. 13128, 10.

4. Luo L, Deng T, Zhao S, et al. Association between HIV infection and prevalence of erectile dysfunction: a systematic review and meta-analysis. J Sex Med 2017;14(9):1125–32.

5. Lee JGL, Griffin GK, Melvin CL. Tobacco use among sexual minorities in the USA, 1987 to May 2007: a systematic review. Tob Control 2009; 18(4):275–82.

6. Meyer IH. Prejudice, social stress, and mental health in lesbian, gay, and bisexual populations: conceptual issues and research evidence. Psychol Bull 2003;129(5):674.

7. World Health Organization. Annual technical report: 2013: Department of Reproductive Health and Research, including UNDP/UNFPA/WHO/World Bank special programme of research training in human Reproduction (HRP). No. WHO/RHR/14.01. World Health Organization; 2014.

8. Boone CA, Lisa B. Structuring sexual pleasure: Equitable access to biomedical HIV prevention for Black men who have sex with men. Am J Public Health 2020;110:157–9.

9. Kantor LM, Laura L. Pleasure and sex education: the need for broadening both content and measurement. Am J Public Health 2020;110(2):145–8.

10. Marrazzo JM. Barriers to infectious disease care among lesbians. Emerg Infect Dis 2004;10(11): 1974.

11. Mishel E. Intersections between sexual identity, sexual attraction, and sexual behavior among a nationally representative sample of American men and women. J Official Stat 2019;35(4):859–84.

12. Bauer GR, Jairam JA. Are lesbians really women who have sex with women (WSW)? Methodological concerns in measuring sexual orientation in health research. Women Health 2008;48(4):383–408.

13. Talley AE, Aranda F, Hughes TL, et al. Longitudinal associations among discordant sexual orientation dimensions and hazardous drinking in a cohort of sexual minority women. J Health Soc Behav 2015; 56(2):225–45.

14. Pathela P, Hajat A, Schillinger J, et al. Discordance between sexual behavior and self-reported sexual identity: a population-based survey of New York City men. Ann Intern Med 2006;145(6):416–25.

15. Diamond M. Sexual identity, attractions, and behavior among young sexual-minority women over a 2-year period. Dev Psychol 2000;36(2): 241.

16. Waldura JF, Arora I, Randall AM, et al. Fifty shades of stigma: exploring the health care experiences of kink-oriented patients. J Sex Med 2016;13(12): 1918–29.

17. Mitchell VE, Mogilski K, Donaldson SH, et al. Sexual motivation and satisfaction among consensually non-monogamous and monogamous individuals. J Sex Med 2020;17(6):1072–85.

18. Brotto LA, Morag Y. Asexuality: sexual orientation, paraphilia, sexual dysfunction, or none of the above? Arch Sex Behav 2017;46(3):619–27.

19. Obedin-Maliver J, Lisha N, Breyer BN, et al. More similarities than differences? An exploratory analysis comparing the sexual complaints, sexual experiences, and genitourinary health of older sexual minority and sexual majority adults. J Sex Med 2019;16(3):347–50.

20. Parish SJ, Hahn SR, Goldstein SW, et al. The International Society for the Study of Women's sexual health process of Care for the Identification of sexual concerns and problems in women. Mayo Clin Proc 2019;94(5):842–56.

21. Althof SE, Rosen RC, Perelman MA, et al. Standard operating procedures for taking a sexual history. J Sex Med 2013;10(1):26–35.

22. Bitzer J, Giraldi A, Pfaus J. Sexual desire and hypoactive sexual desire disorder in women. Introduction and overview. Standard operating procedure (SOP Part 1). J Sex Med 2013;10(1):36–49.

23. Althof SE, McMahon CG, MDWaldinger, et al. An update of the International Society of Sexual Medicine's guidelines for the diagnosis and treatment of premature ejaculation (PE). J Sex Med 2014;11(6): 1392–422.

24. Martin-Tuite P, Shindel AW. Management options for premature ejaculation and delayed ejaculation in men. Sex Med Rev 2019;8(3):473–85.

25. Nehra Ajay, Alterowitz R, Culkin DJ, et al. Peyronie's disease: AUA guideline. J Urol 2015;194(3):745–53.

26. Burnett AL, Nehra A, Breau RH, et al. Erectile dysfunction: AUA guideline. J Urol 2018;200(3): 633–41.

27. American College of Obstetricians and Gynecologists. Female sexual dysfunction: ACOG Practice Bulletin clinical management guidelines for obstetrician-gynecologists, number 213. Obstet Gynecol 2019;134(1):e1–18.

28. Clayton AH, Goldstein I, Kim NN, Althof SE, Faubion SS, Faught BM,, Sadovsky R. The International Society for the Study of Women's Sexual Health process of care for management of hypoactive sexual desire disorder in women. Mayo Clin Proc 2018;93(No. 4):467–87.

29. Goldstein I, Komisaruk BR, Pukall CF, et al. International Society for the Study of Women's Sexual

Health (ISSWSH) Review of Epidemiology and Pathophysiology, and a Consensus Nomenclature and Process of Care for the Management of Persistent Genital Arousal Disorder/Genito-Pelvic Dysesthesia (PGAD/GPD). J Sex Med 2021;18(4):665–97.

30. Ruben MA, Livingston NA, Berke DS, et al. Lesbian, gay, bisexual, and transgender veterans' experiences of discrimination in health care and their relation to health outcomes: a pilot study examining the moderating role of provider communication. Health Equity 2019;3(1):480–8.

31. Lambrechts FJ, Bouwen R, Grieten S, et al. Learning to help through humble inquiry and implications for management research, practice, and education: an interview with Edgar H. Schein. Acad Manag Learn Educ 2011;10(1):131–47.

32. Shindel AW, Parish SJ. CME information: sexuality education in North American medical schools: current status and future directions (CME). J Sex Med 2013;10(1):3–18.

33. Diamant AL, Schuster MA, McGuigan K, et al. Lesbians' sexual history with men: implications for taking a sexual history. Arch Intern Med 1999;159(22):2730–6.

34. Armstrong HL, Reissing ED. Women who have sex with women: a comprehensive review of the literature and conceptual model of sexual function. Sex Relationship Ther 2013;28(4):364–99.

35. Tornello SL, Riskind RG, Patterson CJ. Sexual orientation and sexual and reproductive health among adolescent young women in the United States. J Adolesc Health 2014;54(2):160–8.

36. Xu F, Sternberg MR, Markowitz LE. Women who have sex with women in the United States: prevalence, sexual behavior and prevalence of herpes simplex virus type 2 infection—Results from National Health and Nutrition Examination Survey 2001–2006. Sex Transm Dis 2010;37(7):407–13.

37. Schick V, Rosenberger JG, Herbenick D, et al. Sexual behaviour and risk reduction strategies among a multinational sample of women who have sex with women. Sex Transm infections 2012;88(6):407–12.

38. Laumann EO, Paik A, Rosen RC. Sexual dysfunction in the United States: prevalence and predictors. JAMA 1999;281(6):537–44.

39. Shifren JL, Monz BU, Russo PA, et al. Sexual problems and distress in United States women: prevalence and correlates. Obstet Gynecol 2008;112(5):970–8.

40. Chen J, Sweet G, Shindel A. Urinary disorders and female sexual function. Curr Urol Rep 2013;14(4):298–308.

41. Björkenstam C, Mannheimer L, Löfström M, et al. Sexual Orientation–Related Differences in Sexual Satisfaction and Sexual Problems—A Population-Based Study in Sweden. J Sex Med 2020;17(12):2362–9.

42. Dyar C, Newcomb ME, Mustanski B, et al. A Structural equation model of sexual satisfaction and relationship functioning among sexual and gender minority individuals assigned female at birth in diverse relationships. Arch Sex Behav 2020;49(2):693–710.

43. Scott SB, Ritchie L, Knopp K, et al. Sexuality within female same-gender couples: definitions of sex, sexual frequency norms, and factors associated with sexual satisfaction. Arch Sex Behav 2018;47(3):681–92.

44. Flynn KE, Lin L, Weinfurt KP. Sexual function and satisfaction among heterosexual and sexual minority US adults: a cross-sectional survey. PLoS One 2017;12(4):e0174981.

45. Rosen C, Brown J, Heiman S, et al. The Female Sexual Function Index (FSFI): a multidimensional self-report instrument for the assessment of female sexual function. J Sex Marital Ther 2000;26(2):191–208.

46. Tracy JK, Junginger J. Correlates of lesbian sexual functioning. J Womens Health 2007;16(4):499–509.

47. Boehmer U, Timm A, Izibiff A, et al. Applying the Female Sexual Functioning Index to sexual minority women. J Womens Health 2012;21(4):401–9.

48. Meston CM, Freihart BK, Handy AB, et al. Scoring and interpretation of the FSFI: what can be learned from 20 years of use? J Sex Med 2020;17(1):17–25.

49. Meyer-Bahlburg HFL, Dolezal C. The Female Sexual Function Index: a methodological critique and suggestions for improvement. J Sex Marital Ther 2007;33(3):217–24.

50. van Rosmalen-Nooijens KAWL, Vergeer CM, Lagro-Janssen ALM. Bed death and other lesbian sexual problems unraveled: a qualitative study of the sexual health of lesbian women involved in a relationship. Women Health 2008;48(3):339–62.

51. Cohen JN, Sandra Byers E. Minority stress, protective factors, and sexual functioning of women in a same-sex relationship. Psychol Sex Orientat Gend Divers 2015;2(4):391.

52. Blair KL, Pukall CF, Smith KB, et al. Differential associations of communication and love in heterosexual, lesbian, and bisexual women's perceptions and experiences of chronic vulvar and pelvic pain. J Sex Marital Ther 2015;41(5):498–524.

53. Peixoto MM, Nobre P. Prevalence of sexual problems and associated distress among lesbian and heterosexual women. J Sex Marital Ther 2015;41(4):427–39.

54. Lau JTF, Kim JH, Tsui HY. Prevalence and factors of sexual problems in Chinese males and females having sex with the same-sex partner in Hong Kong: a population-based study. Int J Impotence Res 2006;18(2):130–40.

55. Burri A, Rahman Q, Santtila P, et al. The relationship between same-sex sexual experience, sexual

distress, and female sexual dysfunction. J Sex Med 2012;9(1):198–206.

56. Peixoto MM, Nobre P. Automatic thoughts during sexual activity, distressing sexual symptoms, and sexual orientation: findings from a web survey. J Sex Marital Ther 2016;42(07):616–34.

57. Beaber TE, Werner PD. The relationship between anxiety and sexual functioning in lesbians and heterosexual women. J Homosexuality 2009;56(5): 639–54.

58. Saewyc EM. Research on adolescent sexual orientation: development, health disparities, stigma, and resilience. J Res Adolesc 2011;21(1):256–72.

59. Bostwick WB, Boyd CJ, Hughes TL, et al. Dimensions of sexual orientation and the prevalence of mood and anxiety disorders in the United States. Am J Public Health 2010;100(3):468–75.

60. Eliason MJ. Chronic physical health problems in sexual minority women: review of the literature. LGBT health 2014;1(4):259–68.

61. Szalacha LA, Hughes TL, McNair R, et al. Mental health, sexual identity, and interpersonal violence: findings from the Australian longitudinal Women's health study. BMC Women's Health 2017;17(1): 1–11.

62. Clayton AH, Elia Margarita VJ. Female sexual dysfunction. Med Clin 2019;103(4):681–98.

63. Johnson SD, Phelps DL, Cottler LB. The association of sexual dysfunction and substance use among a community epidemiological sample. Arch Sex Behav 2004;33(1):55–63.

64. Sobecki-Rausch JN, Brown O, Gaupp CL. Sexual dysfunction in lesbian women: a systematic review of the literature. Semin Reprod Med 2017;35(5): 448–59.

65. Williams AD, Bleicher RJ, Ciocca RM. Breast cancer risk, screening, and prevalence among sexual minority women: an analysis of the national health interview survey. LGBT health 2020;7(2): 109–18.

66. Boehmer U, Ozonoff A, Timm A, et al. After breast cancer: sexual functioning of sexual minority survivors. J Sex Res 2014;51(6):681–9.

67. Armstrong C. ACOG guideline on sexual dysfunction in women. Am Fam Physician 2011;84(6): 705–9.

68. Dodge B, Herbenick D, Fu TCJ, et al. Sexual behaviors of US men by self-identified sexual orientation: results from the 2012 National Survey of Sexual Health and Behavior. J Sex Med 2016; 13(4):637–49.

69. Shindel AW, Vittinghoff E, Breyer BN. Erectile dysfunction and premature ejaculation in men who have sex with men. J Sex Med 2012;9(2): 576–84.

70. Richters J, De Visser RO, Rissel CE, et al. Demographic and psychosocial features of participants in bondage and discipline, "sadomasochism" or dominance and submission (BDSM): data from a national survey. J Sex Med 2008;5(7):1660–8.

71. Rosenberger JG, Reece M, Schick V, et al. Sexual behaviors and situational characteristics of most recent male-partnered sexual event among gay and bisexually identified men in the United States. J Sex Med 2011;8(11):3040–50.

72. Rice CE, Maierhofer C, Fields KS, et al. Beyond anal sex: sexual practices of men who have sex with men and associations with HIV and other sexually transmitted infections. J Sex Med 2016;13(3): 374–82.

73. Klein H. Felching among men who engage in barebacking (unprotected anal sex). Arch Sex Behav 2012;41(2):377–84.

74. Prestage G, Hurley M, Brown G. "Cum play" among gay men. Arch Sex Behav 2013;42(7): 1347–56.

75. Bancroft J, Carnes L, Janssen E, et al. Erectile and ejaculatory problems in gay and heterosexual men. Arch Sex Behav 2005;34:285–97.

76. Breyer BN, Smith JF, Eisenberg ML, et al. The impact of sexual orientation on sexuality and sexual practices in North American medical students. J Sex Med 2010;7(7):2391–400.

77. Farrell MR, Corder CJ, Levine LA. Peyronie's disease among men who have sex with men: characteristics, treatment, and psychosocial factors. J Sex Med 2013;10(8):2077–83.

78. Coyne K, Mandalia S, McCullough S, et al. The International Index of Erectile Function: development of an adapted tool for use in HIV-positive men who have sex with men. J Sex Med 2010;7(2 Pt 1): 769–74.

79. Grabski B, Kasparek K, Müldner-Nieckowski Ł, et al. Sexual quality of life in homosexual and bisexual men: the relative role of minority stress. J Sex Med 2019;16(6):860–71.

80. Moreno-Pérez O, Escoín C, Serna-Candel C, et al. Risk factors for sexual and erectile dysfunction in HIV-infected men: the role of protease inhibitors. Aids 2010;24.2:255–64.

81. Augustinavicius JL, Baral SD, Murray SM, et al. Characterizing Cross-Culturally Relevant Metrics of Stigma Among Men Who Have Sex With Men Across 8 Sub-Saharan African Countries and the United States. Am J Epidemiol 2020;189(7):690–7.

82. Dorey G. Is smoking a cause of erectile dysfunction? A literature review. Br J Nurs 2001;10(7):455–65.

83. Štulhofer A, Šević S, Doyle DM. Comparing the prevalence and correlates of sexual health disturbances among heterosexual and nonheterosexual men: an overview of studies. Sex Med Rev 2014; 2(3–4):102–11.

84. Levitan J, Quinn-Nilas C, Milhausen R, et al. The relationship between body image and sexual

functioning among gay and bisexual men. J homosexuality 2018;66(13):1856–81.

85. Li DH, Remble TA, Macapagal K, et al. Stigma on the streets, dissatisfaction in the sheets: is minority stress associated with decreased sexual functioning among young men who have sex with men? J Sex Med 2019;16(2):267–77.

86. Hirshfield S, Chiasson MA, Wagmiller RL, et al. Sexual dysfunction in an Internet sample of US men who have sex with men. J Sex Med 2010; 7(9):3104–14.

87. Symonds T, Perelman MA, Althof S, et al. Development and validation of a premature ejaculation diagnostic tool. Eur Urol 2007;52.2:565–73.

88. Mulhall JP, Trost LW, Brannigan RE, et al. Evaluation and management of testosterone deficiency: AUA guideline. J Urol 2018;200(2):423–32.

89. American Cancer Society. Key Statistics for Prostate Cancer. Available at: https://www.cancer.org/cancer/prostate-cancer/about/key-statistics.html. Accessed March 10, 2021.

90. Saunders CL, Meads C, Abel GA, et al. Associations between sexual orientation and overall and site-specific diagnosis of cancer: evidence from two national patient surveys in England. J Clin Oncol 2017;35(32):3654.

91. Conron KJ, Mimiaga MJ, Landers SJ. A population-based study of sexual orientation identity and gender differences in adult health. Am J Public Health 2010;100(10):1953–60.

92. Ussher JM, Perz J, Kellet A, et al. Health-related quality of life, psychological distress, and sexual changes following prostate cancer: a comparison of gay and bisexual men with heterosexual men. J Sex Med 2016;13(3):425–34.

93. Lee TK, Handy AB, Kwan W, et al. Impact of prostate cancer treatment on the sexual quality of life for men-who-have-sex-with-men. J Sex Med 2015; 12(12):2378–86.

94. Blank TO. Gay men and prostate cancer: invisible diversity. J Clin Oncol 2004;23(12):2593–6.

95. Jägervall D, Carina JB, Johnson E. Gay men's experiences of sexual changes after prostate cancer treatment—a qualitative study in Sweden. Scand J Urol 2019;53(1):40–4.

96. Wassersug RJ, Lyons A, Duncan D, et al. Diagnostic and outcome differences between heterosexual and nonheterosexual men treated for prostate cancer. Urology 2013;82(3):565–71.

97. Fergus KD, Gray RE, Fitch MI. Sexual dysfunction and the preservation of manhood: experiences of men with prostate cancer. J Health Psychol 2002; 7(3):303–16.

98. Thomas B. Homophobia hampers prostate cancer care. Nurs Stand 2018;32(26):29.

99. Ussher JM, Perz J, Rose D, et al. Threat of sexual disqualification: the consequences of erectile dysfunction and other sexual changes for gay and bisexual men with prostate cancer. Arch Sex Behav 2017;46(7):2043–57.

100. Hart TL, Coon DW, Kowalkowski MA, et al. Changes in sexual roles and quality of life for gay men after prostate cancer: challenges for sexual health providers. J Sex Med 2014;11:2308–17.

101. Hartman ME, Irvine J, Currie KL, et al. Exploring gay couples' experience with sexual dysfunction after radical prostatectomy: a qualitative study. J Sex Marital Ther 2014;40:233–53.

102. Pérez-Stable, Eliseo J. "Director's Message for October 6, 2016." National Institute of Minority Health and Health Disparities. Available at: https://www.nimhd.nih.gov/about/directors-corner/messages/message_10-06-16.html. Accessed March 10, 2021.

Pharmaceutical and Energy-Based Management of Sexual Problems in Women

Alexandra Siegal, MD[a], Barbara M. Chubak, MD[b],*

KEYWORDS

- Female sexual dysfunction • Medicalization • Hypoactive sexual desire • Cognitive sexual arousal
- Genital sexual arousal • Laser therapy • Radiofrequency therapy • Electric stimulation therapy

KEY POINTS

- Female sexual dysfunction (FSD) has been inconsistently defined and characterized, so that changes in nomenclature complicate its diagnosis and treatment.
- Whether and how FSD ought to be medicalized is controversial, with associated problems of biomedical nihilism and unregulated proliferation of quack remedies under the aegis of "wellness."
- Because of frequent discordance of cognitive and genital sexuality in females, therapeutic interventions that benefit genital tissue are not necessarily helpful for overall sexual function.
- Medications and energy-based interventions available for FSD provide small, statistically significant improvements in sexual function, as measured by the Female Sexual Function Index; whether these improvements are clinically significant is a question that is most reliably answered by each individual patient.

BACKGROUND TO A NEW ERA

To discuss "a new era" in the management of sexual dysfunction implies progress from a previous norm, so that discussion must begin with an understanding of the historical foundations and associated assumptions undergirding that progress. This is particularly true of the diagnosis of female sexual dysfunction (FSD), which is a prerequisite to application of the novel and experimental therapeutic interventions that are the focus of this article. FSD is a category of diagnoses infamous for its changeability and its constancy over time: in the past three decades, its nomenclature and classification have gone through multiple iterations by various national and international organizations[1]; at the same time, historical and now medically anachronistic terms, such as "frigidity," continue to be used in the context of doctor-patient encounters and popular discourse about female sexuality.

Despite incontrovertible progress in medical science and an evolution of social norms since the early modern period, medical historians describe remarkable continuity in the terms of debate about FSD. These have included argument over whether sexual problems in women deserve significant medical attention (given that they do not necessarily preclude successful reproduction, in contrast with male erectile dysfunction [ED]) and the extent to which they signify a moral or psychological disorder versus a problem of anatomy or physiology.[2] The residue of these debates persists today, in the inequitable distribution of research funding and clinical attention to male sexual dysfunction and FSD, and in the tension between

---

[a] Department of Urology, Icahn School of Medicine at Mount Sinai, 1468 Madison Avenue, 6th Floor, New York, NY 10029, USA; [b] Department of Urology, Icahn School of Medicine at Mount Sinai, 10 Union Square #3A, New York, NY 10003, USA
* Corresponding author.
E-mail address: Barbara.Chubak@mountsinai.org

Urol Clin N Am 48 (2021) 473–486
https://doi.org/10.1016/j.ucl.2021.06.006
0094-0143/21/© 2021 Elsevier Inc. All rights reserved.

different classification systems used to define and diagnose these diseases.

NAVIGATING NOMENCLATURE

The various classification systems currently in use to describe sexual problems have changed over time (**Table 1**) and will likely continue to evolve in response to biomedical research and the bureaucratic structure of medical practice. Practitioners of different medical disciplines preferentially use the nomenclatures with which they are most familiar: psychologists and psychiatrists generally privilege the Diagnostic and Statistical Manual of Mental Disorders terminology[3]; urologists and gynecologists typically use that of the International Classification of Diseases and Statistics (ICD)[4] and/or the International Consultation in Sexual Medicine (ICSM)[5] and International Society for the Study of Women's Sexual Health (ISSWSH) diagnostic systems.[6] The ICSM and ISSWSH nomenclatures are the most recently coined, and

are thus based on the most up-to-date understanding of sexual pathophysiology.[1]

This pathophysiology is interdisciplinary, relying not on traditional Cartesian mind-body dualism, but on biopsychosocial modeling and an integrated view of neuropsychiatry and genital physiology as mutually influential. It is anticipated that the upcoming ICD-11 will base its terminology primarily on the ICSM/ISSWSH classification system, eliminating the ICD's previous distinction between physical and psychological sexual disorders by combining the two groups into a single section titled "Sexual Dysfunctions" within a chapter called "Conditions Related to Sexual Health."[7] It will acknowledge the multifarious and overlapping potential causes of sexual dysfunction, including social and cultural factors, and reinforce the inherent subjectivity of sexuality, proscribing against any normative functional standard.

This subjectivity is a crucial problem in any assessment of female sexual health. It creates space for the use of diagnostic and therapeutic

Table 1
Evolution in female sexual diagnostic nomenclature over the past 25 years

DSM-IV (1994)	ICD-10 (1999)	DSM-5 (2013)	ICSM-5/ISSWSH (2015/2016)
Female hypoactive desire disorder Female arousal disorder	Lack or loss of sexual desire Female sexual arousal disorder	Female sexual interest/ arousal disorder	Hypoactive sexual desire disorder Female genital arousal disorder
Female orgasmic disorder	Female orgasmic dysfunction: failure to reach orgasm	Female orgasmic disorder	Female orgasm disorders Anorgasmia Decreased frequency Muted intensity Premature or delayed Anhedonic
Dyspareunia Vaginismus	Nonorganic dyspareunia Nonorganic vaginismus	Genitopelvic pain/ penetration disorder	Female genital-pelvic pain dysfunction
Sexual aversion disorder Sexual dysfunction caused by a general medical condition	Sexual aversion		
Substance/medication- induced sexual dysfunction		Substance/medication- induced sexual dysfunction	
Sexual dysfunction NOS		Other specified sexual dysfunctions	Female orgasmic illness syndrome Persistent genital arousal disorder
		Unspecified sexual dysfunction	

Abbreviations: DSM, Diagnostic and Statistical Manual of Mental Disorders; ICD, International Classification of Diseases and Statistics; ICSM, International Consultation in Sexual Medicine; ISSWSH, International Society for the Study of Women's Sexual Health; NOS, not otherwise specified.

terminologies that are rich with personal, social, and cultural meaning but lacking in certain scientific or clinical significance. An example of this is the diagnosis of "vaginal laxity" (a term with scant biomedical basis but cultural salience), which may be treated with "vaginal rejuvenation" (again, a term with unclear meaning but strongly positive connotations). This subjectivity complicates the determination of treatment success or failure, because studies of female sexual arousal have shown that vaginal lubrication, tissue engorgement, and other genital changes consistent with arousal are not necessarily associated with subjective arousal by research subjects.[8,9] The epistemology of science is reliant on outcomes that are objectively measured and repeated in diverse individuals; the subjectivity and idiosyncrasy of sexuality is in tension with the premise of evidence-based medicine.

CRITIQUING FEMALE SEXUAL DYSFUNCTION

Some practitioners have responded to this tension with opportunistic quackery, promoting and selling dubious and expensive treatments for FSD under the auspices of promoting "wellness."[10] Others have embraced nihilism: faced with the impossibility of separating sexual science from its biased social, political, and economic contexts, they argue against any medicalization for management of sexual concerns.[11] Feminist scholarship reveals how medicine has historically pathologized the female body[12] and idealized heteronormative, penovaginal intercourse,[13] arguing that FSD diagnosis and treatment is a patriarchal tool of the medical-industrial complex.[14] However, feminism is also vulnerable to commodification: "Even the Score," a seemingly grassroots campaign that agitated for the first Food and Drug Administration (FDA) approval of medication for FSD as an antidote to systemic sex-gender inequity in health care, was ultimately revealed as the creation of the drug manufacturer and owner.[15]

These biases, gendered and financial, explicit and implicit, represent violations of bioethics that merit serious consideration and rectification. Although science may be flawed by bias, it remains an important and helpful source of knowledge. Medical studies, diagnoses, and therapies offer a potentially meaningful and effective structure in which to operationalize that knowledge toward patients' goals of care. Sexual dysfunction, regardless of how and by whom it is defined, has long been and continues to be a source of real suffering for women of all ages worldwide: the rest of this article is devoted to the description and analysis of the currently available treatment options.

PHARMACEUTICAL MANAGEMENT

The ahistorical and biomedically nihilistic narratives about FSD as a disease invented by medical industry to sell its products all begin in 1998, with sildenafil.[16] The commercial success of Viagra for treatment of ED increased enthusiasm for research into female sexual medicine, in hope of identifying a similarly lucrative "female Viagra"; it was this promise and the industry funding that followed from it that enabled the research and medical conferences that were immediate past precursors to ISSWSH.[17] Ultimately, the clinical trials of Viagra in female subjects failed to show clear benefit and in 2004 Pfizer chose not to apply to the FDA for the drug's approval in women. But the "Viagra effect" remains strong, with subsequent medications for FSD consistently compared with it, and the particular way it failed to benefit women provides an important insight into FSD.

Phosphodiesterase-5 Inhibitors

The mechanism through which sildenafil and other phosphodiesterase-5 inhibitors (PDE5i) affect sexual function is by promoting vasodilation within the genital tissues: by preventing degradation of cGMP, the vasodilatory effects of nitric oxide on the genitalia are potentiated.[18] Although this mechanism has been most extensively studied within the male corpora cavernosa and in the context of male erection, it is equally relevant to female sexual function.[19,20] The physiology of female genital arousal also features smooth muscle relaxation and vasocongestion of the cavernous tissues (clitoral and bulbovestibular), which is mediated by nitric oxide. Vasoactive intestinal polypeptide is another vasodilatory neurotransmitter that is also involved in relaying the proarousal signal from the sacral parasympathetic nerves to the genital tissue in both sexes, but its relative significance remains unclear and it has not been instrumentalized for therapeutic purpose.[12] Whereas in men increased genital blood flow manifests with penile erection, in women its most obvious manifestation is swelling and increased lubrication of the vulvovaginal tissues.

Studies of sildenafil in female subjects with various sexual dysfunctions and comorbidities consistently demonstrated physiologic changes of increased genital arousal in response to the medication when compared with placebo. These include increased vaginal lubrication, increased blood flow on Doppler ultrasound, increased fullness on vaginal plethysmography, and decreased genital vibratory perception thresholds.[21–23] However, just as consistent was a disconnect between these objective physical changes and their subjective interpretation by the women who experienced them: whether assessed by simple self-report or validated questionnaire, subjects who were given sildenafil often failed to report improvements in sexual arousal or other aspects of their sexual experience.[24]

This inconsistent relationship of physiologic and psychological response is characteristic of female sexuality, reaffirmed by scientific studies of responsiveness to various interventions and appealing and aversive stimuli. In response to this discordance, the most recent diagnostic nomenclature not only distinguishes between sexual desire and arousal, but also parses female sexual arousal disorder into two distinct problems: female genital arousal disorder, which is a problem of genital physiology; and female cognitive arousal disorder, a problem of mental state, in which genitally erogenous cues are not experienced as being sexually arousing.[6] That a diagnostic classification system purposefully designed to integrate the physical and psychological aspects of sexual problems so readily falls back on Cartesian dualism is ironic evidence of the strength and rhetorical utility of this model. Patients with female genital arousal disorder, especially those with co-morbid diabetes,[25,26] may benefit from treatment with a PDE5i, and it is for this reason that research studies of these medications in women continue to be published more than a decade after Pfizer gave up on sildenafil for women.

Psychoactive Medications

Modulation of genital response has not reliably led to improvement in women's sexual experience. A biomedical approach has, however, had some utility in addressing subjective arousal/libido. The two medications that are FDA-approved for treatment of an FSD, specifically, hypoactive sexual desire disorder (HSDD), act within the brain, according to the logic that where thought and emotion lead, the body and behavior will follow. It is important to keep in mind that just as affective disorders are most effectively treated by a combination of medication and psychotherapy,[27] medications to address sexual dysfunction may work best when used in conjunction with psychotherapeutic sex therapy.[28]

Flibanserin

Flibanserin was discovered serendipitously; initially investigated as an antidepressant, it was ineffective at managing depression but trial participants were incidentally noted to be more sexually active than their placebo-group peers. In this fashion, flibanserin is similar to sildenafil for ED,

which was also a serendipitous discovery. This oral medication is commonly known as "the female Viagra" or "the pink pill," in contrast with sildenafil's (Viagra) blue. These superficialities are where the similarity ends: unlike sildenafil, flibanserin is a psychoactive medication that is intended for chronic use to counter patients' generalized, acquired HSDD by increasing their interest in and receptivity to sexual cues. This standardized 100-mg daily dosing appeals to patients for whom sexual spontaneity is important, because it ensures that the medication will be available to support their libido at all times. As of 2015, flibanserin is only FDA-approved for premenopausal women, but clinical research suggests equivalent efficacy postmenopause.[29]

The mechanism by which flibanserin alters sexual function is incompletely understood; it is a multifunctional serotonin receptor agonist/antagonist, whose complex action has a net result of decreasing serotonin activity within the brain while increasing noradrenergic and dopaminergic activity.[30] All of these neurotransmitters have been implicated in the maintenance of sexual interest within the central nervous system (CNS). Norepinephrine and dopamine stimulate attention, appetite, and reward in response to erotic cues, whereas serotonin (mostly) inhibits sexual interest and responsiveness.[31] The net result of flibanserin's biologic actions is to tilt CNS neurochemistry in a prosexual direction, as one of the many biopsychosocial influences that provide motivation for or against sexual activity according to the Sexual Tipping Point Model.[32]

The prosexual push that flibanserin provides is subtle: in the randomized controlled trials pursuant to its FDA approval,[33–35] the coprimary end points of numerical improvement in numbers of satisfying sexual events per month and in the desire domain for the Female Sexual Function Index (FSFI) measured only a fraction above the placebo response. Trial participants who received flibanserin reported only 0.5 to 1.0 more satisfying sexual events per month and 0.3 to 0.4 additional points in desire domain for the FSFI (on a 1.2- to 6-point scale) compared with placebo group participants.[36,37] Measurements of distress related to low sexual desire, a secondary study end point, were similarly slight, with distress decreased by 0.3 to 0.4 points (on the Revised Female Sexual Distress Scale, a 0- to 4-point scale) with flibanserin compared with placebo.[38] The relevance of these various end points is debatable: increased sexual interest does not necessarily correlate with a rise in sexual activity, and the FSFI, which is a 4-week retrospective inquiry into sexual symptoms, has inherent limitations and biases.[37,39]

Although the improvements in sexual desire and satisfaction, and decreases in distress associated with low sexual desire, associated with flibanserin were statistically significant and are clinically significant for some patients, the question of whether flibanserin's benefits outweigh its risks is controversial. Like many serotonergic medications, it can be sedating, and induce dizziness, hypotension, or syncope; bother from these adverse effects (AEs) is decreased by dosing at bedtime and avoiding combination with other CNS depressants, such as alcohol.[40] It is also important to avoid combination with medications that inhibit CYP3A4, because these interfere with metabolism of flibanserin to increase the risk of AEs. Hepatic disease is a similar contraindication to its use. Various placebo-controlled studies have been done to characterize the degree of AE risk, including assessments of next-day driving performance[41] and of orthostatic hypotension and syncope when flibanserin is combined with alcohol.[42] These risks are confirmed to be low. Nevertheless, these low risks must be weighed against the medication's potential benefit for each individual patient. A robust process of informed shared decision making regarding flibanserin treatment is essential and reinforced by the FDA's risk evaluation and mitigation strategy.[43]

Bremelanotide

The second medication to be FDA-approved for the treatment of HSDD is bremelanotide (Vyleesi), a melanocortin receptor agonist. This agent was incidentally found to increase sexual interest and arousal response in studies intended to determine its dermatologic utility as a sunless tanning agent.[44] Like flibanserin, it is only FDA-approved for the treatment of generalized, acquired HSDD in premenopausal women, but studies of its intranasal spray formulation (also called PT-141) also demonstrated erectogenic properties in male subjects, suggesting its potential utility for treatment of sexual problems in both sexes.[45] Ultimately, the bioavailability of intranasal bremelanotide, and consequent lability in blood pressure, were deemed too variable. The drug was FDA-approved in 2019 in the alternative form of a subcutaneous injection pen, for administration of a standard 1.75-mg dose as needed approximately 45 minutes before sexual activity. Taken this way, randomized controlled trial participants experienced small, statistically significant increases in sexual desire as measured by the FSFI, and decreased distress related to low sexual interest.[46]

Similar to flibanserin, whether the marginal improvement in sexual symptoms with bremelanotide is worth the risk of AEs from taking the medication is an open question that can ultimately only be answered by the patient herself. Some AEs are mitigated by thoughtful dosing: the risk of permanent hyperpigmentation of the skin and gums is substantially reduced by injecting no more than once daily and no more than eight times monthly. Injection is characteristically followed by a transient increase in blood pressure; bremelanotide is therefore contraindicated in patients with uncontrolled hypertension. High rates (up to 40%) of trial participants reported nausea; interestingly, only 8.1% of study participants chose to discontinue use because of nausea.[46] This is an important caution against making assumptions about what ratio of risk-benefit patients with sexual problems will find favorable based on grouped biostatistics, and reinforces the need for individualized and informed choice. The current status of bremelanotide in the form of intranasal PT-141 is a further caution: in the absence of FDA approval, it remains available for online purchase without a doctor's prescription, putting ill-advised customers at substantial risk of harm.

Hormonal Medications: a Blast From the Past

The pharmaceutical industry's most recent forays into treatment of FSD have had somewhat ambiguous results. PDE5i medications target the genitalia to boost arousal response without adequately addressing the cognitive or emotional aspects of sexual function. Flibanserin and bremelanotide target the CNS, to produce only slight improvements in sexual interest and responsiveness when compared with placebo. An alternative to these is off-label use of older, hormonal medications, which act simultaneously on mind and body. It is not surprising that pioneering sexologist William Masters began his clinical research career in the 1940s with a focus on the positive effects of estrogen-replacement therapy on hypogonadal women.[47] At the same time, androgens were also studied and used in women for treatment of various medical problems, including sexual dysfunction.[48] Both sex steroids act within the CNS to stimulate sexual appetite[31] and within the genitalia to maintain vulvovaginal tissue integrity.[49]

Testosterone therapy, in isolation and in combination with estrogen (and sometimes progesterone), has been shown in many randomized controlled trials to increase sexual desire and satisfaction in postmenopausal women with HSDD.[50] Clinical application of these data remains a persistent challenge because it remains uncertain: (1) to what degree testosterone, and not the estrogen into which it may be aromatized, is the relevant actor[51]; (2) whether testosterone supplementation might safely and effectively address sexual problems in premenopausal women[52]; and (3) how to most reliably dose this medication in a regulatory and financial environment that discourages development of testosterone products for women.[53] The risk of AEs, including hirsutism, acne, vocal changes, and clitoromegaly, is necessarily increased when products intended to produce adult male levels of testosterone are prescribed for women.[54] The probability of these AEs is reduced with careful monitoring and dose titration to maintain free testosterone within the normal female range,[55,56] but the optimal testosterone regimen for women has yet to be determined.

ENERGY-BASED MANAGEMENT

Given the concern for systemic AEs and associated uncertainty regarding risk/benefit ratio of the various pharmacotherapies that are used to treat FSD, it is tempting to use more localized treatments. These include various mechanical devices, which apply energy in various forms (eg, light, sound, shockwaves, or electricity) to different tissues (eg, vaginal epithelium, cavernous bodies, or nerves). Enthusiasm for the potential of these devices to improve genital health, including sexual function, is high, to a degree that is currently disproportionate to the quality of the evidence supporting their use for these purposes.

Vaginal Lasers

Various laser technologies are commercially available for vaginal application (**Table 2**).

The IntimaLase by Fotona (Dallas, TX) and Petit Lady by Lutronic, Inc (Fremont, CA) are nonablative erbium-doped yttrium-aluminum-garnet (Er:YAG) lasers[57,58] that heat the tissue to which they are applied, increasing heat shock proteins and collagen production without surface injury.[59] The most popular and aggressively advertised energy-based therapies are tissue ablative fractional CO_2 lasers, including the MonaLisa Touch, developed by DEKA (Calenzano, Italy) and distributed in the United States by Cynosure, Inc (Westford, MA)[60]; the FemiLift, by Alma Lasers (Buffalo Grove, IL)[61]; and the FemTouch, by Lumenis (San Jose, CA).[62] These fractional lasers disperse their energy into microscopic penetration points, such that only a fraction of the treated area is directly affected.[63] Focal injury and resulting areas of thermal necrosis within vaginal epithelial tissue from the laser activate heat shock proteins and growth factors, stimulating tissue remodeling with neoangiogenesis and deposition of collagen and elastin.[64–66]

Proponents of vaginal lasers claim that these tissue changes treat various female genital complaints that are relevant to sexual function, including atrophic vaginitis, vaginal laxity, urinary incontinence, and dyspareunia, in postpartum and postmenopausal contexts.[60–63] Small, single-arm studies of women with genitourinary syndrome of menopause demonstrate compelling improvements in tissue quality and sexual function.[64–68] Evidence from randomized controlled trials, in which laser is compared with sham treatment[69] or vaginal estrogen therapies,[70–72] is more ambiguous: although laser treatment did compare favorably with vaginal hormone therapies in its improving effects on various FSFI subdomains, these subdomain improvements were not consistent across studies, and in one study, patients in the CO_2 laser arm experienced increased vaginal pain.[71] Although CO_2 laser seems to rival vaginal estrogen for treatment of tissue changes related to genitourinary syndrome of menopause/vulvovaginal atrophy, patient expectations should

Table 2 Laser devices		
Device		**Number of Treatments**
MonaLisa Touch, Cynosure	Fractional CO_2	3 treatments at 6-wk intervals
FemiLift, Alma Lasers	Fractional CO_2	3 treatments at 4-6-wk intervals
FemTouch, Lumenis	Fractional CO_2	2–4 treatments at 4-wk intervals
IntimaLase, Fotona	2940-nm nonablative Er:YAG	2 treatments at 8-wk intervals
Petit Lady, Lutronic	2940-nm Er:YAG	3 treatments at 2-wk intervals

Abbreviation: Er:YAG, erbium-doped yttrium-aluminum-garnet.

be set appropriately and potential users advised that these treatments may not fully restore "normal" sexual function.

One part of the appeal of laser treatment is its relative ease: monthly treatments typically last between 10 and 20 minutes, and various probe shapes and sizes are available to accommodate differences in patient anatomy. Most patients do not find the procedure uncomfortable, reporting only a sensation of heat during their treatments, and positive results of three to five monthly treatments are durable up to 12 months afterward.[73] Patients who do not wish to rely on chronic use of medication or are concerned about the potential risks of hormonal therapies might reasonably choose to pay out of pocket for vaginal laser treatments as an alternative. Unfortunately, the purported benefits of vaginal laser therapy claimed in many direct-to-consumer marketing campaigns have scant evidence base, leading the FDA to issue a safety communication in 2018, warning that "the safety and efficacy of energy-based devices to perform vaginal 'rejuvenation'…has not been established."[74]

Since publication of this FDA communication, analyses of the MAUDE (Manufacturer and User Facility Device Experience) and Bloomberg Law databases have discovered only 30 potential AE claims, suggesting that vaginal CO_2 laser procedures are low risk.[75] Er:YAG lasers seem to be similarly safe.[76] The financial considerations germane to this out-of-pocket therapy remain a source of concern. Furthermore, safety in the setting of various potential comorbid conditions and health states, including vulvovaginal infection, pregnancy, postpartum, previous pelvic radiation or surgery with mesh, conditions that impair healing, anticoagulant use, thromboembolic disease, keloid formation, preexisting vaginal or cervical lesions, or POP-Q stage 3 to 4 prolapse,[60] is as yet undefined. The efficacy of vaginal laser treatment of FSD remains an open question in need of further exploration.

Radiofrequency

Radiofrequency (RF) technology has been well-studied for treatment of dermatologic problems, such as cellulitis, laxity, and other age-related changes. RF has also been investigated as a noninvasive tissue-bulking treatment of stress urinary incontinence.[77–79] RF devices use an electromagnetic current, which is transformed into thermal energy as it contacts subcutical tissues. This transformation limits associated epidermal tissue injury and reduces energy loss to scatter, diffraction, or absorption by tissue outside the desired treatment area.[80] Thus, RF heats tissue in a controlled and focused fashion to prompt remodeling through collagen deposition and neo-angiogenesis while avoiding surface tissue injury, in a manner comparable with nonablative laser treatment.[81] Commercially available vaginal RF devices include the Viveve System from Viveve Medical (Sunnyvale, CA) and ThermiVa from ThermiAesthetics (Southlake, TX).[82,83]

The scientific data regarding the effect of vaginal RF on female sexual problems is limited. Small, pilot, single-armed studies have been published, touting the beneficial effects of RF on vaginal laxity (as perceived by the patient); tissue quality (as perceived by the examining health care provider); and associated sexual satisfaction, including improvements of arousal, lubrication, and orgasm.[84–86] The two randomized sham-controlled trials that have been published focus on vulvar appearance (as perceived by the patient and health care provider) and vaginal laxity (as perceived by the patient) as their primary outcomes, with sexual function based on FSFI score a secondary consideration. Both studies describe improvement of genital appearance and self-image in the RF groups; FSFI scores did not substantively differ between the intervention and control groups, but the studies were not powered for robust evaluation of sexual function. Optimal dosing of RF intervention is uncertain: in the VIVEVE I trial, only one course of treatment was administered[87]; in contrast, eight weekly treatments were administered in the Brazilian study using a Tecatherap-VIP device (made by VIP-Eletromedicina, San Martín, Argentina).[88]

Low-Intensity Extracorporeal Shockwave Therapy

Shockwaves are sonic pulsations that can carry energy and propagate through a medium. Focused shockwaves are characterized by a sequential rapid rise in pressure (<10 nanoseconds), high-pressure peak (100 MPa), and short lifecycle (10 microseconds); when they are focused on a particular tissue, their energy creates a high-pressure load that causes mechanical shear stress.[89] This stress on the tissue provokes a healing response,[90–93] so that low-intensity extracorporeal shockwave therapy (LiSWT) holds promise for treatment of various medical problems, including chronic wounds and musculoskeletal disorders.[94,95] Since 2010, LiSWT has been investigated and used for the treatment of male sexual problems, including ED, Peyronie disease, and chronic prostatitis/chronic pelvic pain syndrome.[96] Recent policy statements from the

European Society of Sexual Medicine and Sexual Medicine Society of North America discourage the use of LiSWT for ED outside the context of clinical research, because "its efficacy for the treatment of ED is doubtful and deserves more investigation."[96] There is even less evidence for the benefits of LiSWT for treatment of FSD and no published studies on this subject.

Despite this paucity of evidence, the manufacturers of various sonic-wave generating devices nonetheless advertise themselves for this indication. For example, FemiWave claims to provide increased genital sensitivity, better lubrication with arousal, and orgasmic function, without any evidence to support these or any other claims.[97] Note that the FemiWave device applies radial acoustic waves to tissue, rather than the focused shockwaves used in most of the studies examining the helpfulness of LiSWT for male ED.[98] Thus, any extrapolation from research in men to application in women is doubly tenuous.

Neuromodulation: Sacral and Percutaneous Tibial Nerve Stimulation

Neuromodulatory devices traditionally used to treat voiding dysfunction include sacral neurostimulators (SNS) and percutaneous tibial nerve stimulators (PTNS). SNS stimulates the S3 nerve root via an electrode placed through the S3 foramen, to influence the afferent and efferent spinal nerves to the bladder and bowel.[99] These devices include Medtronic's InterStim (Minneapolis, MN) and the Axonics System (Irvine, CA). Percutaneous (also called posterior or peripheral) tibial nerve stimulation is a form of acupuncture in which electrical stimulation is applied to the posterior tibial nerve at the medial ankle. The posterior tibial nerve originates from the L4-S3 nerve root, so that stimulation of the distal nerve can modulate the afferent and efferent nerves of the sacral plexus (S2-4).[100] SNS devices provide more consistent and effective neuromodulation than 12 sessions of 30 minutes of weekly PTNS, but are more invasive, with a higher risk of bleeding, infection, and surgical complications.

SNS and PTNS devices are principally used to treat symptoms of overactive bladder (OAB), and is helpful for underactive bladder and bowel dysfunction. Epidemiologic data describe comorbidity of sexual and voiding dysfunction, but it is unknown whether their relationship is incidental, causative, or because of a common underlying pathology.[101] It has been hypothesized that fear of coital incontinence and low genital self-image secondary to incontinence motivates comorbid FSD in some women and that improved sexual function is expected after successful treatment of voiding symptoms. Studies comparing sexual function before and after SNS and PTNS demonstrate small, statistically significant improvements across various subdomains of the FSFI, but without consistent subdomain improvements or global improvement of sexual function between studies.[102–106]

The specific effects of neuromodulation on sexual function are uncertain, because all research to assess the influence of SNS or PTNS on sexuality has been conducted in populations that suffer from voiding dysfunction. A study of tibial nerve stimulation in a rat model demonstrated a 500% increase in vaginal blood flow on Doppler ultrasonography following treatment, suggesting that neuromodulation might improve genital arousal response independently of its effects on voiding function.[107] An observational study of women with dry-OAB demonstrated small, statistically significant increases in FSFI score after PTNS treatment, which were independent of lower urinary tract symptom improvement.[108] Research into the sexual benefits of neuromodulation compared with pharmacotherapy for OAB and the correlation of urinary and sexual symptom improvements is ongoing in the STOMP (Sexual function Trial of Overactive bladder Medication vs PTNS) study. At this time, there are no clinical data to support the use of SNS or PTNS to treat patients with isolated FSD.

Neuromodulation: Vagal Nerve Stimulation

The vagus nerve is the tenth cranial nerve and a major component of the parasympathetic nervous system. The vagus nerve mediates a wide variety of bodily functions, including heart rate, digestion, and mood. Surgically implanted vagus nerve stimulators are FDA-approved to apply an electrical stimulus to the vagus nerve at the neck for treatment of medication-refractory epilepsy and depression.[109] Vagal nerve stimulation (VNS) is currently being studied for many other indications, such as pain syndromes, neuropsychiatric disorders, bowel disease, and endometriosis.[110–114] Vagal innervation of the cervix is thought to contribute to female sexual sensation and response, enabling women with a history of spinal cord injury at or higher than the T10 level to have erotic awareness and orgasm with vaginal and/or cervical stimulation.[115] The existence of this proposed genital afferent pathway that bypasses the spine via the vagus nerve is supported by neuroimaging.[116]

Modulation of the vagus nerve is unique among the energy-based interventions discussed in this

Table 3
Clinical care points: medications for HSDD

Medication	Flibanserin	Bremelanotide	Testosterone (1%)
Timing	Routine	As needed	Routine
Route	Oral	Subcutaneous injection	Topical
Dose	100 mg (1 tablet) qHS	1.75 mg (single-dose autoinjector) At least 45 min before sexual activity No more than 1 time/d No more than 8 times/mo	5–10 mg/d Titrate dose to goal serum free T (0.6–0.8 ng/dL)[1]
Side effects	Sedation, hypotension, dizziness, syncope, insomnia	Nausea, flushing, headache, hypertension	Acne, alopecia, hirsutism, vocal change, clitoromegaly
Contraindications	CYP4A4 inhibitors, hepatic impairment	Poorly controlled hypertension, naltrexone	Preexisting symptoms of virilization

Data from[1] Guay A, Munarriz R, Jacobson J, et al. Serum androgen levels in healthy premenopausal women with and without sexual dysfunction: Part A. Serum androgen levels in women aged 20-49 years with no complaints of sexual dysfunction. Int J Imp Res 2004;16:112-20.

article for the scope of its impact: whereas other applications of energy act only on the tissues to which they are applied (vaginal laser, RF, LiSWT, and SNS) or their proximate branches (PTNS), alteration of vagal activity can affect multiple organ systems, and mood and emotional valence. VNS thus has the potential to address FSD in all its biopsychosocial complexity, as described by polyvagal theory.[117] Although this potential is exciting in its promise, there is a great need for caution. The surgically implanted VNS device was approved despite a deficit of research demonstrating its safety, and patients with the implant are at risk of lethal cardiac AEs.[118] Just as PTNS is a less invasive alternative to SNS, auricular acupuncture to stimulate the vagus nerve[113] or meditation to promote parasympathetic tone[119] are safer alternatives that also merit further consideration and evaluation.

SUMMARY

The enthusiasm with which energy-based treatments for sexual dysfunction have been adopted for sale in the medical marketplace is disproportionate to the amount of data that are currently available to support their clinical use. Neuromodulation and focal induction of a healing response hold promise for the improvement of tissue quality, genital arousal response, and related FSD symptoms. Caution and further study are required to determine whether this promise will be fulfilled, and if indeed fulfillment will lead to relief of sexual problems. Given the limited scope of action for most of these devices, the widely ranging

biopsychosocial factors that are implicated in the manifestation of FSD, and the characteristic discordance of female arousal, it is likely that their helpfulness will be specific to defined FSD symptomatology and/or specific populations of women with relevant comorbidities.

Pharmacotherapy for FSD (**Table 3**) has considerably more research evidence to justify its use and the potential to promote sexual desire, cognitive and genital arousal, and orgasmic response. The functional improvements that are produced by these medications are generally small, and their benefits may not outweigh the bother of taking medications and hazarding their potential AEs. There is sufficient demand for medical treatment of sexual dysfunction that studies continue in an effort to expand the demographic for whom the drugs are FDA-approved to include older women and possibly men. It is essential that patients in all of these groups be empowered to make an informed, autonomous determination as to whether the ratio of risk to reward favors the use of pharmacotherapy, energy-based therapy, or some other treatment intervention.

DISCLOSURE

The authors have nothing to disclose.

REFERENCES

1. Parish SJ, Cottler-Casanova S, Clayton AH, et al. The evolution of female sexual disorder/dysfunction definitions, nomenclature, and classifications: a review of DSM, ICSM, ISSWSH, and ICD. Sex Med Rev 2021;9:36–56.

2. Cryle P, Moore A. Frigidity: an intellectual history. Basingstoke, England, UK: Palgrave Macmillan; 2011.

3. American Psychiatric Association (APA). DSM-5: diagnostic and statistical manual of mental disorders. 5th edition. Arlington, VA, USA: American Psychiatric Association; 2013.

4. World Health Organization (WHO). ICD-10: international statistical classification of diseases and related health problems, 10th Revision. 2nd edition. Geneva, Switzerland: World Health Organization; 2004.

5. McCabe M, Sharlip ID, Atalla E, et al. Definitions of sexual dysfunctions in women and men: a consensus statement from the Fourth International Consultation on Sexual Medicine. J Sex Med 2016;13:135–43.

6. Parish S, Meston C, Althof S, et al. Toward a more evidence-based nosology and nomenclature for female sexual dysfunctions – part III. J Sex Med 2019;16:452–62.

7. Reed GM, Drescher J, Krueger RB, et al. Disorders related to sexuality and gender identity in the ICD-11: revising the ICD-10 classification based on current scientific evidence, best clinical practices, and human rights considerations. World Psychiatry 2016;15(3):205–21.

8. Meston CM, Stanton AM. Understanding sexual arousal and subjective genital arousal desynchrony in women. Nat Rev Urol 2019;16:107–20.

9. Chivers ML, Seto MC, Lalumière ML, et al. Agreement of self-reported and genital measures of sexual arousal in men and women. Arc Sex Behav 2010;39(1):5–56.

10. Gunter J. Worshiping the false idols of wellness. New York Times 2018. Available at: https://www.nytimes.com/2018/08/01/style/wellness-industrial-complex.html.

11. Moynihan R. The making of a disease: female sexual dysfunction. BMJ 2003;326:45–7.

12. Lawrence SC, Bendixen K. His and hers: male and female anatomy in anatomy texts for US medical students, 1890-1989. Social Sci Med 1992;35(7):925–34.

13. Irigaray L. In: This sex which is not one. Ithaca, NY, USA: Cornell University Press; 1985. p. 63. Trans. C Porter, C Burke.

14. Tiefer L. Female sexual dysfunction: a case study of disease mongering and activist resistance. Plos Med 2006;3(4):e178.

15. Block J, Canner L. The 'grassroots campaign' for 'female Viagra' was actually funded by its manufacturer. The Cut Sep 8, 2016. Available at: https://www.thecut.com/2016/09/how-addyi-the-female-viagra-won-fda-approval.html. Accessed July 19, 2021.

16. Goldstein I, Lue TF, Padma-Natthan H, et al. Oral sildenafil in the treatment of erectile dysfunction. Sildenafil Study Group. N Engl J Med 1998;338(20):1397–404.

17. Loe M. The rise of Viagra: how the little blue pill changed sex in America. New York, NY, USA: New York University Press; 2004. p. 124–65.

18. Dean RC, Lue TF. Physiology of penile erection and pathophysiology of erectile dysfunction. Urol Clin North Am 2005;32(4):379–95.

19. Levin RJ, Both S, Georgiadis J, et al. The physiology of female sexual function and pathophysiology of female sexual dysfunction (Committee 13A). J Sex Med 2016;13(5):733–59.

20. Graziottin A. Sexual arousal: similarities and differences between men and women. J Mens Health Gend 2004;1(2–3):215–23.

21. Berman J, Berman L, Lin H, et al. Effect of sildenafil on subjective and physiologic parameters of the female sexual response in women with sexual arousal disorder. J Sex Marital Ther 2001;27:411–20.

22. Basson R, Brotto LA. Sexual psychophysiology and effects of sildenafil citrate in oestrogenised women with acquired genital arousal disorder and impaired orgasm: a randomized controlled trial. BJOG 2003;110:1014–24.

23. Laan E, Van Lunsen RH, Everaerd W, et al. The enhancement of vaginal vasocongestion by sildenafil in healthy premenopausal women. J Womens Health Gend Based Med 2002;11:357–65.

24. Chivers ML, Rosen R. Phosphodiesterase type 5 inhibitors and female sexual response: faulty protocols or paradigms? J Sex Med 2009;7:858–72.

25. Caruso S, Rugolo S, Agnello C, et al. Sildenafil improves sexual functioning in premenopausal women with type 1 diabetes who are affected by sexual arousal disorder: a double-blind, crossover, placebo-controlled pilot study. Fertil Steril 2006; 85(5):1496–501.

26. Caruso S, Cicero C, Romano M, et al. Tadalafil 5 mg daily treatment for type 1 diabetic premenopausal women affected by sexual genital arousal disorder. J Sex Med 2012;9(8):2057–65.

27. Cuijpers P, Sijbrandij, Koole SL, et al. Adding psychotherapy to antidepressant medication in depression and anxiety disorders: a meta-analysis. World Psychiatry 2014;13(1):56–67.

28. Kingsberg SA, Althof S, Simon JA, et al. Female sexual dysfunction – medical and psychological treatments, Committee 14. J Sex Med 2017;14:1463–91.

29. Simon JA, Kingsberg SA, Shumel B, et al. Efficacy and safety of flibanserin in postmenopausal women with hypoactive sexual desire disorder: results of the SNOWDROP trial. Menopause 2014;21:633–40.

30. Stahl SM. Mechanism of action of flibanserin, a multifunctional serotonin agonist and antagonist (MSAA), in hypoactive sexual desire disorder. CNS Spectrums 2015;20(1):1–6.

31. Pfaus JG. Pathways of sexual desire. J Sex Med 2009;6(6):1506–33.

32. Perelman M. The sexual tipping point: a mind/body model for sexual medicine. J Sex Med 2009;6(3): 629–32.

33. Thorp J, Simon J, Dattani D, et al. Treatment of hypoactive sexual desire disorder in premenopausal women: efficacy of flibanserin in the DAISY study. J Sex Med 2012;9:793–804.

34. Derogatis LR, Komer L, Katz M, et al. Treatment of hypoactive sexual desire disorder in premenopausal women: efficacy of flibanserin in the VIOLET Study. J Sex Med 2012;9:1074–85.

35. Katz M, Derogatis LR, Ackerman R, et al. Efficacy of flibanserin in women with hypoactive sexual desire disorder: results from the BEGONIA trial. J Sex Med 2013;10:1807–15.

36. Jaspers L, Feys F, Bramer WM, et al. Efficacy and safety of flibanserin for the treatment of hypoactive sexual desire disorder in women: a systematic review and meta-analysis. JAMA Int Med 2016; 176(4):453–62.

37. Sathyanarayana Rao TS, Andrade C. Flibanserin: approval of a controversial drug for a controversial disorder. Indian J Psychiatry 2015;57(3):221–3.

38. Gao Z, Yang D, Yu L, et al. Efficacy and safety of flibanserin in women with hypoactive sexual desire disorder: a systematic review and meta-analysis. J Sex Med 2015;12(11):2095–104.

39. Pyke R, Clayton A. What sexual behaviors relate to decreased sexual desire in women? A review and proposal for end points in treatment of hypoactive sexual desire disorder. Sex Med 2017;5(2):e73–83.

40. Kingsberg SA, McElroy SL, Clayton AH. Evaluation of flibanserin safety: comparison with other serotonergic medications. Sex Med Rev 2019;7(3): 380–92.

41. Kay GG, Hochandel T, Sicard E, et al. Next-day residual effects of flibanserin on simulated driving performance in premenopausal women. Hum Psychopharmacol 2017;32(4):e2603.

42. Simon JA, Clayton AH, Kingsberg SA, et al. Effects of timing of flibanserin administration relative to alcohol intake in health premenopausal women: a randomized, double blind, crossover study. J Sex Med 2019;16(11):1779–86.

43. Food and Drug Administration. Addyi (flibanserin). In: Approved Risk Evaluation and Mitigation Strategies. Available at: https://www.accessdata.fda. gov/scripts/cder/rems/index.cfm? event=IndvRemsDetails.page&REMS=350. Accessed July 19, 2021.

44. Hadley ME. Discovery that a melanocortin regulates sexual functions in male and female humans. Peptides 2005;26(10):1687–9.

45. Ückert S, Bannowsky A, Albrecht K, et al. Melanocortin receptor agonists in the treatment of male and female sexual dysfunctions: results from basic research and clinical studies. Expert Opin Investig Drugs 2014;23(11):1477–83.

46. Kingsberg SA, Clayton AH, Portman D, et al. Bremelanotide for the treatment of hypoactive sexual desire disorder: two randomized phase 3 trials. Obs Gyn 2019;134(5):899–908.

47. Watkins ES. The estrogen elixir: a history of hormone replacement therapy in America. Baltimore, MD, USA: Johns Hopkins University Press; 2007. p. 32–51.

48. Carter AC, Cohen EJ, Schorr E. The use of androgens in women. Vitamins Horm 1947;5:317–91.

49. Pessina MA, Hoyt RF, Goldstein I, et al. Differential effects of estradiol, progesterone, and testosterone on vaginal structural integrity. Endocrinology 2006; 147(1):61–9.

50. Achilli C, Pundir J, Ramanathan P, et al. Efficacy and safety of transdermal testosterone in postmenopausal women with hypoactive sexual desire disorder: a systematic review and meta-analysis. Fertil Steril 2017;107:475–82.

51. Cappelletti M, Wallen K. Increasing women's sexual desire: the comparative effectiveness of estrogens and androgens. Horm Behav 2016;78: 178–93.

52. Islam RM, Bell RJ, Green S, et al. Safety and efficacy of testosterone for women: a systematic review and meta-analysis of randomized controlled trial data. Lancet Diabetes Endocrinol 2019. https://doi.org/10.1016/S2213-8587(19)30189-5.

53. Rowen TS, Davis S, Parish S, et al. Methodological challenges in studying testosterone therapies for hypoactive sexual desire disorder in women. J Sex Med 2020;17(4):585–94.

54. Davis SR, Baber R, Panay N, et al. Global consensus position statement on the use of testosterone therapy for women. J Sex Med 2019;16:1331–7.

55. Guay A, Munarriz R, Jacobson J, et al. Serum androgen levels in healthy premenopausal women with and without sexual dysfunction: part A. Serum androgen levels in women aged 20-49 years with no complaints of sexual dysfunction. Int J Impot Res 2004;16(2):112–20.

56. Braunstein GD, Reitz RE, Buch A, et al. Testosterone reference ranges in normally cycling premenopausal women. J Sex Med 2011;8:2924–34.

57. IntimaLase Laser Vaginal Tightening. Available at: https://www.fotona.com/en/treatments/2054/ intimalase/. Accessed January 1, 2021.

58. Action II Petit Lady. Available at: https://www. lutronic.com.au/action-ii-petit-lady/. Accessed May 17, 2021.

59. Gambacciani M, Levancini M, Cervigni M. Vaginal erbium laser: the second-generation thermotherapy for the genitourinary syndrome of menopause. Climacteric 2015;18(5):757–63.

60. MonaLisa Touch. Available at: https://www.smilemonalisa.com. Accessed January 1, 2021.

61. FemiLift. Available at: https://www.almalasers.com/alma-products/femilift/. Accessed January 1, 2021.

62. FemTouch Laser for Vaginal Health. Available at: https://lumenis.com/aesthetics/products/femtouch/. Accessed January 1, 2021.

63. Karcher C, Sadick N. Vaginal rejuvenation using energy-based devices. Int J Womens Dermatol 2016;2(3):85–8.

64. Salvatore S, Maggiore ULR, Athanasiou S, et al. Histological study on the effects of microablative fractional CO2 laser on atrophic vaginal tissue: an ex vivo study. Menopause 2015;22(8):845–9.

65. Zerbinati N, Serati N, Origoni M, et al. Microscopic and ultrastructural modifications of postmenopausal atrophic vaginal mucosa after fractional carbon dioxide laser treatment. Lasers Med Sci 2015; 30(1):429–36.

66. Samuels JB, Garcia MA. Treatment to external labia and vaginal canal with CO2 laser for symptoms of vulvovaginal atrophy in postmenopausal women. Aesthet Surg J 2019;39(1):83–93.

67. Salvatore S, Nappi RE, Parma M, et al. Sexual function after fractional microablative CO_2 laser in women with vulvovaginal atrophy. Climacteric 2015;18(2):219–25.

68. Salvatore S, Nappi RE, Zerbinati N, et al. A 12-week treatment with fractional CO2 laser for vulvovaginal atrophy: a pilot study. Climacteric 2014; 17(4):363–9.

69. Ruanphoo P, Bunyavejchevin S. Treatment for vaginal atrophy using microablative fractional CO_2 laser: a randomized double-blinded sham-controlled trial. Menopause 2020;27(8):858–63. analysis. Fertil Steril 2017;107:475-82.

70. Politano C, Costa-Paiva L, Aguiar L, et al. Fractional CO_2 laser versus promestriene and lubricant in genitourinary syndrome of menopause: a randomized clinical trial. Menopause 2019;26(8): 833–40.

71. Cruz VL, Steiner ML, Pompei LM, et al. Randomized, double-blind, placebo-controlled clinical trial for evaluating the efficacy of fractional CO_2 laser compared to topical estriol in the treatment of vaginal atrophy in postmenopausal women. Menopause 2018;25(1):21–8.

72. Eftekhar T, Forooghifar T, Khalili T, et al. The effect of CO_2 fractional laser or premarin vaginal cream on improving sexual function in menopausal women: a randomized controlled trial. J Lasers Med Sci 2020;11(3):292–8.

73. Athanasiou S, Pitsouni E, Grigoriadis T, et al. Microablative fractional CO_2 laser for the genitourinary syndrome of menopause: up to 12-month results. Menopause 2019;26(3):248–55.

74. FDA Warns Against Use of Energy-Based Devices to Perform Vaginal 'Rejuvenation' or Vaginal Cosmetic Procedures: FDA Safety Communication. 2018. Available at: https://www.fda.gov/medical-devices/safety communications/fda-warns-against-use-energy-based-devices-perform-vaginal-rejuvenation-or-vaginal-cosmetic. Accessed January 1, 2021.

75. Guo JZ, Souders C, McClelland L, et al. Vaginal laser treatment of genitourinary syndrome of menopause: does the evidence support the FDA safety communication? Menopause 2020;27(10): 1177–84.

76. Photiou L, Lin MJ, Dubin DP, et al. Review of non-invasive vulvovaginal rejuvenation. J Eur Acad Dermatol Venereol 2020;34(4):716–26.

77. Sadick NS, Nassar AH, Dorizas AS, et al. Bipolar and multipolar radiofrequency. Dermatol Surg 2014;40(Suppl 12):S174–9.

78. Sadick NS, Malerich SA, Nassar AH, et al. Radiofrequency: an update on latest innovations. J Drugs Dermatol 2014;13(11):1331–5.

79. Dillon B, Dmochowski R. Radiofrequency for the treatment of stress urinary incontinence in women. Curr Urol Rep 2009;10(5):369–74.

80. Dunbar SW, Goldberg DJ. Radiofrequency in cosmetic dermatology: an update. J Drugs Dermatol 2015;14(11):1229–38.

81. Meyer PF, de Oliveira P, Silva FKBA, et al. Radiofrequency treatment induces fibroblast growth factor 2 expression and subsequently promotes neocollagenesis and neoangiogenesis in the skin tissue. Lasers Med Sci 2017;32:1727–36.

82. Viveve System. Available at: https://us.viveve.com/product-solutions/#VivevesystemFull. Accessed January 29, 2021.

83. ThermiVa. Available at: https://thermiva.com/. Accessed January 29, 2021.

84. Millheiser LS, Pauls RN, Herbst SJ, et al. Radiofrequency treatment of vaginal laxity after vaginal delivery: nonsurgical vaginal tightening. J Sex Med 2010;7(9):3088–95.

85. Sekiguchi Y, Utsugisawa Y, Azekosi Y, et al. Laxity of the vaginal introitus after childbirth: nonsurgical outpatient procedure for vaginal tissue restoration and improved sexual satisfaction using low-energy radiofrequency thermal therapy. J Womens Health (Larchmt) 2013;22(9):775–81.

86. Alinsod RM. Transcutaneous temperature controlled radiofrequency for orgasmic dysfunction. Lasers Surg Med 2016;48(7):64–5.

87. Krychman M, Rowan CG, Allan BB, et al. Effect of single-treatment, surface-cooled radiofrequency therapy on vaginal laxity and female sexual function: the VIVEVE I randomized controlled trial. J Sex Med 2017;14:215–25.

88. Lordêlo P, Leal MRD, Brasil CA, et al. Radiofrequency in female external genital cosmetics and sexual function: a randomized clinical trial. Int Urogynecol J 2016;27:1681–7.

89. Ciampa AR, de Prati AC, Amelio E, et al. Nitric oxide mediates anti-inflammatory action of extracorporeal shock waves. FEBS Lett 2005;579(30):6839–45.

90. Gruenwald I, Kitrey ND, Appel B, et al. Low-intensity extracorporeal shock wave therapy in vascular disease and erectile dysfunction: theory and outcomes. Sex Med Rev 2013;1(2):83–90.

91. Nishida T, Shimokawa H, Oi K, et al. Extracorporeal cardiac shock wave therapy markedly ameliorates ischemia-induced myocardial dysfunction in pigs in vivo. Circulation 2004;110(19):3055–61.

92. Becker M, Goetzenich A, Roehl AB, et al. Myocardial effects of local shock wave therapy in a Langendorff model. Ultrasonics 2014;54(1):131–6.

93. Hayashi D, Kawakami K, Ito K, et al. Low-energy extracorporeal shock wave therapy enhances skin wound healing in diabetic mice: a critical role of endothelial nitric oxide synthase. Wound Repair Rege 2012;20(6):887–95.

94. Zhang L, Weng C, Zhao Z, et al. Extracorporeal shock wave therapy for chronic wounds: a systematic review and meta-analysis of randomized controlled trials. Wound Repair Regen 2017;25(4):697–706.

95. Wang CJ. Extracorporeal shockwave therapy in musculoskeletal disorders. J Orthop Surg Res 2012;7:11.

96. Capogrosso P, Frey A, Jensen CFS, et al. Low-intensity shock wave therapy in sexual medicine: clinical recommendations from the European Society of Sexual Medicine (ESSM). J Sex Med 2019;6(10):1490–505.

97. FemiWave. Available at: https://femiwave.com. Accessed January 7, 2021.

98. Wu SS, Ericson KJ, Shoskes DA. Retrospective comparison of focused shockwave therapy and radial wave therapy for men with erectile dysfunction. Transl Androl Urol 2020;9(5):2122–8.

99. Tam J, Lee W, Kim JK. Female pelvic surgery: neuromodulation for voiding dysfunction. 2nd edition. Cham, Switzerland: Springer; 2020.

100. Farhan BA, Dutta R, Ghoniem G. Percutaneous tibial nerve stimulation in urology: overview. Women's Health Gynecol 2016;5:7–9.

101. Laumann EO, Paik A, Rosen RC. Sexual dysfunction in the United States: prevalence and predictors. JAMA 1999;281(6):537–44.

102. de Oliveira PS, Palma Reis J, de Oliveira TR, et al. The impact of sacral neuromodulation on sexual dysfunction. Curr Urol 2019;12(4):188–94.

103. Kershaw V, Khunda A, McCormick C, et al. The effect of percutaneous tibial nerve stimulation (PTNS) on sexual function: a systematic review and meta-analysis. Int Urogynecol J 2019;30(10):1619–27.

104. Banakhar M, Gazwani Y, Kelini ME, et al. Effect of sacral neuromodulation on female sexual function and quality of life: are they correlated? Can Urol Assoc J 2014;8(11–12):E762–7.

105. Pauls RN, Marinkovic SP, Silva WA, et al. Effects of sacral neuromodulation on female sexual function. Int Urogynecol J Pelvic Floor Dysfunct 2007;18(4):391–5.

106. van Balken MR, Vergunst H, Bemelmans BL. Sexual functioning in patients with lower urinary tract dysfunction improves after percutaneous tibial nerve stimulation. Int J Impot Res 2006;18(5):470–6.

107. Zimmerman LL, Rice IC, Berger MB, et al. Tibial nerve stimulation to drive genital sexual arousal in an anesthetized female rat. J Sex Med 2018;15(3):296–303.

108. Musco S, Serati M, Lombardi G, et al. Percutaneous tibial nerve stimulation improves female sexual function in women with overactive bladder syndrome. J Sex Med 2016;13(2):238–42.

109. Johnson RL, Wilson CG. A review of vagus nerve stimulation as a therapeutic intervention. J Inflamm Res 2018;11:203–13.

110. Yuan H, Silberstein SD. Vagus nerve and vagus nerve stimulation, a comprehensive review: part I. Headache 2016;56(1):71–8.

111. Yuan H, Silberstein SD. Vagus nerve and vagus nerve stimulation, a comprehensive review: part II. Headache 2016;56(2):259–66.

112. Heid M. Science confirms that the vagus nerve is key to well-being. Elemental. 2019. Available at: https://elemental.medium.com/science-confirms-that-the-vagus-nerve-is-key-to-well-being-c23fab90e211. Accessed January 16, 2021.

113. Hu B, Akerman S, Goadsby PJ. Characterization of opioidergic mechanisms related to the anti-migraine effect of vagus nerve stimulation. Neuropharmacology 2021;108375. https://doi.org/10.1016/j.neuropharm.2020.108375.

114. Hao M, Liu X, Rong P, et al. Reduced vagal tone in women with endometriosis and auricular vagus nerve stimulation as a potential therapeutic approach. Sci Rep 2021;11(1):1345.

115. Komisaruk BR, Gerdes CA, Whipple B. 'Complete' spinal cord injury does not block perceptual responses to genital self-stimulation in women. Arch Neurol 1997;54(12):1513–20.

116. Komisaruk BR, Whipple B, Crawford A, et al. Brain activation during vaginocervical self-stimulation and orgasm in women with complete spinal cord

injury: fMRI evidence of mediation by the vagus nerves. Brain Res 2004;1024(1–2):77–88.

117. Porges S. The polyvagal theory: neurophysiological foundation of emotions, attachment, communication, and self-regulation. New York, NY, USA: WW Norton; 2011.

118. Lenzer J. The danger within us: America's untested, unregulated medical device industry and one man's battle to survive it. 1st edition. New York, NY, USA: Little, Brown and Company, Hachette Book Group; 2017.

119. Brotto LA. Better sex through mindfulness: how women can cultivate desire. Vancouver, BC, Canada: GreystoneBooks; 2018.

Managing Female Sexual Pain

Maria Uloko, MD[a],*, Rachel Rubin, MD[b]

KEYWORDS

- Female • Sexual pain disorder • Genito-pelvic pain/penetration disorder • GPPPD

KEY POINTS

- Definition of GPPD.
- Etiology/differential diagnosis.
- Diagnosis.
- Treatment.

INTRODUCTION

With the evolving language regarding gender identity and sexual orientation, the authors believe that it is important to first define gender and sex. Gender refers to the attitudes, feelings, and behaviors that a given culture associates with a person's biological sex. Sex is defined as either of the two main categories (male and female) into which humans and most other living things are divided based on their reproductive functions. The authors of this article will use the terminology.

"Female sexual dysfunction" as defined in the DSM-V[1] to describe anyone assigned female at birth or anyone with female internal or external genitalia.

Female sexual pain disorder or genito-pelvic pain/penetration disorder (GPPPD) is defined as persistent or recurrent symptoms with one or more of the following for at least 6 months:

1. Marked vulvovaginal or pelvic pain during penetrative intercourse or penetration attempts
2. Marked fear or anxiety about vulvovaginal or pelvic pain in anticipation of, during, or as a result of penetration
3. Marked tensing or tightening of the pelvic floor muscles during attempted vaginal penetration.[1]

GPPPD, previously termed dyspareunia and/or vaginismus, first debuted in the Diagnostic and Statistical Manual of Mental Disorders (DSM-5) in 2013. It is classified as either lifelong or acquired and ranges in the degree of distress from mild, moderate to severe. The estimated prevalence of GPPPD in the United States varies between 3% and 25% with causes differing by age group.[2] Women with GPPPD report significantly reduced quality of life and well-being. GPPPD can contribute to a decline in self-esteem, feelings of femininity and is associated with a negative body and genital self-image. GPPPD can pose a significant burden on the couple as well. The disordered cycle of pain can lead to fear, hypervigilance in sexual situations, or complete avoidance of sexual intimacy.[3–5]

Individuals with GPPPD often do not seek care despite the distressing nature of the disorder for a variety of reasons. These reasons include but are not limited to:

1. GPPPD was not previously regarded as a recognized disorder and instead viewed as a culturally taboo subject[6]
2. Feelings of shame and guilt by the individual because of cultural and personal stigmatization[6,7]

[a] San Diego Sexual Medicine, 5555 Resevoir Drive, Suite 300, San Diego, CA 92120, USA; [b] IntimMedicine Specialists, 1850 M St NW, Suite 450, Washington, DC 20036, USA
* Corresponding author.
E-mail address: mariauloko@gmail.com
Twitter: @mariauloko (M.U.)

Urol Clin N Am 48 (2021) 487–497
https://doi.org/10.1016/j.ucl.2021.06.007

3. Lack of appropriately trained health care professionals that do not make an inquiry about sexual health in routine care visits. Provider reluctance to discuss sexuality may stem from a sense that this is not a medical problem, personal discomfort with sexuality, or lack of training/knowledge/time.[8]

Patients with GPPPD who do present for treatment may not receive appropriate treatment/referral, which may lead to a further burden for the individual and partner as well as increased direct health costs. GPPPD symptoms are frequently multifactorial and require a multidisciplinary approach that assesses various factors including biological, psychological, sociocultural, interdependent pathophysiology, critical life events, and relational status.[9–11] A comprehensive biopsychosocial approach should be implemented for assessment and treatment. The treatment plans should focus not only on difficulties with vaginal penetration and muscle tightness associated with sexual intercourse but also the psychological factors that contribute to sexual dissatisfaction and couple dynamics.[12–14] Psychological factors that may contribute to dyspareunia include anxiety or guilt about intercourse, memories of distressing early sexual experiences, fear of penetration, unresolved anger, feelings of shame or guilt, and inadequate precoital stimulation.

Pathophysiology

Genitourinary Syndrome of Menopause: Genitourinary Syndrome of Menopause (GSM), previously described as vulvovaginal atrophy/atrophic vaginitis, is mediated by depletion of androgens and estrogens and subsequently decreased blood flow to the vagina and vulva. GSM is characterized by genital symptoms (eg, dryness, burning, and irritation), sexual symptoms (eg, lack of lubrication, discomfort or pain, and decreased libido and difficulty with arousal and orgasm), and/or urinary symptoms (eg, urgency, dysuria, and recurrent urinary tract infections).[15] GSM may occur in hormone-depleted states outside of menopause including breastfeeding, oral contraceptive use, adjuvant hormonal deprivation therapy for various disorders, gender-affirming hormone therapy, thyroid disorders, and pituitary tumors[16–18] (**Fig. 1**).

Vestibulodynia: Vestibulodynia (VD), previously known as vulvar vestibulitis syndrome, is defined as vulvar vestibule pain lasting more than 3 months unrelated to infection, skin disorders, or other identifiable factors. It is often characterized as burning, stinging, itching, pain with penetration, and/or rawness of the vestibule/vagina. The most common factors associated with VD are hormonal changes, hypertonic pelvic floor dysfunction (PFD), and/or an increased number of nerve endings in the mucosa of the vestibule termed neuroproliferative VD.[19]

Clitorodynia: Clitorodynia is a form of vulvodynia localized to the clitoris. It is characterized by frequent and intense pain episodes that can be either provoked or unprovoked. Clitorodynia may cause significant impairment in both activities of daily living and sexual activity. It may be associated with other chronic pain disorders, lichen sclerosus, multiple sclerosis, pelvic surgery, and vaginal delivery.[20] Physical examination may show clitoral adhesions, phimosis, balanitis, or skin changes associated with lichen sclerosus.

Pelvic Floor Dysfunction: PFD is an umbrella term encompassing the constellation of symptoms secondary to the nonrelaxing and spastic pelvic

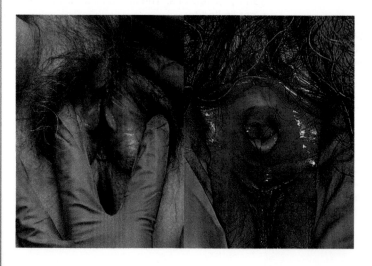

Fig. 1. (A) The 50% resorbed and thin labia minora. (B) The protruding urethra, pallor, and erythema of the vestibule. Patient's vaginal pH was 7.5, whereas the goal should be 4.5. Image courtesy of Rachel Rubin, MD, NW, Washington.

floor musculature. The presenting symptoms of PFD depend on the particular muscle(s) in spasm. Common manifestations include dyspareunia, voiding dysfunction, incontinence, urinary retention, constipation, and dyschezia.

Anatomy/Physiology

A detailed understanding of female genital anatomy is crucial in providing comprehensive evaluation and optimizing treatment. The anatomic female sexual organs include the clitoris (glans and crura), labia major and minora, the vulvar vestibule, the vagina, the cervix, the vestibular bulbs, and the pelvic floor muscles.

Vulva

The vulva is a complicated anatomic structure intricately involved in the sexual response cycle. It includes the mons pubis, labia majora, labia minora, vestibule, and clitoris.

Vestibule

The vulvar vestibule is located between the labia minora and the hymen. This tissue originates from endoderm and is hormonally regulated by testosterone.[21] The medial border is the hymen and lateral border is "Hart's Line," which marks the change from the vulva skin to the smooth transitional skin of the vulva located inside the labia minora. The vestibule contains the external urethral meatus, the openings of the two greater (Bartholin's) glands, and the perivestibular/Skeene's glands (respectively analogous to Cowper's glands and glands of Littre in male anatomy). The vulvar vestibule can become painful due to changes in hormones (ie, low androgen states like menopause or use of oral contraceptive pills), inflammation, muscle hypertonicity, or more rarely congenital neuroproliferation.[22] The vestibule is an area of significance in patients presenting with vulvar pain and GPPPD (**Fig. 2**).

Clitoris

The clitoris consists of spongy vascular tissue that engorges with blood during arousal. The body of the clitoris is surrounded by the tunica albuginea and consists of two paired corpora cavernosa composed of trabecular smooth muscle and lacunar sinusoids. The glans clitoris is the component of the clitoris that is, visible but often covered by a "hood" of preputial skin, particularly in the unaroused state. The preputial skin can develop phimosis and/or balanitis, which may contribute to clitoral pain (clitorodynia) and/or anorgasmia.[23]

Vagina

The vagina is an elastic, muscular canal that extends from the vulva to the cervix. The vaginal wall consists of three layers: (1) an inner mucous type stratified squamous cell epithelium supported by a thick lamina propia, that undergoes hormone-related cyclical changes, (2) the muscularis, composed of outer longitudinal smooth muscle fibers and inner circular fibers, and (3) an outer fibrous layer, rich in collagen and elastin, which provides structural support to the vagina.[24] It serves a multitude of functions in response to hormonal changes and plays a vital role in the reproductive system and sexual pleasure. The vaginal mucosa contains a high concentration of estrogen and androgen receptors.[25]

Pelvic floor

The female pelvic floor muscles support the bladder, uterus, and colon and play a vital role in sexual function as well as bladder and bowel control. A clock face can be used as a reference when describing the location of the pelvic structures.

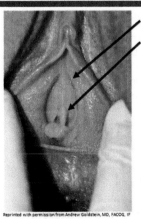

Reprinted with permission from Andrew Goldstein, MD, FACOG, IF   AR= androgen receptor; ER= estrogen receptor

- Lateral border is Hart's line
- Medial border is the hymen and urethra
- Ostia of the Bartholin's, Skene's, and minor vestibular glands
- Derived from the primitive urogenital sinus
- Different blood supply from the vagina
- Rich in AR (> ER)

Fig. 2. The vestibule. Courtesy of Irwin Goldstein, MD, San Diego, California, with permission

The 12- and 6-o'clock positions correspond to the anterior and posterior midline, or pubic symphysis and anus, respectively. (10) The obturator internus and externus can be palpated by sweeping from the pubic ramus downward along the muscle belly behind the pubic ramus at 1- and 11-o'clock. At 3- and 9-o'clock, the levator ani complex is present, and at 5- and 7-o'clock, the iliococcygeus muscle (distal) is palpable. Approximately, a finger-length depth into the vagina around 4- and 8-o'clock, the ischial spines are palpated as bony prominences. The ischial spines serve as the anatomic marker for the pudendal nerve, which runs approximately 2 cm posteromedial to the ischial spine and innervates the clitoris, vulva, and anus.[26]

Lymphovascular

Arterial

The internal pudendal artery is the dominant blood supply to the female external genitalia. The internal pudendal artery is a branch of the internal iliac artery. The labia majora is also supplied by the superficial external pudendal artery, a branch of the femoral. This anatomic distinction is important to note as the dual blood supply makes it a useful flap in reconstructive surgeries.[27]

Venous

The venous drainage of the external female genitalia is via the external and internal pudendal veins. The external pudendal vein drains to the great saphenous vein, which in turn drains into the femoral vein and from there to the external iliac vein after ascending past the inguinal ligament. The internal pudendal vein drains back into the internal iliac vein. Both the external and internal iliac veins will ascend and merge to form the common iliac veins, which merge to form the inferior vena cava.[27]

Lymphatic

The lymphatic drainage of the external female genitalia is primarily by the superficial inguinal lymph nodes; the exception to this is the clitoris, which drains toward the deep inguinal lymph nodes. The superficial and deep inguinal lymph nodes conjoin and drain into the common iliac lymph nodes. All of this lymph will ascend toward the inferior part of the thoracic duct known as the cisterna chyli.[27]

Neuroanatomy and Physiology

Autonomic Nervous System

Sexual response is the result of coordinated activity of the parasympathetic, sympathetic, and somatic nervous system. The reproductive organs receive preganglionic parasympathetic innervation from the sacral spinal cord, sympathetic innervation from the outflow of the lower thoracic and upper lumbar spinal cord segments, and somatic motor innervation from α-motor neurons in the ventral horn of the lower spinal cord segments.[28] During genital stimulation, afferent somatic sensory endings in the dorsal roots of S2–S4 are relayed centrally to the somatic sensory cortex. This is the region of the cerebral cortex concerned with processing sensory information from the body surface, subcutaneous tissues, muscles, and joints. Activation of the somatic sensory cortex leads to decreased sympathetic input and increased parasympathetic activity via the pelvic nerve causing a release of nitric oxide resulting in vasodilation. This in turn leads to a rise in clitoral cavernosal artery inflow and increased clitoral intracavernosal pressure. Increasing pressure leads to clitoral engorgement, extrusion of the glans clitoris from the prepuce, and enhanced sensitivity. Increased blood flow to the vagina leads to vasocongestion within the vaginal submucosa, increasing oncotic pressure, which leads to the production of a fluid transudate (lubrication) that passes into the vaginal lumen via aquaporins located in the vaginal mucosa.[29,30]

The lumbar sympathetic pathway to the sexual organs originates in the thoracolumbar segments (T11–L2) and reaches the target organs via the corresponding sympathetic chain ganglia and the inferior mesenteric and pelvic ganglia in the hypogastric nerve. The sympathetic nervous system produces rhythmic smooth muscle contractions of the vagina during orgasm.

The somatic nervous system is composed of the pudendal nerve (S2–S4). The pudendal nerve reaches the perineum through Alcock's canal and provides sensory and motor innervation to the external genitalia. Excitatory input leads to muscle contraction of the bulbocavernosus and ischiocavernosus muscles that accompany orgasm.[31]

Hormonal Physiology

Estrogens (E) are the primary "female" sex steroids and act by binding to widely distributed estrogen receptors within the body.[32,33] Three estrogens are naturally produced in the female body.[34] In premenopausal women, 17β-estradiol (Estradiol or E_2) produced by the ovary is the estrogen present in the largest quantity; circulating estradiol levels fluctuate from 40 to 200–400 pg/mL across the menstrual cycle.[35] Owing to its high affinity for the estrogen receptor, it is the most potent of the three estrogens. Estrone (E1) is a less potent estrogen that can be synthesized via E2 by the enzyme 17-beta hydroxysteroid dehydrogenase or through the conversion of androstenedione in adipose tissue via aromatase. The third endogenous estrogen, estriol (E_3), is also a metabolite of estradiol in the periphery. Estriol is the principle estrogen produced by the placenta during pregnancy but is found in smaller quantities than either estradiol or estrone in nonpregnant individuals. In postmenopausal women, estradiol levels drop to less than 20 pg/mL. The ovary ceases producing estradiol, but the adrenal gland continues making androstenedione, the immediate precursor to estrone, so the levels of estrone remain unchanged despite the dramatic fall of estradiol.[36]

At the target organ, estrogens diffuse into the cell and through the nuclear membrane. Inside the nucleus, estrogens attach to an estrogen receptor to form a ligand-receptor complex, which binds to DNA and initiates gene transcription. Gene transcription in turn leads to the production of specific proteins that trigger estrogenic effects in the target tissue (eg, maintenance of tissue integrity and thickness in the vaginal wall).[37]

Androgen receptors are also common and extensive throughout the female genitourinary tract. Androgens (ie, dehydroepiandrosterone [DHEA], androstenedione, and testosterone), which are produced in the adrenal cortex and ovaries, are necessary precursors for the biosynthesis of estrogens and play important direct roles in the physiology and homeostasis of the vagina.[38] Their production is significantly greater than that of estrogens in premenopausal and postmenopausal women.[39]

EVALUATION
History

Providers should provide an open and compassionate approach with patients when addressing sexual health to increase patient's comfort on such a sensitive subject matter. The most important goal during the introductory discussion is to provide validation of the patient's pain and distress. This will aid in establishing rapport and trust between the patient and provider. This should be done while the patient is fully dressed and ideally not in an examination room.

Open-ended questions, affirming statements, and reflective listening should be used to obtain a comprehensive history. Generalizing statements are helpful tools to engage the patient; an example of this would be "Many women with (a specified condition) experience (a specific or generalized issue with sex); Do you experience this?". The use of validated self-reported questionnaires such as the Female Sexual Function Index, the McGill Pain Questionnaire, or the Patient-Reported Outcomes Measurement Information System (PROMIS) vulvar discomfort scale can also provide objective information when quantifying pain and the impact it has on the patients' life.[40] A focused sexual history should review the following:

1. Pain characteristics (location, duration, exacerbating factors, alleviating factors)
2. Associated symptoms such as bowel, bladder, or musculoskeletal symptoms
3. Sexual activity and behavior
4. Past medical history
5. Surgical history
6. Medication history (use of hormonal birth control, SSRIs, etc)
7. Mental health history
8. Obstetrics and gynecologic history including onset of menstruation, characteristics of periods, and onset of menopause
9. History of physical or sexual abuse
10. Previous interventions

Physical Examination

Many objective findings on physical examination can be seen in a patient with sexual complaints. A full vulvar and vaginal examination will aid in finding the proper treatment for the patient. Important anatomy to assess includes:

- Labia majora and minora.
- Clitoris, including glans and hood.
- Urethra and periurethral glands.
- Vestibule.
- Vaginal vault.
- Cervix.
- Pelvic floor levator ani muscles.

Important factors to evaluate in the focused genital examination include:

- Distribution of hair.
- Symmetry and size of genital tissues.
- Evidence of atrophy or stenosis.
- Areas of provoked pain.
- Color uniformity, erythema, or other discoloration.
- Visible lesions, excoriations, or scars.
- Pelvic organ prolapse.
- Pelvic floor muscle tone and voluntary control.
- Presence of vaginal discharge.
- Presence or absence of vaginal rugae.

Each examination should begin with an explanation of each step and a real-time discussion of the examination findings with the patient. The examination should include an external and internal musculoskeletal evaluation, external visual and sensory examination, and a bimanual examination if tolerated by the patient. It is empowering for patients to visualize their anatomy either with a vulvoscope or mirror as a means to better understand and feel comfortable with their anatomy. The external musculoskeletal examination should include evaluation of posture/gait, symmetry/asymmetry, palpation of abdominal, gluteal, back, and lower extremity muscles. Assessment should include areas of tension and/or pain, muscle strength, range of motion, sensation, and reflexes.

Examination of the vulva is performed by inspecting the external genitalia, perineum, perianal areas, and the mons pubis. The clinician should evaluate for signs of infection, trauma, atrophy, fissures, and dermatologic changes. A cotton swab should be used to assess allodynia and/or hyperalgesia by light palpation of the vulvar structures. The vestibule should be examined making sure to note areas of hyperemia or erythema and assessment/presence of the periurethral and perivestibular glands. A sensory test should be performed using a cotton swab to palpate the vestibule in 7 anatomic sites (12 o'clock, 1 o'clock, 3 o'clock, 5 o'clock, 7 o'clock, 9 o'clock, and 11 o'clock).

The internal pelvic muscles should be examined through the vagina. The examination should start with light palpation for general tone, then deeper pressure to assess for trigger points, which are hallmark diagnostic indicators of PFD. Using the index finger, the examiner can palpate the lateral, anterior, and posterior walls of the vagina, the urethra, and pelvic floor muscles assessing for tone, tenderness, or involuntary contractions. Clinical criteria that indicate presence of a trigger point include (1) a palpable taut band, (2) an extremely tender nodule in the taut band, (3) ability to reproduce the pain with palpation of the tender nodule, and (4) painful limit to stretch or full range of motion.[41] If pain or hypertonic muscles are noted during this examination, a pelvic floor physical therapy referral may be warranted.

A bimanual examination should be performed to evaluate the uterus and adnexa for any masses or tenderness. Internal examination of the vagina and cervix should follow using a warmed small-sized Grave's or Pederson speculum. The speculum should be inserted slowly ensuring to avoid the urethra or vestibule as these areas can provoke pain. During the speculum examination, the internal vaginal tissue, cervix, and vaginal secretions are examined. Cultures or biopsies can be collected at this time to rule out infections, dermatoses, or abnormal cellular dysplasia that can cause dyspareunia or vulvodynia.

TREATMENT
Genitourinary Symptoms of Menopause

The primary goals for treating GSM are alleviation of symptoms, restoring vaginal pH, and preventing recurrent urinary tract infections. A multimodal approach can be used to optimize results.

Local Vaginal Therapy

Low-dose vaginal estrogen
Life-long low-dose vaginal hormone therapy is the mainstay treatment for GSM (eg, vaginal creams, intravaginal tablets, or intravaginal rings). It is recommended by the American Urologic Association for the treatment of recurrent urinary tract infections in premenopausal and postmenopausal women as data show it prevents urinary tract infection by restoring vaginal flora and pH.[42] Topical low dose vaginal estrogen restores hormone levels within the tissue without significant systemic absorption. This results in rapid improvement of vaginal symptoms within 2 to 3 weeks but may take 2 months for maximal benefit. Systemic estrogen therapy can be considered in addition to topical estrogen if there are concomitant vasomotor symptoms. Its use as monotherapy, however, has not been shown to treat symptoms of GSM. The American College of Obstetricians and Gynecologists recommends the use of nonhormonal options as the first choice for the treatment of vaginal atrophy in women with current or a history of estrogen-dependent breast cancer. Vaginal estrogen therapy is deemed appropriate for patients with a history of estrogen-dependent breast cancer who are unresponsive to nonhormonal remedies but only after a thorough discussion of risks and benefits with their oncologist.[43]

Androgen/testosterone
Vaginal DHEA suppositories (Intrarosa) are FDA approved for the treatment of moderate to severe GPPPD. DHEA is converted by enzymes in the vulva, vestibule, and vagina into estrogen and testosterone. This results in significant improvements in vaginal epithelial cells and integrity, vaginal pH, parabasal cells, increased vaginal secretions, all without affecting serum levels of estradiol and testosterone or endometrial tissues.[44,45]

Lubricants and moisturizers
Several over-the-counter vaginal lubricants (water-, silicone-, or oil-based) and moisturizers are commonly used for supplemental/symptomatic treatment of postmenopausal women with vulvovaginal symptoms. Moisturizers are used as daily therapy and lubricants are used as needed

typically for sexual activity but can be used independently of sexual activity. Patients should choose a product that is physiologically most similar to natural vaginal secretions and will not disturb the vaginal pH.[46] Water-based lubricants are often preferred over oil-based lubricants as they are nonstaining and associated with fewer genital symptoms, although they often need to be reapplied. Caution should be used with oil-based lubricants as this can lead to condom breakage.[47]

Oral Therapy

Selective estrogen receptor modulators
Selective estrogen receptor modulators (SERMs) are systemic nonhormonal therapy delivered orally. Ospemifene is the only SERM approved by the US Food and Drug Administration (FDA) for the treatment of moderate to severe dyspareunia.[48] Several studies have shown that it increases vaginal maturation index and lubrication and normalizes vaginal pH. Common side-effects include hot flashes, vaginal discharge, and muscle spasm. Contraindications include estrogen-dependent neoplasms, history of venous thromboembolism, previous stroke or MI, or active heart disease (see **Table 1**).[48,49]

Nonsurgical/Nonmedical Treatments

Vaginal dilators
Women with GSM may see benefit from gentle stretching of the vagina with the use of lubricated, sequential dilators. Dilators have been shown to increase vaginal elasticity, which in turn decreases pain with penetration. Pelvic floor muscle therapy may also be useful in patients with nonrelaxing or high-tone pelvic floor muscle dysfunction triggered by painful sexual activity related to GSM.[50] Patients and providers can find pelvic floor physical therapists through numerous online resources including https://aptapelvichealth.org/.

Lasers: fractional CO_2 laser or erbium:YAG laser can be used as a nonhormonal treatment option for GSM.[51] Several small studies have shown restoration of the vaginal epithelium, increase in premenopausal vaginal flora, and subjective improvement in symptoms of GSM, including lower urinary tract symptoms.[52] At this time, these therapies are not FDA approved and should not be considered a standard of care. Readers interested in more detail on these therapies are referred to the chapter in this volume on energy-based and pharmaceutical treatments for sexual concerns in women.

VD treatment
The treatment of VD requires a multidisciplinary biopsychosocial approach as most cases are multifactorial. In terms of medical management, hormone therapy with vaginal estrogen and testosterone are the mainstay of medical management for hormonally mediated VD; options include DHEA vaginal inserts or compounded estrogen/testosterone creams. We recommend compounded estradiol 0.03% and testosterone 0.1% in a methyl cellulose or versa base applied to the vestibule 1 to 2 per day. Studies have shown

Table 1
Pharmacologic treatments for genitourinary syndrome of menopause (GSM)

Treatment	Product Name	Dose
Vaginal Cream		
17-beta-estradiol cream	Estrace, generic	0.5–1 g daily for 2 wk, and then 0.5–1 g 1–3× per wk
Conjugated equine estrogens cream	Premarin	0.5–1 g daily for 2 wk, and then 0.5–1 g 1–3× per wk
Vaginal Inserts		
Estradiol vaginal tablets	Vagifem®, Yuvafem®,	10 mcg inserts daily for 2 wk, and then 2× per wk
Estradiol soft gel capsules	ImVexxy®	4, 10 mcg inserts daily for 2 wk, and then 2× per wk
DHEA (prasterone) inserts	Intrarosa®	6.5 mg capsules daily
Vaginal Ring		
17-beta-estradiol ring	Estring®	1 ring inserted every 3 mo
SERM		
Ospemifene oral tablets	Osphena®	60 mg tablet daily

improvement in 50% of people with VD symptoms over 12 weeks.[53] Discontinuation of oral hormonal contraception is a consideration if the onset of symptoms is linked to the initiation of this treatment. Patients should be counseled on long-acting reversible contraception, which may have lesser hormonal effects on the vestibule.[54]

Cognitive behavioral therapy and sex therapy facilitated by a licensed professional play a key role not only in the treatment of VD but also in all causes of GPPD. Resources for sex therapy include the American Association of Sex Educators, Councilors, and Therapists (www.aasect.org/) and the Society for Sex Therapy and Research (www.sstarnet.org/).

Topical steroids may be indicated in cases of VD associated with dermatologic conditions, that is, Lichen Sclerosus. Pelvic floor physical therapy, biofeedback, OnabotulinumtoxinA injection, compounded vaginal valium suppositories, pudendal nerve blocks, and neuromodulation are other adjuvant therapies that have been shown to be beneficial in the treatment of some cases of VD.[41] In refractory cases or for those with persistent pain despite correction with hormone therapy, a vulvar vestibulectomy with vaginal flap advancement, may be offered. A high success rate can be expected for appropriately selected patients cared for by an experienced surgeon (**Fig. 3**).

Clitorodynia treatment

The treatment for clitorodynia is determined by the underlying cause. If clitorodynia is secondary to phimosis or lichen sclerosis, potent topical steroids may be used for management.[20,55] Surgical treatment can be offered if the pain is associated with correctable physical examination findings such as clitoral pearl or adhesions refractory to medication. Either office-based lysis of adhesions or surgical dorsal slit may be considered dependent on patient tolerance and severity of disease (**Fig. 4**).

Pelvic floor rehabilitation

Pelvic floor rehabilitation (PFR) is most typically a multimodal treatment plan developed in consultation with a licensed physical therapist with expertise in the management of PFD. The mainstay of PFR is pelvic floor physical therapy, which includes manual techniques of massage, myofacial and trigger point release, and joint mobilization. Adjunct therapies include trigger point injections with steroids or OnabotulinumtoxinA for pelvic floor tightness or spasticity, intravaginal diazepam

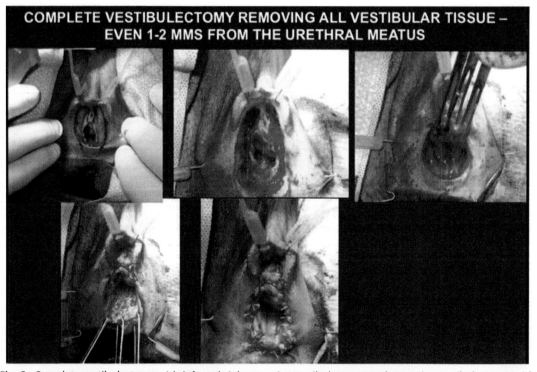

COMPLETE VESTIBULECTOMY REMOVING ALL VESTIBULAR TISSUE – EVEN 1-2 MMS FROM THE URETHRAL MEATUS

Fig. 3. Complete vestibulectomy with left and right anterior vestibulectomy and posterior vestibulectomy with vaginal advancement flap reconstruction. (Photos courtesy of Irwin Goldstein MD)

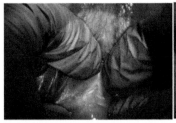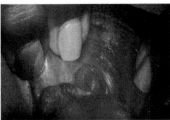

Fig. 4. Phimosis of the clitoris and clitoral lysis of adhesions. Courtesy of Rachel Rubin, MD, NW, Washington.

suppositories, transcutaneous electrical nerve stimulation, and neuromodulation.

SUMMARY

GPPPD is a complex often multifactorial disorder that significantly impacts patients' physical health, mental health, and overall quality of life. Owing to the complex nature of sexual response, GPPPD is typically best managed using a multidisciplinary approach that includes medical, surgical, behavioral, and musculoskeletal interventions.

CLINICS CARE POINTS

- Female sexual pain disorder or genito-pelvic pain/penetration disorder (GPPPD), previously known as dyspareunia, is defined as persistent or recurrent symptoms with one or more of symptoms for over 6 months.

- The estimated prevalence of GPPPD in the United States varies between 3% and 25% with causes differing by age groups.

- GPPPD is frequently multifactorial and requires a multidisciplinary approach that includes biological, psychological, sociocultural, and relational factors.

- An understanding of female genital anatomy is essential to provide comprehensive evaluation and optimize treatment outcomes for women with sexual concerns.

DISCLOSURE

The authors have nothing to disclose.

REFERENCES

1. Diagnostic and Statistical manual of mental disorders. 5th Edition. https://doi.org/10.1176/appi.books.9780890425596.893619.

2. Hayes RD, Dennerstein L, Bennett CM, et al. What is the "true" prevalence of female sexual dysfunctions and does the way we assess these conditions have an impact? J Sex Med 2008;5(4). https://doi.org/10.1111/j.1743-6109.2007.00768.x.

3. Cherner RA, Reissing ED. A comparative study of sexual function, behavior, and cognitions of women with lifelong vaginismus. Arch Sex Behav 2013;42(8). https://doi.org/10.1007/s10508-013-0111-3.

4. Farmer MA, Meston CM. Predictors of genital pain in young women. Arch Sex Behav 2007;36(6). https://doi.org/10.1007/s10508-007-9199-7.

5. Reissing ED, Binik YM, Khalif S, et al. Etiological correlates of vaginismus: sexual and physical abuse, sexual knowledge, sexual self-schema, and relationship adjustment. J Sex Marital Ther 2003;29(1). https://doi.org/10.1080/713847095.

6. Bergvall L, Himelein MJ. Attitudes toward seeking help for sexual dysfunctions among us and Swedish college students. Sex Relationship Ther 2014;29(2). https://doi.org/10.1080/14681994.2013.860222.

7. Donaldson RL, Meana M. Early dyspareunia experience in young women: confusion, consequences, and help-seeking barriers. J Sex Med 2011;8(3). https://doi.org/10.1111/j.1743-6109.2010.02150.x.

8. Hinchliff S, Gott M. Seeking medical help for sexual concerns in mid- and later life: a review of the literature. J Sex Res 2011;48(2–3). https://doi.org/10.1080/00224499.2010.548610.

9. Granot M, Lavee Y. Psychological factors associated with perception of experimental pain in vulvar vestibulitis syndrome. J Sex Marital Ther 2005;31(4). https://doi.org/10.1080/00926230590950208.

10. Pazmany E, Bergeron S, Van Oudenhove L, et al. Body image and genital self-image in pre-menopausal women with dyspareunia. Arch Sex Behav 2013;42(6). https://doi.org/10.1007/s10508-013-0102-4.

11. Ayling K, Ussher JM. "If sex hurts, am i still a woman?" the subjective experience of vulvodynia in hetero-sexual women. Arch Sex Behav 2008;37(2). https://doi.org/10.1007/s10508-007-9204-1.

12. Bergeron S, Lord M-J. The integration of pelvi-perineal re-education and cognitive behavioural therapy in the multidisciplinary treatment of the sexual pain

disorders. Sex Relationship Ther 2010;25(3). https://doi.org/10.1080/14681994.2010.496968.

13. Aerts L, Bergeron S, Pukall CF, et al. Provoked vestibulodynia: does pain intensity correlate with sexual dysfunction and dissatisfaction? J Sex Med 2016; 13(6). https://doi.org/10.1016/j.jsxm.2016.03.368.

14. Binik YM, Meana M. The future of sex therapy: specialization or marginalization? Arch Sex Behav 2009;38(6). https://doi.org/10.1007/s10508-009-9475-9.

15. Sarrel PM. Ovarian hormones and vaginal blood flow: using laser Doppler velocimetry to measure effects in a clinical trial of post-menopausal women. Int J Impot Res 1998;10(suppl. 2).

16. Tan O, Bradshaw K, Carr BR. Management of vulvovaginal atrophy-related sexual dysfunction in postmenopausal women. Menopause 2012;19(1). https://doi.org/10.1097/gme.0b013e31821f92df.

17. Nappi RE, Seracchioli R, Salvatore S, et al. Impact of vulvovaginal atrophy of menopause: prevalence and symptoms in Italian women according to the eves study. Gynecol Endocrinol 2019;35(5). https://doi.org/10.1080/09513590.2018.1563883.

18. Kingsberg SA, Kellogg S, Krychman M. Treating dyspareunia caused by vaginal atrophy: a review of treatment options using vaginal estrogen therapy. Int J Womens Health 2009;1(1). https://doi.org/10.2147/ijwh.s4872.

19. Bornstein J, Goldstein AT, Stockdale CK, et al. 2015 issvd, isswsh, and ipps consensus terminology and classification of persistent vulvar pain and vulvodynia. J Sex Med 2016;13(4). https://doi.org/10.1016/j.jsxm.2016.02.167.

20. Parada M, D'Amours T, Amsel R, et al. Clitorodynia: a descriptive study of clitoral pain. J Sex Med 2015; 12(8). https://doi.org/10.1111/jsm.12934.

21. Maseroli E, Vignozzi L. Testosterone and vaginal function. Sex Med Rev 2020;8(3). https://doi.org/10.1016/j.sxmr.2020.03.003.

22. Dalley AF. The american association of clinical anatomists (aaca): the other american anatomy association. Anat Rec 1999;257(5). https://doi.org/10.1002/(sici)1097-0185(19991015)257:5<154::aid-ar3>3.0.co;2-2.

23. O'connell HE, Sanjeevan KV, Hutson JM. Anatomy of the clitoris. J Urol 2005;174(4 part 1). https://doi.org/10.1097/01.ju.0000173639.38898.cd.

24. Gold JM, Shrimanker I. Physiology, vaginal. Stat Pearls; 2019. p. 45–60.

25. Bachmann G, Lobo RA, Gut R, et al. Efficacy of low-dose estradiol vaginal tablets in the treatment of atrophic vaginitis. Obstet Gynecol 2008;111(1). https://doi.org/10.1097/01.aog.0000296714.12226.0f.

26. Maldonado PA, Chin K, Garcia AA, et al. Anatomic variations of pudendal nerve within pelvis and pudendal canal: clinical applications. Am J Obstet Gynecol 2015;213(5). https://doi.org/10.1016/j.ajog.2015.06.009.

27. Nguyen J, Duong H. Anatomy, Abdomen and Pelvis. Female External Genitalia 2020. PMID: 31613483.

28. Purves D, Augustine G, Fitzpatrick D, et al. Neuroscience. 2nd edition. Sunderland (MA): Sinauer Associates; 2001. 2(40–56).

29. Manson JE, Chlebowski RT, Stefanick ML, et al. Menopausal hormone therapy and health outcomes during the intervention and extended poststopping phases of the women's health initiative randomized trials. JAMA 2013;310(13). https://doi.org/10.1001/jama.2013.278040.

30. Simon J, Nachtigall L, Gut R, et al. Effective treatment of vaginal atrophy with an ultra–low-dose estradiol vaginal tablet. Obstet Gynecol 2008;112(5). https://doi.org/10.1097/aog.0b013e31818aa7c3.

31. Meston CM. Sympathetic nervous system activity and female sexual arousal. Am J Cardiol 2000; 86(2). https://doi.org/10.1016/s0002-9149(00)00889-4.

32. Levin RJ. The physiology of sexual arousal in the human female: a recreational and procreational synthesis. Arch Sex Behav 2002;31(5). https://doi.org/10.1023/a:1019836007416.

33. Yang CC, Cold CJ, Yilmaz U, et al. Sexually responsive vascular tissue of the vulva. BJU Int 2006;97(4). https://doi.org/10.1111/j.1464-410x.2005.05961.x.

34. Glass RH, Kase NG. Clinical gynecologic endocrinology and infertility. Endocrinologist 1991;1(1). https://doi.org/10.1097/00019616-199102000-00012.

35. M. S. Menopause practice: a clinician's guide. Can Fam Physician 2012;50–9.

36. Jones KP. Estrogens and progestins: what to use and how to use it. Clin Obstet Gynecol 1992;35(4). https://doi.org/10.1097/00003081-199212000-00021.

37. Cato ACB, Nestl A, Mink S. Rapid actions of steroid receptors in cellular signaling pathways. Sci STKE 2002;2002(138). https://doi.org/10.1126/stke.2002.138.re9.

38. Traish AM, Botchevar E, Kim NN. Biochemical factors modulating female genital sexual arousal physiology. J Sex Med 2010;7(9). https://doi.org/10.1111/j.1743-6109.2010.01903.x.

39. Simon JA, Goldstein I, Kim NN, et al. The role of androgens in the treatment of genitourinary syndrome of menopause (gsm): international society for the study of women's sexual health (isswsh) expert consensus panel review. Menopause 2018;25(7). https://doi.org/10.1097/gme.0000000000001138.

40. Ader DN. Developing the patient-reported outcomes measurement information system (promis). Med Care 2007;45(5). https://doi.org/10.1097/01.mlr.0000260537.45076.74.

41. Zoorob D, South M, Karram M, et al. A pilot randomized trial of levator injections versus physical therapy for treatment of pelvic floor myalgia and sexual pain. Int Urogynecol J 2015;26(6). https://doi.org/10.1007/s00192-014-2606-4.

42. Anger J, Lee U, Ackerman AL, et al. Recurrent uncomplicated urinary tract infections in women: aua/cua/sufu guideline. J Urol 2019;202(2). https://doi.org/10.1097/ju.0000000000000296.

43. Farrell R. Acog committee opinion no. 659 summary: the use of vaginal estrogen in women with a history of estrogen-dependent breast cancer. Obstet Gynecol 2016;127(3). https://doi.org/10.1097/aog.0000000000001349.

44. Archer DF, Labrie F, Bouchard C, et al. Treatment of pain at sexual activity (dyspareunia) with intravaginal dehydroepiandrosterone (prasterone). Menopause 2015;22(9). https://doi.org/10.1097/gme.0000000000000428.

45. Labrie F, Archer DF, Koltun W, et al. Efficacy of intravaginal dehydroepiandrosterone (dhea) on moderate to severe dyspareunia and vaginal dryness, symptoms of vulvovaginal atrophy, and of the genitourinary syndrome of menopause. Menopause 2016;23(3). https://doi.org/10.1097/gme.0000000000000571.

46. Herbenick D, Reece M, Hensel D, et al. Association of lubricant use with women's sexual pleasure, sexual satisfaction, and genital symptoms: a prospective daily diary study. J Sex Med 2011;8(1). https://doi.org/10.1111/j.1743-6109.2010.02067.x.

47. Edwards D, Panay N. Treating vulvovaginal atrophy/genitourinary syndrome of menopause: how important is vaginal lubricant and moisturizer composition? Climacteric 2016;19(2). https://doi.org/10.3109/13697137.2015.1124259.

48. Portman DJ, Goldstein SR, Kagan R. Treatment of moderate to severe dyspareunia with intravaginal prasterone therapy: a review. Climacteric 2019;22(1). https://doi.org/10.1080/13697137.2018.1535583.

49. Di Donato V, Schiavi MC, Iacobelli V, et al. Ospemifene for the treatment of vulvar and vaginal atrophy: a meta-analysis of randomized trials. Part ii: evaluation of tolerability and safety. Maturitas 2019;121. https://doi.org/10.1016/j.maturitas.2018.11.017.

50. Faubion SS, Sood R, Kapoor E. Genitourinary syndrome of menopause: management strategies for the clinician. Mayo Clin Proc 2017. https://doi.org/10.1016/j.mayocp.2017.08.019.

51. Arunkalaivanan A, Kaur H, Onuma O. Laser therapy as a treatment modality for genitourinary syndrome of menopause: a critical appraisal of evidence. Int Urogynecol J 2017;28(5). https://doi.org/10.1007/s00192-017-3282-y.

52. Naumova I, Castelo-Branco C. Current treatment options for postmenopausal vaginal atrophy. Int J Womens Health 2018;10. https://doi.org/10.2147/ijwh.s158913.

53. Burrows LJ, Goldstein AT. The treatment of vestibulodynia with topical estradiol and testosterone. Sex Med 2013;1(1). https://doi.org/10.1002/sm2.4.

54. Goldstein I. Hormonal factors in women's sexual pain disorders. In: Female sexual pain disorders. Wiley; 2009. p. 180–94. https://doi.org/10.1002/9781444308136.ch28.

55. Flynn KE, Carter J, Lin L, et al. Assessment of vulvar discomfort with sexual activity among women in the United States. Am J Obstet Gynecol 2017;3:45–50. https://doi.org/10.1016/j.ajog.2016.12.006.

Oncology Survivorship and Sexual Wellness for Women

Mindy Goldman, MD[a,*], Mary Kathryn Abel, AB[b]

KEYWORDS

- Sexual health • Sexual dysfunction • Cancer • Survivorship
- Genitourinary syndrome of menopause • Hyposexual desire disorder

KEY POINTS

- Sexual dysfunction is common in cancer survivors due to both cancer-specific and treatment-related issues.
- The discomfort and stigma surrounding sexual dysfunction in cancer survivors should be eliminated, and sexual concerns should be discussed like any other aspect of cancer care.
- It is essential to ask about sexual concerns openly and frequently in a nondiscriminatory, culturally competent way.
- Treatment of sexual dysfunction in cancer survivors is multifaceted, and care teams should include appropriate specialists, including gynecologists, psychologists, physical therapists, and sexual health specialists.

INTRODUCTION

Sexual problems are common in the general population and may be even higher in cancer survivors.[1] Sexual dysfunction occurs when there is personal distress associated with a sexual problem. There are different types of sexual dysfunction, including problems with sexual desire, impaired arousal, inability to achieve orgasm, or pain associated with sexual activity. The types of sexual dysfunction seen in cancer survivors vary depending on the type of the cancer, the treatments of the cancer, the status of the cancer, and the physical and psychosocial well-being of the individual.

With advances in detection and treatment, cancer survivors are living longer, and the long-term effects of treatment are important to address as part of overall care. There are published guidelines from national organizations like the National Cancer Comprehensive Network (NCCN) and the American Society of Clinical Oncology (ASCO) that address various aspects of survivorship, including sexual functioning.[2,3] Each discusses the importance of regularly discussing any sexual concerns that survivors may have and offering specific treatments and referrals as indicated. The NCCN guidelines offer a user-friendly algorithm format that can guide providers through the evaluation process and specific treatment and referral recommendations (**Figs. 1–3**).[4]

This review discusses a general overview of sexual dysfunction as it pertains to women who are survivors of cancer and articulate areas in which further research is required. We devote particular attention to sexual functioning in women who are a part of a minority group, who are at the extremes of age, and/or who have metastatic disease.

How Cancer Affects Sexuality in Women

Sexual dysfunction in cancer survivors is similar in many respects to sexual dysfunction in the general population. The physical and psychological

[a] Department of Obstetrics, Gynecology, and Reproductive Sciences, University of California, San Francisco, 2356 Sutter Street, San Francisco, CA 94143, USA; [b] University of California, San Francisco School of Medicine, 2356 Sutter Street, San Francisco, CA 94143, USA
* Corresponding author.
E-mail address: mindy.goldman@ucsf.edu

Urol Clin N Am 48 (2021) 499–512
https://doi.org/10.1016/j.ucl.2021.06.008

National Comprehensive Cancer Network® NCCN NCCN Guidelines Version 2.2020
Survivorship: Hormone-Related Symptoms (Female)

NCCN Guidelines Index
Table of Contents
Discussion

MENOPAUSE SYMPTOM	TREATMENT

Vaginal dryness ⟶	• Non-hormonal treatments
	  ‣ Vaginal moisturizers, vaginal gels, oils (category 2B)
	• Lubricants for sexual activity[n]
	• Local estrogen treatment[o] (ie, rings, suppositories, creams) (category 2B)
	  ‣ Limited data in breast cancer survivors suggest minimal systemic absorption with rings and suppositories. Therefore, if estrogen-based treatment is warranted, rings and suppositories are preferred over creams for survivors of hormonally sensitive tumors.
	• Other topical hormones (ie, testosterone,[p] DHEA[o,q])
	• Consider referral to appropriate specialist for management
	• For vaginal pain or discomfort, see SSF-2

Urogenital complaints (females) ⟶	• Local estrogen treatment[o] • Referral to appropriate specialist for management

[n]Survivors should be cautioned that some lubricants may be irritating to the area of application.
[o]Vaginal estrogen and vaginal testosterone preparations can be used in managing vaginal atrophy, but safety has not been established for use in patients with or survivors of estrogen-dependent cancers.
[p]Although compounded testosterone vaginal creams are often used, there is a lack of data showing efficacy or safety in cancer survivors.
[q]DHEA should be used with caution in survivors with a history of estrogen-dependent cancers.

Note: All recommendations are category 2A unless otherwise indicated.
Clinical Trials: NCCN believes that the best management of any patient with cancer is in a clinical trial. Participation in clinical trials is especially encouraged.

SMP-5

Fig. 1. NCCN algorithm addressing management of vaginal dryness. (Referenced with permission from the NCCN Clinical Practice Guidelines in Oncology (NCCN Guidelines®) for Survivorship V.2.2020. © National Comprehensive Cancer Network, Inc. 2020. All rights reserved. Accessed [Month and Day, Year]. To view the most recent and complete version of the guideline, go online to NCCN.org.)

burden of cancer and its treatment can pose unique sexual challenges. There are also little published data on how sexual function concerns may differ between patients with local, advanced, and metastatic disease. Common sexual problems in female cancer survivors include:

- Cancer survivors treated with pelvic surgery or radiation may have vaginal or vulvar scarring that can lead to pain with touch or penetration as well as difficulty with lubrication.
- Women treated with chemotherapy may experience neuropathy that influences genital sensitivity and impairs arousal.
- Surgical-, radiation-, and chemotherapy-induced disruption of ovarian function may result in menopause, thereby leading to vaginal dryness, sexual pain, and decreased desire.
- Cancer surgeries (eg, mastectomy, gynecologic organ resection, ostomy creation) alter the body, potentially leading to changes in body image, well-being, and sense of sexual identity.
- Stem cell transplants may cause graft-versus-host disease, leading to scarring, stenosis, sexual pain, and decreased arousal or desire.
- Cancer treatments or cancer itself may cause pain, which can make any activity (including sex) difficult or impossible
- Cancer-related stress, anxiety, and depression can affect well-being and overall interest in sex.

Assessment of Sexual Concerns

All cancer survivors should be asked about distress as it relates to their sexual functioning at regular intervals during their follow-up care. Open-ended, nonjudgmental questions such as "Do you have any sexual concerns?" should be used when possible. If patients perceive that their providers are uncomfortable talking about sex, they are less likely to discuss sexual concerns.[5,6]

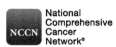

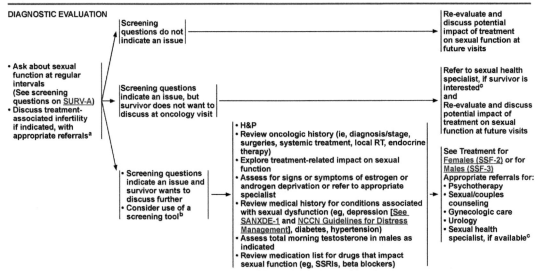

Fig. 2. NCCN sexual functioning guidelines regarding diagnostic evaluation. (Referenced with permission from the NCCN Clinical Practice Guidelines in Oncology (NCCN Guidelines®) for Survivorship V.2.2020. © National Comprehensive Cancer Network, Inc. 2020. All rights reserved. Accessed [Month and Day, Year]. To view the most recent and complete version of the guideline, go online to NCCN.org.)

Providers should prioritize sexual concerns as they would any other medical concern related to cancer and its treatment (eg, pain, fatigue, and hair loss).

For some patients and providers, validated assessment scales may help to "break the ice" and facilitate conversations about sexual wellness. Some common tools that may be useful for screening sexual concerns include:

- Brief Symptom Checklist[7]
- Arizona Sexual Experience Scale[8]
- Female Sexual Functioning Index (FSFI), including a breast-specific adaptation of the FSFI[9]
- PROMIS Sexual Function and Satisfaction Measure (SexFs)[10]

The FSFI has been validated in cancer survivors but requires users to have been sexually active in the last 4 weeks.[11] The PROMIS measure was specifically developed in cancer survivors, and Version 2.0 has been expanded in this population

and may be a better tool because it has a broader assessment of overall sexual function and satisfaction. Providers should decide who in the practice will do the screen and what specific screening tool they will use. These tools should be easily accessible during patient visits. If there are concerning responses from a specific tool or from answers to open-ended questions, then a comprehensive evaluation should be performed to address factors that could be affecting sexual functioning. However, no scale can take the place of a sensitive and thorough inquiry and evaluation by a trained provider.

Relevant factors to assess when evaluating for sexual dysfunction

- Past medical and psychological history, particularly any history of trauma or interpersonal violence
- Gynecologic history with a review of prior problems or surgeries

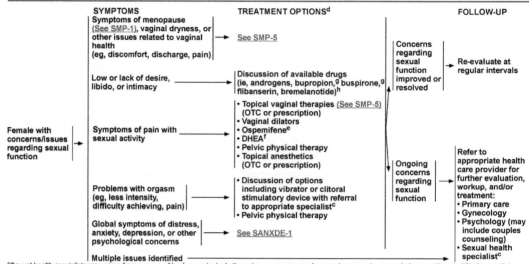

Fig. 3. NCCN sexual functioning guidelines regarding symptoms, treatment options, and follow-up. (Referenced with permission from the NCCN Clinical Practice Guidelines in Oncology (NCCN Guidelines®) for Survivorship V.2.2020. © National Comprehensive Cancer Network, Inc. 2020. All rights reserved. Accessed [Month and Day, Year]. To view the most recent and complete version of the guideline, go online to NCCN.org.)

- Psychological status
- Current medications
- Current side effects from cancer treatments
- Habits such as smoking, alcohol, or any illicit drug use
- Relationship issues, including assessment of partner and any issues affecting partner's sexual function
- Physical examination, with a focus on how the specific cancer could be affecting sexual health
- Gynecologic examination and selected laboratory test results if indicated

An important part of this assessment is addressing both prescriptions and over-the-counter (OTC) medications that could be contributing to sexual dysfunction. In particular, selective serotonin reuptake inhibitors (SSRIs), which are commonly used in cancer survivors, can have effects on arousal and ability to climax.[12] Narcotic, drug, and alcohol use should be assessed, as well as mood and anxiety disorders, because all can affect sexual functioning. If providers have concerns about one or more of these factors, they should have appropriate referrals available; these may include referrals to psychology, gynecology, primary care, physical therapy, and sexual health specialists.

An important part of assessment includes a discussion regarding contraception (when indicated) as well as fertility desires or concerns. Unplanned pregnancy rates are approximately 3 times higher in cancer survivors compared with the general population.[13] For patients concerned with future fertility, referrals should be made to specialists who can make plans for preserving the ability to have children in the future. ASCO has published guidelines regarding fertility preservation in cancer survivors.[14]

Assessment of sexual concerns is an iterative process. The topic of sexual function should be raised at each visit, because sexual issues often become more concerning to patients as time passes since their initial treatments.

Treatment of Sexual Dysfunction

Sexual dysfunction in cancer survivors is multifactorial, and treatments should be broad to encompass the many factors that could be contributing to the type of dysfunction. In general, there is limited high-quality evidence for specific types of treatments in cancer survivors. Treatment recommendations should be based on what is known in the general population, taking into account treatment- and disease-induced effects that may make certain therapies inadvisable (eg, hormone therapy in patients with hormone-sensitive malignancies).

Genitourinary syndrome of menopause

Chemotherapy, radiation, or other treatment-induced menopause can lead to vaginal dryness, resulting in pain with touch or penetration. The term *genitourinary syndrome of menopause* (GSM) was coined in 2014 as the condition used to describe the effects of hypoestrogenism on the vagina, vulva, and urinary tract.[15] This broad condition describes the symptoms of vaginal and vulvar dryness, burning, irritation, lack of lubrication, dyspareunia, urinary urgency, frequency, dysuria, and frequent urinary tract infections (UTIs). Severe GSM symptoms are commonly seen in breast cancer survivors who are taking aromatase inhibitors due to suppression of all peripheral estrogen production.[16]

Specific treatment options to address GSM include OTC topical agents and vaginal hormonal therapies, including vaginal estrogens, the selective estrogen receptor modulator (SERM) ospemifene, vaginal dehydroepiandrosterone (DHEA), and vaginal testosterone. There are reviews and published guidelines from national organizations including North American Menopause Society, the International Society for the Study of Women's Sexual Health, and the NCCN that discuss specific recommendations (see **Fig. 1**).[17–19] All expert groups recommend OTC topical agents as first-line therapy. These agents include lubricants for sexual activity, vaginal moisturizers, pH-balanced gels, topical oils, and topical anesthetics for introital pain. Lubricants are meant to be used to decrease friction associated with sexual activity, whereas products such as moisturizers retain water and are recommended to be used more regularly to provide longer-term relief from dryness not necessarily related to sexual activity. Oils penetrate thin tissue and can be particularly helpful for vulvar thinning and discomfort. Although there are limited studies that suggest a specific moisturizer called Replens may provide similar relief to vaginal estrogen, most of these products have relatively limited data.[20,21] Most of these products provide relief but require long-term administration.

Vaginal estrogens are thought to more effectively treat GSM by improving blood supply, tone, and lubrication; normalizing the vaginal pH; and helping prevent UTIs. Formulations include creams, rings, and suppositories, and all have been found to be equally efficacious.[22] For women without hormone-dependent cancer, any formulation can be used, and choices should be based on patient preference, convenience, and cost. Although there are some historical concerns about the safety of vaginal estrogens in patients with hormone-dependent cancers, vaginal estrogen is not thought to increase the risk of breast cancer recurrence.[23] Limited data in breast cancer survivors suggest that the ring and suppository formulations have minimal systemic absorption and generally should be used if vaginal estrogen therapy is being prescribed.[24–26] This is particularly important for those survivors on aromatase inhibitors, because these drugs function to suppress all estrogen production. It is crucial not to use any vaginal formulations that would lead to an increase in systemic estrogen levels. The typical dose of estrogen creams that are used in the vagina may potentially cause an increase in systemic estradiol and should be avoided in women with hormone-dependent cancers. However, focal amounts applied directly to areas of vulvar discomfort should not cause similar increases in estradiol. The formulations and recommended doses of vaginal estrogens are given in **Table 1**.

Some survivors choose to obtain vaginal estrogens from compounding pharmacies. There can be some confusion between these formulations and what are known as "bioidentical hormones." Bioidentical hormones are molecularly similar to those produced by the body and include US Food and Drug Administration (FDA)-regulated forms of hormones like estradiol. Compounded formulations, on the other hand, may include bioidentical hormones as well as other hormones in nonstandard preparations and dosages. The safety and efficacy of these formulations is less clear due to the lack of regulation by the FDA. Although there may be transient increases in serum estradiol with the initial use of vaginal hormonal therapies, there is no evidence that routine serum estradiol level assessment is required in cancer survivors using these therapies.[27]

DHEA (trade name Prasterone) is a precursor to androgens. DHEA as a vaginal insert is approved by the FDA as a treatment of dyspareunia associated with GSM. Although there are no safety or efficacy data comparing DHEA directly with vaginal

Table 1
Estrogen formulations

Formulation	Brand Name	Dosing
Estradiol insert	Vagifem	10 μg nightly for 2 wk,[a] followed by twice per week
	Imvexxy	4 and 10 μg nightly for 2 wk,[a] then twice per week
Estradiol vaginal ring	Estring	2 mg estradiol every 3 mo
Estradiol cream	Estrace	0.01%–1 g nightly for 2 wk followed by three times per week
Conjugated equine estrogen cream	Premarin	0.625 CE/g–1g nightly for 2 wk followed by 3 times per week

[a] For patients with hormone-positive breast cancer, consider avoiding loading dose of estradiol inserts and start with twice-weekly dosing.

estrogens in patients (including cancer survivors), it is not thought to lead to increases in systemic levels of either estrogens or androgens. This fact makes DHEA of particular interest for survivors of hormone-dependent cancers, including breast cancer survivors on aromatase inhibitors. A recent trial of vaginal DHEA in women with hormone receptor-positive breast cancer and endometrial cancer showed serum levels of estrogens and androgens in the postmenopausal range, including those who were on aromatase inhibitors.[28] There was a dose-dependent small increase in total testosterone levels. The significance of this finding is unknown, and as such vaginal DHEA should be considered investigational rather than a current standard of care in survivors of hormone-dependent cancers.

Although testosterone is not approved by the FDA for use in women, vaginal testosterone may be compounded as a cream for off-label use in GSM, because the vagina is rich in androgen receptors. There are little data about the use of testosterone in female cancer survivors and some concerns about the safety for women with hormone-sensitive breast cancer because of the possibility of testosterone in serum being aromatized to estrogen.[26] Vaginal testosterone should be used only with caution and a full discussion of potential risks in survivors of hormone-dependent cancers.

The oral SERM ospemifene is another FDA-approved treatment of GSM. Ospemifene may be preferred by patients who cannot or choose not to use vaginal therapy. This drug is associated with systemic side effects, including hot flashes, and can increase the risk of blood clots.[29] Although the drug is not thought to have estrogenic effects on the breast, its safety has not been established for breast cancer survivors.

Given concerns of estrogenlike activity in the uterus ospemifene should not at this time be used for survivors of hormone-dependent cancers.

Given the lack of safety and efficacy data regarding the use of vaginal hormonal therapy for those with hormone-sensitive breast cancer or high-risk endometrial cancers, there is growing interest in nondrug options, including vaginal lasers or other energy devices. Although the mechanisms are different for these nonablative lasers and radiofrequency devices, all cause microtrauma to the tissue and result in the formation of new blood supply and connective tissue, thereby causing vaginal remodeling. There are small trials of the fractional CO_2 laser device in breast cancer survivors that suggest efficacy without significant adverse effects.[30] None of these devices are approved by the FDA and are associated with significant out-of-pocket costs. Although there are many small published trials with varying end points reporting success in noncancer populations, the FDA issued a warning statement in 2018 regarding the potential for burns.[31] Expert groups like the NCCN state that larger trials are needed before recommending the use of these devices in cancer survivors. Readers who are interested in more information about these therapies should refer to the Alexandra Siegal and Barbara M. Chubak's article, "Pharmaceutical and Energy-Based Management of Sexual Problems in Women," in this issue.

An important part of GSM treatment also includes referral to qualified therapists for cognitive behavioral therapy (CBT) and sexual therapy when indicated. Although these forms of therapy are not used solely for GSM, discomfort associated with GSM can lead to avoidance of sexual activity and associated personal distress. Sex therapy, CBT, and/or couples counseling may be used in conjunction with other therapies to help women overcome any of these negative thoughts.

Cancer and sexual pain

Sexual pain in cancer survivors is common. In a cross-sectional survey of 109 patients with gynecologic cancer and 109 patients with breast cancer, 39% (n = 84) reported vaginal pain.[32] Sexual pain may be both a sexual disorder and a pain disorder. Cancer pain may be acute or chronic, related to either the treatments or diagnostic testing for the cancer, as well as a direct result of the cancer itself. There are several cancer pain syndromes, and each of these can affect sexual functioning. Neuropathic pain is often associated with decreased sensation. Pain from tumors may make certain sexual positions uncomfortable. Sexual pain can also be caused by cancer surgeries and radiation. Gynecologic or anal cancer surgeries may lead to genital scarring. Pelvic radiation can lead to vaginal mucositis, ulceration, and stenosis. GSM can also cause vaginal and vulvar pain. The myriad risks that patients with cancer face makes development of both generalized and sex-specific pain very common.

When assessing pain, it is important for the symptoms to be clarified and the underlying source to be identified so that treatments can be tailored.[33] It is essential to assess whether pain was present before cancer. Eliciting whether pain is associated with touching of the genitals or with penetration or whether there is anxiety associated with anticipated sexual activity is important for treatment recommendations. Treatments should be multifactorial, and setting realistic goals is important. General and neuropathic pain should be addressed to improve comfort, function, and general quality of life. Any issues related to GSM should be addressed as well. The medications ospemifene and Prasterone are specifically approved by the FDA for dyspareunia. A small trial of ospemifene in cervical cancer survivors showed improvement in overall sexual enjoyment, and a randomized controlled trial in 464 survivors with breast and gynecologic cancers showed that vaginal DHEA improved sexual pain.[28] Given these beneficial results, this drug may be a useful option in women with hormone-dependent cancers once additional safety data are available.

Topical anesthetics can be useful for introital pain and are recommended to be applied 10 to 15 minutes before planned penetrative sex. Lidocaine can be obtained OTC or as a prescription, and formulations range from a 2% to 5% concentration. A small trial in breast cancer survivors showed that the use of topical lidocaine improved symptoms of dyspareunia.[34]

For survivors with pelvic floor dysfunction, pelvic floor physical therapy (PFPT) can be helpful. It is crucial to refer to physical therapists who are experienced in myofascial release and pelvic floor rehabilitation. A small trial in gynecologic cancer survivors showed improved sexual functioning with PFPT, and another trial showed success with PFPT and vaginal dilators.[35,36] Vaginal dilators can be used for postradiation stenosis to help regain vaginal length, capacity, and flexibility by allowing for gentle stretching of the tissue. Moreover, use of vaginal dilators can help women determine what type of penetration does and does not hurt in nonsexual setting without the presence of a partner.

An often underutilized treatment is sex therapy, which is a specialized form of psychotherapy focused on sexual functioning. This subspecialty takes into account the impact of cancer treatment on the functional, psychological, and relationship aspects of the cancer experience. Treatments often include counseling, education, communication skills training, and specific sensate-focused exercises that can improve intimacy and connection. The American Association of Sexuality Educators, Counselors and Therapists (aasect.org) and the Society for Sexuality Therapy and Research (sstarnet.org) provide information on certified sex therapists.[37] As cancer survivors can benefit from a multimodal approach to their sexual wellness, a qualified sex therapist should be part of the treatment team if available.

Integrative therapies such as yoga, meditation, and mindfulness may have some benefits on improving sexual functioning, partly by improving pain and overall well-being.[38]

Hypoactive sexual desire disorder

Hypoactive sexual desire disorder (HSDD) is the most common form of female sexual dysfunction, including in cancer survivors. Sexual desire is thought to be regulated by key regions within the brain through the action of specific neurotransmitters. The drugs used to treat HSDD are shown in **Table 2**. Two drugs are currently approved by the FDA for HSDD in premenopausal women. Flibanserin (Addyi) is a novel nonhormonal, multifunctional serotonin agonist antagonist that acts in the central nervous system to increase dopamine and norepinephrine (both responsible for sexual excitement) while decreasing serotonin (responsible for sexual satiety and inhibition). It is taken as a daily oral pill. A meta-analysis in noncancer populations showed modest improvements in sexual desire and an increase of one additional sexual satisfying event per month. Adverse events are primarily dizziness, somnolence, and hypotension.[39] Low libido is a common menopausal complaint, and the SNOWDROP trial showed improvements in sexual functioning for postmenopausal women using flibanserin versus placebo.[40] Despite these data, the drug is not approved by the FDA for postmenopausal women and must be used off-label in this population. Although there are no published trials of flibanserin in cancer survivors, it is reasonable to consider using it in those who have low desire given its mechanism of action.

Bremelanotide (Vyleesi) was approved by the FDA in 2019 to treat HSDD in premenopausal women. Bremelanotide is a peptide agonist of the melanocortin receptors and acts centrally in the brain to reduce inhibition and increase excitation. This drug comes in a push pen injectable form that is injected into the abdomen or thigh at least 45 minutes before anticipated sexual activity. Bremelanotide was found to improve desire and satisfaction compared with placebo after 24 weeks in 2 randomized controlled trials in noncancer populations. Despite the high frequency of adverse events like nausea and vomiting, headache, flushing, and transient increases in blood pressure, there was low discontinuation of the medication. However, it should not be used in patients with uncontrolled hypertension and/or known cardiovascular disease.[41] There are no published trials studying bremelanotide in cancer survivors, but this drug may be an option for premenopausal women with HSDD or for off-label use in postmenopausal women. At present, both flibanserin and bremelanotide can only be obtained from specialized pharmacies.

Although testosterone is not FDA approved for use in women, there is evidence to support androgen supplementation in select women with low biochemical androgen levels and symptoms possibly attributable to low androgen levels.[42,43] There are limited data on both safety and efficacy in the general menopausal population and in cancer survivors.[44–46] Common formulations include a 1% compounded cream, gel, or ointment, with limitations in purity and quality due to a lack of oversight in compounded formulations. Other ways of prescribing include small doses of male preparations with the goal of approximating hormone concentrations of premenopausal women, which are about 10% of male levels. Lipids and liver function should be monitored when using androgen therapies. Owing to limited data, testosterone should be used with caution, particularly for those with hormone-dependent cancers.

Small trials in noncancer populations have shown mild benefits in sexual desire with the antidepressant bupropion and the anxiolytic buspirone.[47] However, data on buspirone are limited to posthoc analysis only. There are no specific contraindications for the use of these medications in cancer survivors, but the FDA-approved medications flibanserin and bremelanotide have more robust data and should be considered first-line agents of choice for appropriately selected patients.

Sildenafil citrate (Viagra) is a phosphodiesterase (PDE-5) inhibitor that is very effective in treating male erectile dysfunction. Sildenafil citrate has not been approved by the FDA for any use in women, and studies looking at the use of sildenafil in women have shown conflicting results. The primary benefit of sildenafil has been seen in women with sexual dysfunction due to SSRI use and possibly in those with specific impairment of genital arousal responses.[48–50] Cancer survivors with HSDD who need SSRIs to control depression or anxiety may experience some enhancement of genital response (not necessarily subjective arousal or satisfaction) with sildenafil citrate off-label use (**Table 2**).

Impaired arousal

Historically, "sexual arousal" may refer to both subjective/cognitive arousal and genital arousal. With arousal disorders, there is a lack of response to sexual stimulation. There is little information published evaluating impaired arousal in cancer survivors specifically. Often, it is difficult to distinguish between low desire and impaired arousal. The term female sexual interest/arousal disorder was adopted by the recent *Diagnostic and Statistical Manual of Mental Disorders* (Fifth Edition).[51] The decision to combine issues of desire and arousal has not been universally accepted; the International Society for the Study of Women's Sexual Health recently proposed a classification system that distinguished HSDD from female genital arousal disorders, a specific form of arousal disorder specific to genital sexual responses in women.[52]

Similar to other types of sexual dysfunction, impairment of arousal is often multifactorial, and the treatments should be based on what is known in the general population and considerations for disease and treatment-related effects. Any modifiable factors relating to impaired arousal such as GSM or sexual pain should be treated. Covariables should be addressed as well, including treatment of sleep issues, vasomotor symptoms, mood and anxiety disorders, and relationship concerns. The drugs previously discussed that work on either

Table 2
Medications to treat HSDD

Formulation	Brand Name	Dosing
Flibanserin: multifunctional serotonin agonist antagonist	Addyi	100 mg at bedtime
Bremelanotide: peptide agonist of the melanocortin receptors	Vyleesi	1.75 mg subcutaneous injection 45 min before planned sexual activity
Testosterone: androgen		1% compounded formulation or 10% of standard male dosage
Bupropion: antidepressant	Wellbutrin	150–300 mg daily
Buspirone: anxiolytic	Buspar	15–60 mg daily
Sildenafil citrate: PDE-5 inhibitor	Viagra	50–100 mg 1–2 h before sexual activity

arousal or genital responses may be of benefit in women with specific problems attaining genital arousal.

Inability to achieve orgasm

Inability to achieve orgasm is defined by a marked delay in, frequency of, or absence of orgasm or markedly decreased intensity of orgasm sensation following sexual arousal and adequate sexual stimulation.[52] Orgasmic disorders can be lifelong or acquired and may occur in all or select situations.[51] There is limited literature on this type of sexual dysfunction in cancer survivors, and treatment should be the same as in noncancer populations. Options include education; exercises to increase comfort with sexual intimacy; sensate focus exercises; directed masturbation with or without sexual enhancement devices (eg, vibrators, clitoral stimulators); psychosocial interventions, such as cognitive behavioral sex therapy; and anxiety reduction exercises/techniques. Clinical trials of efficacy of many of these treatments are limited. Sildenafil may have a small benefit in women using SSRIs based on a small, randomized study, but evidence remains limited.[48] It is important to set realistic and clear goals, and referral to a sexual therapist should be offered.

Herbal products and sexual dysfunction

Many cancer survivors may choose to use herbal therapies for treatment of sexual dysfunction. However, there are no definitive data regarding the use of these therapies in patients with cancer, and there may be components of these products that could cause adverse effects. Herbal supplements are only loosely regulated, and quality control is variable. As such, herbal products and supplements cannot be recommended for treatment of sexual concerns.

Sexual Health in Minority Populations

An exceedingly important but often overlooked area of care in oncology survivorship literature (including that pertaining to sexuality) is the sexual wellness in gender, sexual, racial, and/or ethnic minority people.

Sexual and gender minority patients

Literature regarding sexual health in cancer survivors who identify as sexual and gender minority (SGM) is limited, in part because large, national cancer registries do not ask about sexual and gender identity. This fact limits robust research and improved understanding of the unique needs of SGM cancer survivors.[53] There is evidence that SGM individuals may be at an elevated risk of certain cancers like breast and cervical cancers, partly due to lower rates of screening and other barriers to care.[53,54] However, the NCCN guidelines do not address the clinical management considerations for these patients, and only 1.8% of SGM-focused research from the National Institutes of Health (NIH) is directed toward cancer.[55,56] This lack of research is concerning, because SGM cancer survivors often report lower satisfaction with their overall care than heterosexual cis-gender cancer survivors, even after controlling for important demographic and clinical characteristics.[57]

The handful of studies about sexual health in SGM patients focuses on comparing perspectives between lesbian, bisexual, and heterosexual women. Two studies have found no differences in engagement in sexual activity, sexual satisfaction, or initiation of sexual activity before and following breast cancer diagnosis.[58,59] However, concerns have been raised about comparing sexual functioning in SGM and heterosexual, cisgender women with cancer given differences in sexual expression. A more appropriate comparison may be evaluating sexual functioning in SGM women with and without cancer.[60,61] For example, a case-control study comparing sexual minority breast cancer survivors and sexual minority individuals without cancer found that although the 2 groups did not differ in the overall level of sexual functioning, cancer survivors had lower sexual frequency, desire, and ability to orgasm and higher pain scores compared with noncancer survivors.[61] To our knowledge, there are no studies that address sexual health following cancer diagnosis or treatment in transgender or intersex individuals.

At present, there are limited resources available that address cancer survivorship issues in SGM populations.[62] Ultimately, to promote better understanding and research about sexual health in SGM populations for both patients and providers, national organizations like NCCN and ASCO will need to explicitly address these issues and devote resources to this research. However, until there are specific published guidelines on management, the recommendations discussed in this review should be applied to these patients in a nondiscriminatory, culturally competent way.

Racial and ethnic minority patients

Similar to the SGM literature, there is limited research about sexual functioning in racial and ethnic minority individuals with cancer. Gynecologic and breast cancer survivors identifying as racial and ethnic minorities seem to have similar desire to address sexual issues as an aspect of survivorship.[63] Whether racial/ethnic minorities are more likely to experience sexual concern after cancer treatment remains unclear. One study found that individuals with gynecologic cancers who self-reported as black or Hispanic were more likely to report sexual dysfunction (based on FSFI score) compared with white individuals.[64] However, another study reported no differences in the Sexual Quality of Life scores by race among breast cancer survivors.[65] It is vital that research continues to explore the impact of race on sexual functioning in patients with cancer.

Sexual Health in Young and Older Populations with Cancer

Although cancers diagnosed in adolescents and young adults (AYA) between the ages 15 and 39 years only represent 5% of all cancer diagnoses in the United States, evidence suggests that many AYA patients will present with sexual dysfunction due to their diagnosis and/or treatment.[66] Compared with AYA men diagnosed with cancer, AYA women may be more likely to report sexual dysfunction.[67] In a systematic review, issues regarding sexual desire in AYA women diagnosed with cancer were the most common; as such, providers should ask about this regularly.[68]

Limited evidence suggests that AYA women with cancer are more likely to experience and report sexual dysfunction compared with older women with cancer. In a pivotal study, young survivors of cancer were found to report poorer sexual function compared with older survivors, with nearly half of young patients reporting decreased sexual functioning, arousal, lubrication, orgasm, and frequency of sexual activity.[69] Moreover, young women with cancer may be more interested in receiving care to address sexual issues and more willing to be contacted for a formal program about sexual health and cancer compared with older women.[63]

The reasons for these differences are not well understood. Abrupt onset of treatment-induced menopause and the accompanying symptoms like hot flashes and vaginal dryness may account for the greater number of problems experienced by AYA patients with cancer.[69] Moreover, body image issues have been found to be higher in younger patients as well, which may also impact sexual functioning.[70] Providers should treat menopausal symptoms and provide support and appropriate referrals for any body image changes for AYA cancer survivors.

Importantly, despite the fact that sexual dysfunction is more common in AYA cancer survivors, it is well established that older women also desire sexual intimacy and struggle with sexual dysfunction.[71] In fact, one study found that 1 in 5 patients with cancer older than 65 years were still interested in receiving information about sexual health.[63] These findings highlight that sexual health issues should be addressed in all women with cancer, regardless of age.

Sexual Health in Metastatic Disease

Sexual health and functioning in the setting of cancer has largely focused on patients with early-stage disease and not in those with metastatic disease or individuals receiving palliative care. There is a misconception that survivorship issues like sexual health only apply to those who are likely to have long life expectancies.[72] However, patients with metastatic cancer desire sexual intimacy and may have concerns about sexual functioning. Sexual health issues should be addressed regardless of cancer stage or life expectancy.[73,74]

Across the limited existing literature, sexuality has been described as vitally important by individuals with advanced cancers. However, interactions with the health care team about sexuality in end-of-life care appear to be minimal and suboptimal. A qualitative study of 10 patients with a variety of advanced cancers receiving palliative care found that only one patient was asked about sexuality in the context of their clinical care despite all subjects indicating that these topics should have been discussed.[75] Others found barriers to expressing sexuality in the palliative care units or hospice centers because of shared rooms, regular staff intrusions, and a lack of privacy.[75]

It is also important to appreciate that the definition of sexuality may differ by person.[72,75] For example, some individuals may prioritize physical sexual activity, whereas others may feel that intimate emotional connection is a more important component of sexuality that takes precedence over physical sexual acts.[75,76] Providers may not appreciate that emotional connection to a partner may be more important than the physical act of sex in women with metastatic disease; in fact, one study found that women who raised concerns about their sexual health were commonly offered vaginal lubricants that did not fully address their concerns.[72]

Patients with metastatic disease often choose to address sexual health concerns with their nonprimary oncology providers (eg, with home care nurses) because they have established strong relationships with these individuals.[77] Oncology providers should ask open-ended questions to patients with metastatic disease about how they express their sexuality, and treatments and strategies should be targeted to their specific expression.

There are few centers in the United States that are devoted specifically to sexual dysfunction in general and even fewer for those with cancer-related sexual dysfunction. As cancer survivorship programs evolve and survivorship issues become a standard part of overall cancer care, sexual wellness should be a routine part of this care.

CLINICS CARE POINTS

- Sexual dysfunction is common in female cancer survivors. Although there may be limited trials addressing evaluation and treatment of sexual dysfunction in specific cancer populations, this lack of research should not imply that sexual functioning is not an essential part of oncologic care.

- Cancer survivors are less likely to bring up the topic of sexual dysfunction if they sense discomfort on the part of the oncology provider. Sexual dysfunction should be discussed in the same way as any other side effect of cancer treatment.

- The types of sexual dysfunction in cancer survivors are similar to the general population, but the causes are often broader and include both direct cancer effects and effects related to treatment. As such, clinical evaluation and treatment need to consider this nuance.

- Treatments should include the same options as those in the general population but should be considered in the context of specific cancer treatments and their potential effects on sexual dysfunction. The risks and benefits of hormonal therapies need to be discussed for survivors with hormone dependent cancers.

SUMMARY

Sexual dysfunction is common in cancer survivors. Open-ended questions about sexual functioning should be asked about regularly. Conversations about sexual health should be normalized, and any stigma should be addressed. Providers should treat any issues that may be related to sexual dysfunction, including menopausal symptoms, stress, fatigue, mood or relationship issues, pain, lymphedema, and sleep dysfunction. As with other aspects of survivorship, patients should be encouraged to engage in regular exercise and maintain a healthy diet. Treatments of sexual dysfunction in cancer survivors should be multidimensional and include psychologists, gynecologists, sex therapists, and pelvic floor physical therapists who are knowledgeable about sexual issues in cancer survivors.

DISCLOSURE

Neither author reports any commercial or financial conflicts of interest or any funding sources.

REFERENCES

1. Maiorino MI, Chiodini P, Bellastella G, et al. Sexual dysfunction in women with cancer: a systematic review with meta-analysis of studies using the female sexual function index. Endocrine 2016;54(2):329–41.

2. Sanft T, Denlinger CS, Armenian S, et al. NCCN guidelines insights: survivorship, version 2.2019. J Natl Compr Cancer Netw 2019;17(7):784–94.

3. American Society of Clinical Oncology. Cancer care initiatives. Available at: https://www.asco.org/practice-policy/cancer-care-initiatives/prevention-survivorship/survivorship-compendium-0. Accessed January 18, 2021.

4. Referenced with permission from the NCCN clinical practice guidelines in oncology (NCCN Guidelines®) for survivorship V.2.2020. National Comprehensive Cancer Network, Inc; 2020. All rights reserved. Accessed January 31, 2021.

5. Flynn KE, Reese JB, Jeffery DD, et al. Patient experiences with communication about sex during and after treatment for cancer. Psychooncology 2012; 21(6):594–601.

6. Reese JB, Sorice K, Lepore SJ, et al. Patient-clinician communication about sexual health in breast cancer: a mixed-methods analysis of clinic dialogue. Patient Educ Couns 2019;102(3):436.

7. Hatzichristou D, Rosen RC, Derogatis LR, et al. Recommendations for the clinical evaluation of men and women with sexual dysfunction. J Sex Med 2010;7: 337–48.

8. McGahuey CA, Gelenberg AJ, Laukes CA, et al. The arizona sexual experience scale (Asex): reliability and validity. J Sex Marital Ther 2000;26(1):25–40.

9. Rosen R, Brown C, Heiman J, et al. The female sexual function index (FSFI): a multidimensional self-report instrument for the assessment of female sexual function. J Sex Marital Ther 2000;26(2):191–208.

10. PROMIS sexual function and satisfaction manual. Available at: http://www.healthmeasures.net/images/PROMIS/manuals/PROMIS_Sexual_Function_and_Satisfaction_Measures_User_Manual_v1.0_and_v2.0.pdf. Accessed January 31, 2021.

11. Baser RE, Li Y, Carter J. Psychometric validation of the female sexual function index (FSFI) in cancer survivors. Cancer 2012;118(18):4606–18.

12. Lorenz T, Rullo J, Faubion S. Antidepressant-induced female sexual dysfunction. Mayo Clin Proc 2016;91(9):1280–6.

13. Quinn MM, Letourneau JM, Rosen MP. Contraception after cancer treatment: describing methods, counseling, and unintended pregnancy risk. Contraception 2014;89(5):466–71.

14. Oktay K, Harvey BE, Partridge AH, et al. Fertility preservation in patients with cancer: ASCO clinical practice guideline update. J Clin Oncol 2018; 36(19):1994–2001.

15. Portman D, Gass M. Vulvovaginal Atrophy Terminology Consensus Conference Panel. Genitourinary syndrome of menopause: new terminology for vulvovaginal atrophy from the International Society for the Study of Women's Sexual Health and the North American Menopause Society. Maturitas 2014; 79(3):349–54.

16. Morales MM, Olsen J, Johansen P, et al. Viral infection, atopy and mycosis fungoides: a European multicentre case-control study. Eur J Cancer 2003. https://doi.org/10.1016/S0959-8049(02)00773-6.

17. Crean-Tate KK, Faubion SS, Pederson HJ, et al. Management of genitourinary syndrome of menopause in female cancer patients: a focus on vaginal hormonal therapy. Am J Obstet Gynecol 2020; 222(2):103–13.

18. Faubion SS, Larkin LC, Stuenkel CA, et al. Management of genitourinary syndrome of menopause in women with or at high risk for breast cancer: consensus recommendations from the North American Menopause Society and the International Society for the Study of Women's Sexual Health. Menopause 2018;25(6):596–608.

19. Denlinger CS, Sanft T, Baker KS, et al. Survivorship, Version 2.2017: clinical practice guidelines in oncology. J Natl Compr Cancer Netw 2017;15(9):1140–63.

20. Bygdeman M, Swahn ML. Replens versus dienoestrol cream in the symptomatic treatment of vaginal atrophy in postmenopausal women. Maturitas 1996;23(3):259–63.

21. Nachtigall LE. Comparative study: Replens versus local estrogen in menopausal women. Fertil Steril 1994;61(1):178–80.

22. The 2020 genitourinary syndrome of menopause position statement of The North American Menopause Society. Menopause 2020;27(9):976–92.

23. Le Ray I, Dell'Aniello S, Bonnetain F, et al. Local estrogen therapy and risk of breast cancer recurrence among hormone-treated patients: a nested case-control study. Breast Cancer Res Treat 2012; 135(2):603–9.

24. American College of Obstetricians and Gynecologists. Committee opinion number 659: the use of vaginal estrogen in women with a history of estrogen-dependent breast cancer. Obstet Gynecol 2016;127(3):618–9.

25. Wills S, Ravipati A, Venuturumilli P, et al. Effects of vaginal estrogens on serum estradiol levels in postmenopausal breast cancer survivors and women at risk of breast cancer taking an aromatase inhibitor or a selective estrogen receptor modulator. J Oncol Pract 2012;8(3):144–8.

26. Melisko ME, Goldman ME, Hwang J, et al. Vaginal testosterone cream vs estradiol vaginal ring for vaginal dryness or decreased libido in women receiving aromatase inhibitors for early-stage breast cancer a randomized clinical trial. JAMA Oncol 2017;3:313–9.

27. Santen RJ. Vaginal administration of estradiol: effects of dose, preparation and timing on plasma estradiol levels. Climacteric 2015;18(2):121–34.

28. Barton DL, Shuster LT, Dockter T, et al. Systemic and local effects of vaginal dehydroepiandrosterone (DHEA): NCCTG N10C1 (Alliance). Support Care Cancer 2018;26(4):1335–43.

29. Simon JA, Altomare C, Cort S, et al. Overall safety of ospemifene in postmenopausal women from placebo-controlled phase 2 and 3 trials. J Womens Health (Larchmt) 2018;27(1):14–23.

30. Knight C, Logan V, Fenlon D. A systematic review of laser therapy for vulvovaginal atrophy/genitourinary

syndrome of menopause in breast cancer survivors. Ecancermedicalscience 2019;13:988.

31. U.S. Food and Drug Administration. Statement from FDA Commissioner Scott Gottlieb, M.D., on efforts to safeguard women's health from deceptive health claims and significant risks related to devices marketed for use in medical procedures for "vaginal rejuvenation." Silver Spring (MD): FDA; 2018. Available at: https://www.fda.gov/news-events/press-announcements/statement-fda-commissioner-scott-gottlieb-md-efforts-safeguard-womens-health-deceptive-health-claims.

32. Stabile C, Goldfarb S, Baser RE, et al. Sexual health needs and educational intervention preferences for women with cancer. Breast Cancer Res Treat 2017; 165(1):77–84.

33. Coady D, Kennedy V. Sexual health in women affected by cancer. Obstet Gynecol 2016;128(4): 775–91.

34. Goetsch MF, Lim JY, Caughey AB. A practical solution for dyspareunia in breast cancer survivors: a randomized controlled trial. J Clin Oncol 2015; 33(30):3394–400.

35. Yang EJ, Lim JY, Rah UW, et al. Effect of a pelvic floor muscle training program on gynecologic cancer survivors with pelvic floor dysfunction: a randomized controlled trial. Gynecol Oncol 2012;125(3): 705–11.

36. Carter J, Stabile C, Seidel B, et al. Vaginal and sexual health treatment strategies within a female sexual medicine program for cancer patients and survivors. J Cancer Surviv 2017;11(2):274–83.

37. American Association of Sexuality Educators. Counselors and Therapists. Available at: https://www.aasect.org/. Accessed January 18, 2021.

38. Brotto LA, Erskine Y, Carey M, et al. A brief mindfulness-based cognitive behavioral intervention improves sexual functioning versus wait-list control in women treated for gynecologic cancer. Gynecol Oncol 2012;125(2):320–5.

39. Vallejos X, Wu C. Flibanserin: a novel, nonhormonal agent for the treatment of hypoactive sexual desire disorder in premenopausal women. J Pharm Pract 2017;30(2):256–60.

40. Simon JA, Kingsberg SA, Shumel B, et al. Efficacy and safety of flibanserin in postmenopausal women with hypoactive sexual desire disorder: results of the SNOWDROP trial. Menopause 2014;21(6): 633–40.

41. Mayer D, Lynch SE. Bremelanotide: new drug approved for treating hypoactive sexual desire disorder. Ann Pharmacother 2020;54(7):684–90.

42. Islam RM, Bell RJ, Green S, et al. Safety and efficacy of testosterone for women: a systematic review and meta-analysis of randomised controlled trial data. Lancet Diabetes Endocrinol 2019;7(10):754–66.

43. Davis SR, Baber R, Panay N, et al. Global consensus position statement on the use of testosterone therapy for women. J Clin Endocrinol Metab 2019;104(10):4660–6.

44. Gouveia M, Sanches R, Andrade S, et al. The role of testosterone in the improvement of sexual desire in postmenopausal women: an evidence-based clinical review. Acta Med Port 2018;31(11):680–90.

45. Vegunta S, Kling JM, Kapoor E. Androgen therapy in women. J Womens Health (Larchmt) 2020;29(1): 57–64.

46. Barton DL, Wender DB, Sloan JA, et al. Randomized controlled trial to evaluate transdermal testosterone in female cancer survivors with decreased libido; North Central Cancer Treatment Group Protocol N02C3. J Natl Cancer Inst 2007;99(9):672–9.

47. Goldstein I, Kim NN, Clayton AH, et al. Hypoactive sexual desire disorder: international society for the study of women's sexual health (ISSWSH) expert consensus panel review. Mayo Clin Proc 2017; 92(1):114–28.

48. Nurnberg HG, Hensley PL, Heiman JR, et al. Sildenafil treatment of women with antidepressant-associated sexual dysfunction: a randomized controlled trial. JAMA 2008;300(4):395–404.

49. Caruso S, Rugolo S, Agnello C, et al. Sildenafil improves sexual functioning in premenopausal women with type 1 diabetes who are affected by sexual arousal disorder: a double-blind, crossover, placebo-controlled pilot study. Fertil Steril 2006; 85(5):1496–501.

50. DasGupta R, Wiseman OJ, Kanabar G, et al. Efficacy of sildenafil in the treatment of female sexual dysfunction due to multiple sclerosis. J Urol 2004; 171(3):1189–93.

51. American Psychiatric Association. Diagnostic and Statistical Manual of Mental Disorders. 5th ed. Washington: American Psychiatric Association; 2013.

52. Parish SJ, Cottler-Casanova S, Clayton AH, et al. The evolution of the female sexual disorder/dysfunction definitions, nomenclature, and classifications: a review of DSM, ICSM, ISSWSH, and ICD. Sex Med Rev 2021;9:36–56.

53. Obedin-Maliver J. Time to change: Supporting sexual and gender minority people - An underserved, understudied cancer risk population. J Natl Compr Cancer Netw 2017;15(11):1305–8.

54. Potter J, Peitzmeier SM, Bernstein I, et al. Cervical cancer screening for patients on the female-to-male spectrum: a narrative review and guide for clinicians. J Gen Intern Med 2015;30(12):1857–64.

55. Pratt-Chapman M, Potter J. Cancer care considerations for sexual and gender minority patients. Oncol Issues 2019;34(6):26–36.

56. NIH FY 2016–2020 strategic plan to advance research on the health and well-being of sexual

and gender minorities. Bethesda, Maryland: National Institutes of Health; 2015.

57. Jabson JM, Kamen CS. Sexual minority cancer survivors' satisfaction with care. J Psychosoc Oncol 2016;34(1):28–38.

58. Fobair P, O'Hanlan K, Koopman C, et al. Comparison of lesbian and heterosexual women's response to newly diagnosed breast cancer. Psychooncology 2001;10(1):40–51.

59. Arena PL, Carver CS, Antoni MH, et al. Psychosocial responses to treatment for breast cancer among lesbian and heterosexual women. Womens Health (Lond) 2006;44(2):81–102.

60. Boehmer U, Potter J, Bowen DJ. Sexual functioning after cancer in sexual minority women. Cancer 2009; 15(1):65–9.

61. Boehmer U, Ozonoff A, Timm A, et al. After breast cancer: sexual functioning of sexual minority survivors. J Sex Res 2014;51(6):681–9.

62. National LGBT cancer network. Available at: https://cancer-network.org/cancer-information/cancer-and-the-lgbt-community/cancer-survivorship-issues/. Accessed January 18, 2021.

63. Hill EK, Sandbo S, Abramsohn E, et al. Assessing gynecologic and breast cancer survivors' sexual health care needs. Cancer 2011;117(12):2643–51.

64. Frimer, Turker LB, Shankar V, et al. The association of sexual dysfunction with race in women with gynecologic malignancies. Gynecol Oncol Rep 2019;30: 100495.

65. Canzona MR, Fisher CL, Wright KB, et al. Talking about sexual health during survivorship: understanding what shapes breast cancer survivors' willingness to communicate with providers. J Cancer Surviv 2019;13(6):932–42.

66. National Cancer Institute. Adolescents and young adults with cancer. Available at: https://www.cancer.gov/types/aya. Accessed January 18, 2021.

67. Acquati C, Zebrack BJ, Faul AC, et al. Sexual functioning among young adult cancer patients: a 2-year longitudinal study. Cancer 2018;124(2):398–405.

68. Stanton AM, Handy AB, Meston CM. Sexual function in adolescents and young adults diagnosed with cancer: a systematic review. J Cancer Surviv 2018; 12(1):47–63.

69. Champion VL, Wagner LI, Monahan PO, et al. Comparison of younger and older breast cancer survivors and age-matched controls on specific and overall quality of life domains. Cancer 2014; 120(15):2237–46.

70. Avis NE, Crawford S, Manuel J. Quality of life among younger women with breast cancer. J Clin Oncol 2005;23(15):3322–30.

71. Lindau ST, Schumm LP, Laumann EO, et al. A study of sexuality and health among older adults in the United States. N Engl J Med 2007;357(8):762–74.

72. McClelland SI, Holland KJ, Griggs JJ. Vaginal dryness and beyond: the sexual health needs of women diagnosed with metastatic breast cancer. J Sex Res 2015;52(6):604–16.

73. Silverman M, Rabow M. Sexual health in young women with metastatic breast cancer: the state of the science. J Clin Oncol 2018;223.

74. Basson R. Sexual function of women with chronic illness and cancer. Womens Health (Lond) 2010; 6(3):407–29.

75. Lemieux L, Kaiser S, Pereira J, et al. Sexuality in palliative care: Patient perspectives. Palliat Med 2004;18(7):630–7.

76. Vitrano V, Catania V, Mercadante S. Sexuality in patients with advanced cancer: a prospective study in a population admitted to an acute pain relief and palliative care unit. Am J Hosp Palliat Med 2011; 28(3):198–202.

77. Stausmire JM. Sexuality at the end of life. Am J Hosp Palliat Med 2004;21(1):33–9.

Physiology of Erection and Pathophysiology of Erectile Dysfunction

Susan M. MacDonald, MD[a],*, Arthur L. Burnett, MD, MBA[b]

KEYWORDS

- Erection • Physiology • Erectile dysfunction • Pathophysiology • Impotence

KEY POINTS

- Erections can be classified as psychogenic, reflexogenic, or nocturnal. Psychogenic erections are a result of cortical processing, whereas reflexogenic erections are mediated by a reflex arc involving the sacral spinal cord.
- Any alteration in the neuronal pathways coursing from the cerebral cortex, limbic system, and spinal cord to the peripheral nerves may result in erectile dysfunction.
- Nitric oxide is a key mediator of vasodilation for erections, and the RhoA calcium sensitization pathway is paramount for maintaining flaccidity.
- Arteriogenic erectile dysfunction has been strongly correlated with cardiovascular disease and is thought to be due to endothelial dysfunction, alterations of smooth muscle function, autonomic dysregulation, and concomitant hypogonadism.
- Erectile dysfunction resulting from a clinical comorbidity (hypertension, diabetes, and so forth) may be classified systematically by dysfunction (ie, vasculogenic, neurogenic, endocrine, or psychogenic).

INTRODUCTION

The complex pathway from sexual arousal to penile erection has been elucidated in great detail. Advances in neuroimaging have delineated the cortical and limbic system involvement in erections. The molecular biology underlying erections has been expanded on, identifying several potential therapeutic targets. Furthermore, the intricate interplay of molecular biology and physiology underlying erectile dysfunction (ED) has been associated with common medical comorbidities, such as cardiovascular disease and diabetes. This article discusses advances in the science of erections and the pathophysiology associated with their dysfunction.

PHYSIOLOGY OF PENILE TUMESCENCE AND DETUMESCENCE

At baseline, the penis is primarily under sympathetic tone and flaccid. The smooth muscle within the cavernosal sinusoids and the penile arteries is tonically contracted, maintaining the unerect state. This sympathetic tone is mediated by the release of noradrenaline, which maintains flaccidity for 23 hours a day, on average.[1] In response to sexual stimulation, a series of physiologic changes occur—the stages of tumescence:

1. Sexual or tactile stimulation leads to a release of nitric oxide (NO) from the cavernous nerves that induces smooth muscle relaxation. This

[a] Division of Urology, Penn State Health Milton S. Hershey Medical Center, Mail Code H055, 500 University Drive, Hershey, PA 17033, USA; [b] James Buchanan Brady Urological Institute, Johns Hopkins School of Medicine, 600 North Wolfe Street, Marburg 407, Baltimore, MD 21287, USA
* Corresponding author.
E-mail address: smacdonald@pennstatehealth.psu.edu
Twitter: @smacdonald_md (S.M.M.)

Urol Clin N Am 48 (2021) 513–525
https://doi.org/10.1016/j.ucl.2021.06.009
0094-0143/21/© 2021 Elsevier Inc. All rights reserved.

relaxation results in dilation of arterioles and arteries within the corpora cavernosa.[2]

2. Blood accumulates within the cavernosal sinusoids, which compress the subtunical venous plexus and decreases venous outflow (latent phase).

3. Expansion of the corpora cavernosa stretches the tunica albuginea. The emissary veins draining the corporal bodies are compressed between the inner circular and outer longitudinal layers of the tunica albuginea (tumescent phase).

4. Intracavernosal pressure (up to 100 mm Hg) and oxygen content (up to 90 mm Hg) increase as blood is trapped in the corpora and penile erection occurs (full erection phase).

5. Intracavernosal pressure is increased further with contraction of the ischiocavernosus and bulbocavernosus muscles, leading to glans engorgement and a rigid erection, which can be associated with suprasystolic intracorporal pressures (rigid phase).

The process of detumescence occurs when sexual stimulation resolves or after orgasm; detumescence has been studied in canine models and a similar process is thought to mediate loss of erection in humans[3]:

1. Intracavernosal pressure transiently rises as cavernous arteries vasoconstrict due to smooth muscle cell contraction.

2. Intracavernosal pressure decreases slowly as arterial inflow returns to baseline and venous outflow begins.

3. Rapid intracavernosal pressure decreases (80% overall pressure) due to decompression of the emissary veins and full restoration of venous outflow.

CORPUS SPONGIOSUM AND GLANS PENIS

During an erection, the pressure within the corpus spongiosum and glans penis rises one-half that of the corpora cavernosa despite similar arterial flow; this lesser degree of tumescence stems from the thinner tunical covering of the corpus spongiosum and subsequently weaker venous occlusion. The deep dorsal and circumflex veins are compressed between Buck fascia and the turgid corpora cavernosa. During the rigid erection phase, the spongiosum is compressed by the ischiocavernosus and bulbocavernosus muscles, markedly increasing pressure and turgidity of the spongosium and glans. In most adult men, this corresponds to the period immediately preceding ejaculation/orgasm.

TYPES OF ERECTIONS

Penile erection may be induced by several stimuli, both external and internal. Broadly speaking, erections are classified into 3 types, which are not necessarily mutually exclusive:

- Psychogenic—triggered by auditory, visual, or nongenital tactile stimulation that involves cortical processing of the stimulus as erotic. This type of erection is mediated by cortical inhibition of sympathetic tone from the spinal cord and may be preserved in patients with lower spinal cord injury (ie, below T11).[4]
- Reflexogenic—triggered by tactile stimulation of the genitals via a reflex arc through the autonomic nuclei to the cavernous nerves. Reflexogenic erections typically are maintained in patients with upper spinal cord injury (ie, above T11).[4]
- Nocturnal—occur involuntarily, primarily during rapid eye movement sleep

NEUROANATOMY OF AN ERECTION
Cortex to Spinal Cord

Advances in positron emission tomography and functional magnetic resonance imaging (fMRI) have permitted imaging of the brain areas activated during sexual arousal via changes in regional blood flow. Allen and colleagues[5] used fMRI to create a somatosensory map of the brain in response to sexual and nonsexual touch of genital areas. Gentle touch of the glans or shaft resulted in activation of the superficial paracentral lobule whereas forceful touch activated deeper cortex within the same region.[5]

Poeppl and colleagues[6] compiled a meta-analysis of 20 brain imaging studies during psychosexual (mental) and physiosexual (physical) arousal. Activation in the bilateral insular cortices, bilateral claustra, right putamen, anterior midcingulate gyrus, and subgenual anterior cingulate gyrus were found to correlate positively with penile erection.[6] The investigators hypothesized a complex sequence of brain activation with sexual stimulus leading to arousal and then penile erection.[6] The lateral prefrontal cortex and hippocampus appear to be involved in a cognitive and memory-guided evaluation of a particular sexual stimulus. Next, the sensory processing of this stimulus occurs in temporo-occipital cortex and superior parietal lobes.[6] The investigators speculated that an autonomic response mediated by the hypothalamus then results in both a sexual urge created by the amygdala and the awareness of sexual arousal with activation of the anterior insular cortex.[6] Portions of the temporal and parietal lobes, areas involved inself-awareness or introspection, appear to be deactivated during sexual arousal.[6]

Animal studies have identified structures within the limbic system to be control centers for sexual arousal (remove this comma) including the medial amygdala, medial preoptic aprea (MPOA) and paraventricular nucleus (PVN) within the hypothalamus, nucleus accumbens, hippocampus, periaqueductal gray, and ventral tegmentum.[7–10] Direct electrical stimulation of the MPOA and the PVN have been shown to elicit an erection in rats.[11,12] In rats, lesions of the amygdala abolish psychogenic erections, and lesions of the PVN delay and decrease the number of psychogenic erections. Reflexogenic erections are preserved in both of these model systems.[13,14]

Human fMRI studies suggest the limbic system coordinates the autonomic response to sexual stimuli. The amygdala activates in response to a visual sexual stimulus, perhaps gauging its potency.[6,15] Redoute and colleagues[16] first noted increased blood flow in the anterior and middle cingulate gyrus during psychogenic erections with audiovisual stimulation. Georgiadis and colleagues[17] confirmed activation of the anterior middle cingulate cortex and the lateral hypothalamus during penile erection with tactile stimulation. Poeppl and colleagues[6] further hypothesized that the putamen may act as a command center, linking corticostriatal loops that coordinate subjective sexual arousal, penile erection, and eventually ejaculation.

In summary, activation of the cerebral cortex appears to occur with processing tactile stimulation to the penis (paracentral lobule) or audiovisual stimuli (inferior temporal lobes bilaterally). Areas of the limbic system then appear to be involved in the contextual or emotional processing of these stimuli and the motivation to act on them. Impulses then travel to the spinal erection centers (T11-L2 and S2-4) to activate initiation of a psychogenic erection through the peripheral nerves (**Fig. 1**).

Spinal Cord to the Peripheral Nerves

Within the spinal cord, 3 types of neurons travel to the genitalia to coordinate erection and ejaculation: sympathetic (thoracolumbar), parasympathetic (sacral), and somatic (motor and sensory) (**Fig. 2**).[18]

Autonomic pathway

- **Sympathetic**: the intermediolateral cell column and dorsal gray column contain sympathetic preganglionic neuronal cell bodies.[19] Presynatic sympathetic nerve fibers extend from T11 to L2 to the sympathetic chain ganglia. Fibers then pass to the pelvic (inferior hypogastric) plexus via the hypogastric and pelvic nerves. This pathway is responsible for detumescence and flaccidity.
- **Parasympathetic**: the cell bodies of parasympathetic neurons innervating the phallus are found within the intermediolateral cell column of sacral segments S2-4.[19] Preganglionic parasympathetic neurons traverse from this location via the pelvic nerve to the pelvic (inferior hypogastric) plexus. They then travel via the cavernous nerves, along with sympathetic fibers, to innervate the cavernous smooth muscle. Parasympathetic input is responsible for initiating tumescence and rigidity.

Somatic pathway

- **Motor**: somatic motor neuron cell bodies are located within Onuf nucleus in the ventral horn of the sacral segments, primarily S2.[19] These fibers travel via the pudendal nerve to innervate the ischiocavernosus and bulbospongiosus muscles.
- **Sensory**: sensory receptors along the penile skin, glans, urethra, and corpora cavernosa coalesce to form the dorsal nerve of the penis. Receptors sensitive to touch and temperature, and less commonly pressure sensitive receptors, connect to thinly myelinated A_δ and C fibers.[20] Sensory fibers originate in the glans and coalesce to form the dorsal nerve of the penis that travels in 2 or more anastomosing main branches along the dorsum of the phallus.[21] The dorsal nerve then joins with other peripheral branches to become the pudendal nerve, which connects to the spinal cord via S2-4 nerve roots. Sensory afferents also travel via the hypogastric nerve to the thoracolumbar dorsal roots. Sensory afferents terminate in the medial dorsal horn and dorsal gray column of the lumbosacral spinal cord.[19] Pain, temperature, and touch are transmitted by these sensory neurons via the spinothalamic and spinoreticular pathways to the thalamus and sensory cortex for sensory perception.[22]

MOLECULAR MECHANISM

The smooth muscle cells of the corpora cavernosa are maintained in a tonically contracted state via intracellular calcium (Ca^{2+}) and Rho kinase activation. Norepinephrine and other vasoconstrictor agonists (endothelin 1, prostaglandin $2F_\alpha$, angiotensin II, and TXA_2) act on their receptors to activate their respective G proteins. Angiotensin

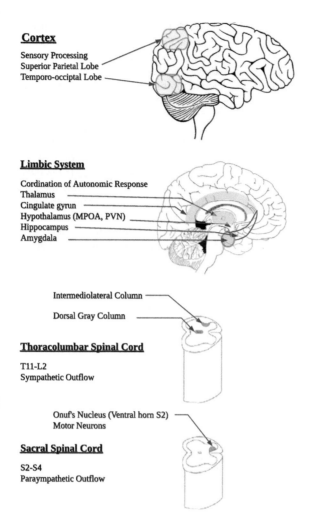

Fig. 1. Overview of neuroanatomy of an erection.

II binds to angiotensin type I receptors activating the RhoA/Rho-associated protein kinase (ROCK) pathway (described later) as well as NADPH oxidase, creating reactive oxygen species, which decreases NO availability.[23] Norepinephrine binds to postsynaptic α-adrenergic receptors and activates Gq/11 protein, as do endothelin 1 and prostaglandin 2F$_\alpha$ released from endothelial cells. Gq/11 activates phospholipase C, creating inositol triphosphate (IP$_3$) and 1,2-diacylglycerol. IP$_3$ binds to the endoplasmic reticulum releasing Ca^{2+}. Increased intracellular Ca^{2+} leads to Ca^{2+} binding to calmodulin. This causes a change in configuration of the complex that increases its affinity to bind with myosin light chain kinase (MLCK). Now activated and in combination with available ATP, MLCK phosphorylates the myosin light chain, which leads to actin and myosin initiating cross-bridge cycling, leading to contraction of muscle fibers.

The enzyme myosin light chain phosphatase (MLCP), which dephosphorylates (deactivates) myosin light chain is regulated by ROCK. ROCK phosphorylates MLCP, inhibiting its phosphatase activity and promoting smooth muscle contraction (and thus flaccidity) by sensitizing actin myosin to lower levels of intracytosolic Ca^{2+} (**Fig. 3**).[24]

An erection is triggered by stimulation of the cavernous nerves generating Ca^{2+}-dependent (depolarization) and Ca^{2+}-independent (sensitization) mechanisms for the neurogenic response. The Ca^{2+} sensitization mechanism is understood to drive a sustained neuronal NO release by phosphorylation of neuronal NO synthase (nNOS) involving cyclic adenosine monophosphate production and activation of protein kinase A. NO triggers guanylate cyclase to create cyclic guanosine monophosphate (cGMP). The amount of available cGMP is a balance between the activity of guanylate cyclase, which creates the molecule, and

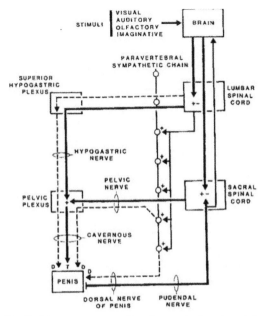

Fig. 2. Diagram representing the central and peripheral pathways governing an erection. Synaptic excitatory and inhibitory mechanisms are indicated by + and –, respectively. D, penile detumescence; T, penile tumescence. (With permission from deGroat W. C. and Steers W. D.: Neuroanatomy and neurophysiology of penile erection. In: Contemporary Management of Impotence and Infertility. Edited by E.A. Tanagho, T.F. Lue and R.D. McClure. Baltimore: Williams and Wilkins, Chapter 1, pp. 3–27. 1988.)

phosphodiesterase type 5 (PDE5), which degrades it. PDE5 inhibitors, such as sildenafil, essentially inhibit the off switch for cavernous relaxation, thus potentiating erection.

Protein kinase G is activated by cGMP, inducing smooth muscle relaxation via multiple mechanisms, including the inhibition of ROCK and stimulation of MLCP.[25] Serine protein kinase AKT then is up-regulated by shear force from increased blood flow, subsequently phosphorylating vascular endothelial NO synthase (eNOS). Phosphorylated eNOS and nNOS prolong NO production and sustain erection[2,26,27] (**Fig. 4**).

PATHOPHYSIOLOGY OF ERECTILE DYSFUNCTION
Introduction

ED often is the end result of multiple pathophysiologic processes. Once a man has experienced ED, it is impossible to rule out at least some psychological component, given the anxiety-provoking nature of the disease. Although classification schemes differ, for the purposes of this article, conditions known to be associated with organic ED are grouped into vasculogenic, neurogenic, and hormonal categories (**Fig. 5**).[28]

Vasculogenic

Arteriogenic (arterial insufficiency)
Cardiovascular disease, the leading cause of death in the United States, clearly has been associated with arteriogenic ED. In 2003,

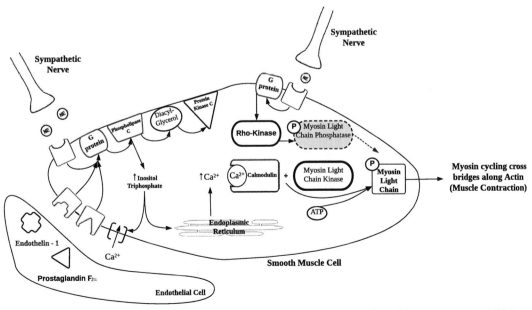

Fig. 3. Flaccidity: molecular activity—bold lines represent activation; gray or dotted lines represent inhibition.

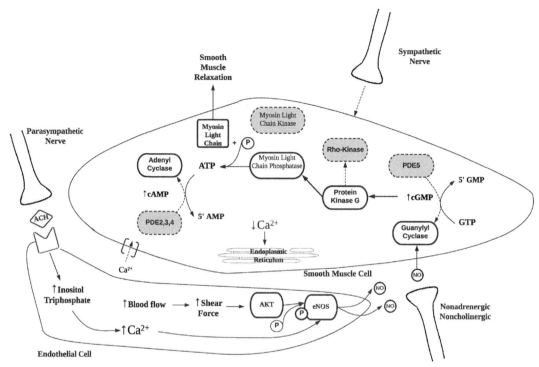

Fig. 4. Erection: molecular activity—bold lines represent activation; gray or dotted lines represent inhibition. ACH, acetylcholine; AMP, adenosine monophosphate; CGMP, cyclic guanosine monophosphate; P, phosphate.

Montorsi and colleagues[29] examined 300 patients with acute chest pain and angiographically proved coronary artery disease (CAD) and found a 49% prevalence of ED. A majority of patients (67%) reported that ED preceded CAD on average by 38 months. Vasculopathy of the cavernosal arteries manifesting as ED may serve as a harbinger of future cardiac disease. Thompson and colleagues[30] determined that the risk for a future cardiovascular event conferred by ED is equivalent to smoking, hyperlipidemia, or a family history of MI. Ponholzer and colleagues[31] correlated the degree of ED with CAD risk. Mild ED was associated with a small (2%–11%) increased risk, whereas moderate ED and severe ED were associated with a 65% increased relative risk of CAD at 10 years.

ED categorized as "arteriogenic" is due to diminished arterial inflow and thus decreased perfusion pressure. This manifests as decreased maximal rigidity and delayed time to a full erection. The etiology of arteriogenic ED may be atherosclerotic disease or trauma to the hypogastric-cavernous-helicine arterial tree. In young patients with a history of blunt pelvic or perineal trauma, focal stenosis of the common penile or cavernosal artery may be the etiology.[32] Arteriogenic ED, which accounts for a majority of cases, has been strongly linked to the following conditions:

hypertension, hyperlipidemia, tobacco use, metabolic syndrome/obesity, sedentary lifestyle, diabetes, and pelvic radiation.[33–38] Doppler ultrasound has been used to correlate decreased peak systolic velocity of the cavernosal arteries with underlying vascular disease and risk of cardiovascular events.[39,40]

The pathologic mechanism underlying arteriogenic ED is likely multifactorial, including 1 or more of the following, as suggested by Musicki and colleagues[41] in a 2015 review: (1) endothelial dysfunction, (2) smooth muscle alterations, (3) autonomic dysregulation (discussed later), (4) hypogonadism (see endocrine section), and (5) metabolic defects. Endothelial dysfunction typically is described as decreased reactivity to vasodilators or increased reactivity to vasoconstrictors; other factors, such as oxidative stress, may play a role. Hypercholesterolemia-induced atherosclerosis in the penis is associated with endothelial dysfunction as indicated by reduced NO production, impaired relaxation in response to muscarinic stimulation, and increased lipid peroxidation.[42] Diabetes manifests such changes as decreased nNOS expression, reduced eNOS activity, reduced vascular endothelial growth factor release, and increased reactive oxygen species production in the corpora cavernosa in animal models.[43]

Organic
I. Vasculogenic
  A. Arteriogenic
  B. Cavernosal
  C. Mixed

II. Neurogenic
III. Anatomic
IV. Endocrinologic

Psychogenic
I. Generalized
  A. Generalized unresponsiveness
    1. Primary lack of sexual arousability
    2. Aging-related decline in sexual arousability

  B. Generalized inhibition
    1. Chronic disorder of sexual intimacy

II. Situational
  A. Partner-related
    1. Lack of arousability in specific relationship
    2. Lack of arousability owing to sexual object preference
    3. High central inhibition owing to partner conflict or threat

  B. Performance-related
    1. Associated with other sexual dysfunction/s (eg, rapid ejaculation)
    2. Situational performance anxiety (e.g. fear of failure)
  C. Psychological distress-related or adjustment-related
    1. Associated with negative mood state (eg, depression) or major life stress (eg, death of partner)

Fig. 5. Traditional classification scheme created by the International Society for Impotence Research.

Alterations of vascular smooth muscle content and function have been suggested as contributing factors to ED. In a rabbit model of ED due to atherosclerosis in the iliac artery, increased contraction of cavernosal smooth muscle was noted in response to electrical impulses.[44] The investigators hypothesized that the ischemia may interfere with full relaxation of the smooth muscle tissue required for inflow and thus the dilation of trabeculae required for veno-occlusion.[44]

Cavernosal dysfunction
ED due to cavernosal dysfunction is the inability to maintain adequate vascular tension for a rigid erection due to a variety of structural defects including enlarged veins, fibrosis, increased smooth muscle tone, or impaired sinusoidal endothelial-dependent relaxation. Previously, this category was referred to as *venous leak*; however, this term did not adequately encompass the wide array of ultrastructural changes that lead to ED. Large congenital or ectopic superficial dorsal, deep dorsal, or crural veins may elevate end diastolic velocity or outflow.[45,46] More commonly, fibrosis of the tunica albuginea and/or corpora (as in Peyronie disease or other scar tissue conditions) leads to insufficient compression of the emissary veins. Inadequate relaxation of the trabecular smooth muscle due to decreased fibroelasticity or increased adrenergic tone, as well as persistent venous shunts (eg, related to prior treatment of priapism) also may cause

cavernosal dysfunction.[44] Animal models of diabetes have demonstrated significantly less smooth muscle contractility via decreased mRNA and protein expressions of smooth muscle α-actin and M myosin heavy chain required for function in cavernosal tissue.[47] A 50% decrease in maximal contraction of cavernosal smooth muscle was demonstrated at 8 weeks in diabetic rats in response to phenylephrine.[48]

The classic history in patients with congenitally enlarged or anomalous venous drainage is an insufficient erection or duration of erection since initial sexual encounters.[49] Ye and colleagues[50] examined 139 patients with venous leakage with CT cavernosography and showed that excess outflow was isolated to the deep dorsal vein alone in 15.8%, whereas 84.2% were classified as complex. It is unclear whether or not the investigators used a redosing regimen for erectogenic agent is typically as recommended for such testing, so the results must be interpreted with caution.[50] Significant anatomic variation was noted with single, double, and complex branching patterns of the deep dorsal vein and similar variation in the prostatic venous plexus as well.[50] Penile Doppler ultrasound (PDUS) is a modality utilized more commonly to make a diagnosis of venous leak. Performance of PDUS is dependent on induction of an adequate arterial erection response to characterize end-diastolic velocity accurately.[51]

Neurogenic

It is difficult to provide a true estimate of neurogenic ED because this category includes a broad range of etiologies at multiple levels of the nervous system. In broad terms, cortical impairment, traumatic injury of the spinal cord, iatrogenic peripheral nerve injury during pelvic surgery, and autonomic dysfunction and/or demyelination due to conditions, such as diabetes, all may be conceptualized as sources of neurogenic ED.

Cerebral cortex

Any disease that interferes with cortical processes involved in the registration, processing, and physical reactivity to sexual stimuli may result in neurogenic ED. Conditions include Parkinson disease, Alzheimer disease, dementia, cerebrovascular accidents or stroke, encephalitis, Shy-Drager syndrome, temporal lobe epilepsy, tumors, and traumatic brain injury. Consistent with the understanding that the MPOA, PVN, and hippocampus are crucial for sexual arousal and erection, lesions in the thalamus due to cerebrovascular accidents correlate with ED as determined by insufficient rigidity on RigiScan (Gesiva Medical LLC. Eden Prairie, MN) during audiovisual sexual stimulation.[52–54]

Spinal cord

Injury to the spinal cord often leads to ED. The extent of erection impairment, however, is determined by the location and nature of the injury. Aside from trauma, multiple sclerosis, spina bifida, syringomyelia, and disc herniation all may result in neurogenic ED. Lesions above T11 damage communication between the thoracolumbar nerves impairing psychogenic erections. The sacral pathway, however, is intact and thus most retain reflexogenic erections.[55] Patients with lesions below T11 but above the sacral pathway may have some preservation of function due to maintenance of both reflexogenic as well as psychogenic erections.[55] Lesions involving the sacral parasympathetic pathway but sparing the cauda equina often result in loss of reflexogenic erections.[55] Reflexogenic erections typically are of shorter duration and require constant stimulation to maintain. Reflexogenic erections are present in up to 95% of patients with complete upper spinal cord lesions, but only 25% of patients with complete lower cord lesions.[56,57]

Peripheral nerves

The parasympathetic nerve fibers responsible for erections synapse in the pelvic plexus along the anterolateral aspect of the middle third of the rectum, posterior to the bladder, and then travel alongside the prostate down to the penis via the cavernous nerves. There is a high likelihood of iatrogenic injury to the pelvic and cavernous nerves during surgery on the bladder, prostate, or rectum. Factors, such as age, preoperative erectile function, cancer stage, comorbidities, and degree of nerve sparing all significantly affect a patient's postoperative potency. A majority of patients undergoing an abdominoperineal resection or radical prostatectomy experience transient loss of function (weeks to months), if not permanent impairment.

Autonomic dysregulation

Increased contractions due to adrenergic stimulation and decreased relaxation due to acetylcholine stimulation have been shown in spontaneously hypertensive rats.[58] In a hyperglycemic rat model characterize by elevated norepinephrine release, sympathetic nervous dysfunction was demonstrated.[59] As demonstrated by abnormalities in corneal nerve fibers on confocal microscopy and altered cardiovascular responses to deep breathing or prolonged standing in type 1 diabetes mellitus patients, there may be an association between autonomic neuropathy and ED.[60,61] Increased sympathetic tone or decreased transmission of parasympathetic nerve impulses may contribute to neurogenic ED.

Endocrine

Hypogonadism

There is a complex relationship between ED and serum testosterone levels. ED is a well-known potential consequence of androgen deprivation therapy.[62] In a population of men with ED ages 25 years to 80 years, 7% were found to have serum testosterone levels less than 200 ng/dL, 23% less than 300 ng/dL, and 33% less than 346 ng/dL.[63] In men with low testosterone, supplementation increases sexual desire and may improve erectile response.[64,65] Supplementation of hypogonadal men with testosterone was shown to improve responses to PDE5 inhibitor therapy for ED.[66] Further support for the androgen-dependent extent of erectile function includes a threshold testosterone value of 200 ng/dL for regular nocturnal erections.[67] In a population of 52 male patients without significant comorbidities who underwent PDUS as part of a work-up for ED, free testosterone levels were associated positively with peak systolic velocity and resistive index and negatively associated with end diastolic velocity.[68] Although the significance is as yet unknown, there may be locally mediated acute effect of testosterone because levels vary at the time of erection within serum and the corpora cavernosa.[69,70]

The correlation between low testosterone and decreased erectile function has been studied in animal models to elucidate the physiologic mechanism. In rats castrated for 2 weeks, a prolonged latency period and decreased filling rate of the cavernosa as well as decreased intracavernosal pressure were observed.[71] Overall, a 50% decrease in erectile response was noted, which was restored with testosterone or dihydrotestosterone (DHT) supplementation.[71,72] Dai and colleagues[73] demonstrated reduced veno-occlusion in electrically induced erections in castrate rats, which was restored with testosterone supplementation. This effect appeared to be mediated by NO.[73] Studies have demonstrated that testosterone and DHT stimulate nNOS gene expression and increase NO in the corpora during erections.[72,74] Van den Broeck and colleagues[75] confirmed dose-dependent relaxation of human corpora cavernosal tissue with increasing testosterone and DHT.

Hyperprolactinemia

Hyperprolactinemia results in reproductive as well as sexual dysfunction. Symptoms associated with hyperprolactinemia include loss of libido, ED, galactorrhea, gynecomastia, and infertility. These symptoms typically occur only at severely elevated levels (>35 ng/mL or 735 mU/L).[76] Hyperprolactinemia may be idiopathic, drug induced, secondary to a pituitary adenoma, or related to chronic renal failure.[77] Concomitant low testosterone most likely is mediated by prolactin induced inhibition of gonadotropin-releasing hormone secretion by the pituitary gland.[77]

Thyroid dysfunction

Hyperthyroidism or hypothyroidism also may be associated with ED. In a small study of patients with hyperthyroidism and hypothyroidism (71 total patients), 70% and 84% of patients reported at least mild ED, with a Sexual Health Inventory for Men (SHIM) score of less than 21, respectively, compared with 34% of the control group.[78] With treatment, statistically significant mean increases in SHIM scores of 7 points in the hyperthyroidism cohort and 8.5 points in the hypothyroidism cohort were noted.[78] Thyroid hormone effects may be mediated by secondary effects on other hormones known to be associated with sexual function. Hypothyroidism is associated with increased serum prolactin and decreased serum testosterone whereas hyperthyroidism is associated with increased estrogen levels.[79–81] A direct effect of thyroxine may also be at play in thyroid hormone ED, because both alpha and beta thyroxine receptors have been shown to be present in endothelial and smooth muscle cells from human corpora cavernosa.[82] Impairment in NO-dependent relaxation of the corpora cavernosa has been reported in animal models of hyperthyroidism.[83,84]

Psychogenic

Historically, psychogenic issues were thought to be the principal etiology for the vast majority of ED presentations. Pscyhogenic ED may not be a primary etiology in most cases but it is a contributing factor in virtually all cases. There are conflicting data as to whether purely psychogenic ED may be more common among younger patients (<40 years old), with the reported incidence varying from 13% to 83%.[85–87] The degree to which ED is psychogenic versus physiologic is difficult to parse out; isolated psychogenic ED is considered a diagnosis of exclusion clinically.

As discussed previously, erections are tonically inhibited by the sympathetic nervous system, which then can be modulated by cortical impulses that are excitatory or inhibitory.[6] Cera and colleagues[88] found gray matter atrophy in the bilateral nucleus accumbens and the left hypothalamus on fMRI in patients with psychogenic ED. These areas previously have been correlated to the motivational process in sexual arousal, suggesting abnormal evaluation of erotic stimuli and compromised processing thereof. Research repeatedly has demonstrated a link between depression/anxiety and ED. It is possible that repeated intrusive thoughts distract the attentional aspect of sexual arousal as well.

SUMMARY

Advances in neuroimaging and understanding of molecular physiology have clarified the biological processes underlying penile erection. This information contributes to the understanding of the scientific basis of ED. Comorbidities that predispose to ED cause concomitant physiologic changes within multiple categories of ED (ie, vasculogenic, neurogenic, endocrine, and psychogenic). An array of disruptions at the molecular (cell signaling and responsiveness to neurotransmitters) and structural (changes in the tunica albuginea, smooth muscle, or vasculature) levels may contribute to ED. Evolving understanding of the science of erections and the pathophysiology of ED helps clinicians guide current and future therapy for patients.

DISCLOSURE STATEMENT

Susan MacDonald is a consultant for Boston Scientific.

Arthur Burnett has the following disclosures: American Medical Systems/Boston Scientific—investigator for study or trial; *Andrology*—associate editor; Astellas—consultant, advisor for trial or study; Comphya—consultant, advisor for trial or study; Futura Medical—consultant, advisor for trial or study; *International Urology and Nephrology*—associate editor; Lilly, LLC—consultant, advisor for trial or study; Myriad Genetics—consultant, advisor; MHN Biotech—owner, product development; National Institutes of Health—investigator for trial or study; Novartis Pharmaceuticals—consultant, advisor for trial or study; Pfizer—investigator for trial or study; Reflexonic, LLC—consultant, advisor; *The Canadian Journal of Urology*—associate editor; UroMissionsWorks, Inc.—leadership position; *Urology Practice*—patient care editor; and *Urology Times* Editorial Council—consultant, advisor.

REFERENCES

1. Anele UA, Burnett AL. Nitrergic Mechanisms for Management of Recurrent Priapism. Sex Med Rev 2015;3(3):160–8.

2. Hurt KJ, Sezen SF, Lagoda GF, et al. Cyclic AMP-dependent phosphorylation of neuronal nitric oxide synthase mediates penile erection. Proc Natl Acad Sci U S A 2012;109(41):16624–9.

3. Bosch RJ, Benard F, Aboseif SR, et al. Penile detumescence: characterization of three phases. J Urol 1991;146(3):867–71.

4. Giuliano F, Rampin O. Neural control of erection. Physiol Behav 2004;83(2):189–201.

5. Allen K, Wise N, Frangos E, et al. Male Urogenital System Mapped Onto the Sensory Cortex: Functional Magnetic Resonance Imaging Evidence. J Sex Med 2020;17(4):603–13.

6. Poeppl TB, Langguth B, Laird AR, et al. The functional neuroanatomy of male psychosexual and physiosexual arousal: a quantitative meta-analysis. Hum Brain Mapp 2014;35(4):1404–21.

7. Marson L, Platt KB, McKenna KE. Central nervous system innervation of the penis as revealed by the transneuronal transport of pseudorabies virus. Neurosci 1993;55(1):263–80.

8. Mallick HN, Manchanda SK, Kumar VM. Sensory modulation of the medial preoptic area neuronal activity by dorsal penile nerve stimulation in rats. J Urol 1994;151(3):759–62.

9. Andersson KE. Mechanisms of penile erection and basis for pharmacological treatment of erectile dysfunction. Pharmacol Rev 2011;63(4):811–59.

10. Melis MR, Argiolas A. Central control of penile erection: a re-visitation of the role of oxytocin and its interaction with dopamine and glutamic acid in male rats. Neurosci Biobehav Rev 2011;35(3): 939–55.

11. Chen KK, Chan SH, Chang LS, et al. Participation of paraventricular nucleus of hypothalamus in central regulation of penile erection in the rat. J Urol 1997; 158(1):238–44.

12. Courtois FJ, Macdougall JC. Higher CNS control of penile responses in rats: the effect of hypothalamic stimulation. Physiol Behav 1988;44(2):165–71.

13. Kondo Y, Sachs BD, Sakuma Y. Importance of the medial amygdala in rat penile erection evoked by remote stimuli from estrous females. Behav Brain Res 1998;91(1–2):215–22.

14. Liu YC, Salamone JD, Sachs BD. Impaired sexual response after lesions of the paraventricular nucleus of the hypothalamus in male rats. Behav Neurosci 1997;111(6):1361–7.

15. Pessoa L, Adolphs R. Emotion processing and the amygdala: from a 'low road' to 'many roads' of evaluating biological significance. Nat Rev Neurosci 2010;11(11):773–83.

16. Redoute J, Stoleru S, Gregoire MC, et al. Brain processing of visual sexual stimuli in human males. Hum Brain Mapp 2000;11(3):162–77.

17. Georgiadis JR, Farrell MJ, Boessen R, et al. Dynamic subcortical blood flow during male sexual

activity with ecological validity: a perfusion fMRI study. Neuroimage 2010;50(1):208–16.

18. D. dWCaSW. Neuroanatomy and neurophysiology of penile erection. In: Tanagho EA, TFLaRDM, editors. Contemporary Management of Impotence and Infertility. Baltimore: Williams and Wilkins; 1988. p. 3–27.

19. Giuliano F. Neurophysiology of erection and ejaculation. J Sex Med 2011;8(Suppl 4):310–5.

20. Halata Z, Munger BL. The neuroanatomical basis for the protopathic sensibility of the human glans penis. Brain Res 1986;371(2):205–30.

21. Kozacioglu Z, Kiray A, Ergur I, et al. Anatomy of the dorsal nerve of the penis, clinical implications. Urologiia 2014;83(1):121–4.

22. McKenna KE. Central control of penile erection. Int J impotence Res 1998;10(Suppl 1):S25–34.

23. Jin LM. Angiotensin II Signaling and Its Implication in Erectile Dysfunction. J Sex Med 2009;6:302–10.

24. Sopko NA, Hannan JL, Bivalacqua TJ. Understanding and targeting the Rho kinase pathway in erectile dysfunction. Nat Rev Urol 2014;11(11):622–8.

25. Francis SH, Busch JL, Corbin JD, et al. cGMP-dependent protein kinases and cGMP phosphodiesterases in nitric oxide and cGMP action. Pharmacol Rev 2010;62(3):525–63.

26. Dimmeler S, Fleming I, Fisslthaler B, et al. Activation of nitric oxide synthase in endothelial cells by Akt-dependent phosphorylation. Nature 1999; 399(6736):601–5.

27. Hurt KJ, Musicki B, Palese MA, et al. Akt-dependent phosphorylation of endothelial nitric-oxide synthase mediates penile erection. Proc Natl Acad Sci U S A 2002;99(6):4061–6.

28. Burnett AL, Nehra A, Breau RH, et al. Erectile Dysfunction: AUA Guideline. J Urol 2018;200(3): 633–41.

29. Montorsi F, Briganti A, Salonia A, et al. Erectile dysfunction prevalence, time of onset and association with risk factors in 300 consecutive patients with acute chest pain and angiographically documented coronary artery disease. Eur Urol 2003; 44(3):360–4. discussion 364-365.

30. Thompson IM, Tangen CM, Goodman PJ, et al. Erectile dysfunction and subsequent cardiovascular disease. J Am Med Assoc 2005;294(23):2996–3002.

31. Ponholzer A, Temml C, Obermayr R, et al. Is erectile dysfunction an indicator for increased risk of coronary heart disease and stroke? Eur Urol 2005; 48(3):512–8. discussion 517-518.

32. Munarriz RM, Yan QR, A ZN, et al. Blunt trauma: the pathophysiology of hemodynamic injury leading to erectile dysfunction. J Urol 1995;153(6):1831–40.

33. Feldman HA, Goldstein I, Hatzichristou DG, et al. Impotence and its medical and psychosocial correlates: results of the Massachusetts Male Aging Study. J Urol 1994;151(1):54–61.

34. Giugliano F, Maiorino M, Bellastella G, et al. Determinants of erectile dysfunction in type 2 diabetes. Int J Impotence Res 2010;22(3):204–9.

35. Levine FJ, Greenfield AJ, Goldstein I. Arteriographically determined occlusive disease within the hypogastric-cavernous bed in impotent patients following blunt perineal and pelvic trauma. J Urol 1990;144(5):1147–53.

36. Goldstein I, Feldman MI, Deckers PJ, et al. Radiation-associated impotence. A clinical study of its mechanism. J Am Med Assoc 1984;251(7):903–10.

37. Kupelian V, Araujo AB, Chiu GR, et al. Relative contributions of modifiable risk factors to erectile dysfunction: results from the Boston Area Community Health (BACH) Survey. Prevent Med 2010; 50(1–2):19–25.

38. Martin-Morales A, Sanchez-Cruz JJ, Saenz de Tejada I, et al. Prevalence and independent risk factors for erectile dysfunction in Spain: results of the Epidemiologia de la Disfuncion Erectil Masculina Study. J Urol 2001;166(2):569–74. discussion 574-565.

39. Corona G, Monami M, Boddi V, et al. Male sexuality and cardiovascular risk. A cohort study in patients with erectile dysfunction. J Sex Med 2010;7(5): 1918–27.

40. Montorsi P, Ravagnani PM, Galli S, et al. Association between erectile dysfunction and coronary artery disease: Matching the right target with the right test in the right patient. Eur Urol 2006;50(4):721–31.

41. Musicki B, Bella AJ, Bivalacqua TJ, et al. Basic Science Evidence for the Link Between Erectile Dysfunction and Cardiometabolic Dysfunction. J Sex Med 2015;12(12):2233–55.

42. Baumhäkel M, Custodis F, Schlimmer N, et al. Improvement of endothelial function of the corpus cavernosum in apolipoprotein E knockout mice treated with irbesartan. J Pharmacol Exp Ther 2008;327(3):692–8.

43. Yang J, Wang T, Yang J, et al. S-allyl cysteine restores erectile function through inhibition of reactive oxygen species generation in diabetic rats. Andrologie 2013;1(3):487–94.

44. Azadzoi KM, Krane RJ, Saenz de Tejada I, et al. Relative roles of cyclooxygenase and nitric oxide synthase pathways in ischemia-induced increased contraction of cavernosal smooth muscle. J Urol 1999;161(4):1324–8.

45. Ebbehoj J, Wagner G. Insufficient penile erection due to abnormal drainage of cavernous bodies. Urol 1979;13(5):507–10.

46. Stief CG, Gall H, Scherb W, et al. Erectile dysfunction due to ectopic penile vein. Urol 1988;31(4): 300–3.

47. Wei AY, He SH, Zhao JF, et al. Characterization of corpus cavernosum smooth muscle cell phenotype

in diabetic rats with erectile dysfunction. Int J impotence Res 2012;24(5):196–201.

48. Elçioğlu HK, Kabasakal L, Özkan N, et al. A study comparing the effects of rosiglitazone and/or insulin treatments on streptozotocin induced diabetic (type I diabetes) rat aorta and cavernous tissues. Eur J Pharmacol 2011;660(2–3):476–84.

49. Rahman NU, Dean RC, Carrion R, et al. Crural ligation for primary erectile dysfunction: a case series. J Urol 2005;173(6):2064–6.

50. Ye T, Li J, Li L, et al. Computed tomography cavernosography combined with volume rendering to observe venous leakage in young patients with erectile dysfunction. The British journal of radiology 2018;91(1091):20180118.

51. Teloken PE, Park K, Parker M, et al. The false diagnosis of venous leak: prevalence and predictors. J Sex Med 2011;8(8):2344–9.

52. Jeon SW, Yoo KH, Kim TH, et al. Correlation of the erectile dysfunction with lesions of cerebrovascular accidents. J Sex Med 2009;6(1):251–6.

53. Chen KK, Chan JY, Chang LS. Dopaminergic neurotransmission at the paraventricular nucleus of hypothalamus in central regulation of penile erection in the rat. J Urol 1999;162(1):237–42.

54. McKenna KE. Some proposals regarding the organization of the central nervous system control of penile erection. Neurosci biobehavioral Rev 2000;24(5): 535–40.

55. DeRoo EM, Mellon MJ. Sexual Dysfunction in Male Spinal Cord Injury Patients. Curr Bladder Dysfunct Rep 2014;9(4):268–74.

56. Biering-Sorensen F, Sonksen J. Sexual function in spinal cord lesioned men. Spinal cord 2001;39(9): 455–70.

57. Chapelle PA, Durand J, Lacert P. Penile erection following complete spinal cord injury in man. Br J Urol 1980;52(3):216–9.

58. Shimizu S, Tsounapi P, Honda M, et al. Effect of an angiotensin II receptor blocker and a calcium channel blocker on hypertension associated penile dysfunction in a rat model. Biomed Res (Tokyo, Japan) 2014;35(3):215–21.

59. Thackeray JT, Radziuk J, Harper ME, et al. Sympathetic nervous dysregulation in the absence of systolic left ventricular dysfunction in a rat model of insulin resistance with hyperglycemia. Cardiovasc diabetology 2011;10:75.

60. Azmi S, Ferdousi M, Alam U, et al. Small-fibre neuropathy in men with type 1 diabetes and erectile dysfunction: a cross-sectional study. Diabetologia 2017;60(6):1094–101.

61. Pavy-Le Traon A, Fontaine S, Tap G, et al. Cardiovascular autonomic neuropathy and other complications in type 1 diabetes. Clin Auton Res 2010;20(3): 153–60.

62. Fode M, Sønksen J. Sexual Function in Elderly Men Receiving Androgen Deprivation Therapy (ADT). Sex Med Rev 2014;2(1):36–46.

63. Köhler TS, Kim J, Feia K, et al. Prevalence of androgen deficiency in men with erectile dysfunction. Urol 2008;71(4):693–7.

64. Corona G, Isidori AM, Buvat J, et al. Testosterone supplementation and sexual function: a meta-analysis study. J Sex Med 2014;11(6):1577–92.

65. Mulhall JP, Trost LW, Brannigan RE, et al. Evaluation and Management of Testosterone Deficiency: AUA Guideline. J Urol 2018;200(2):423–32.

66. Buvat J, Montorsi F, Maggi M, et al. Hypogonadal men nonresponders to the PDE5 inhibitor tadalafil benefit from normalization of testosterone levels with a 1% hydroalcoholic testosterone gel in the treatment of erectile dysfunction (TADTEST study). J Sex Med 2011;8(1):284–93.

67. Granata AR, Rochira V, Lerchl A, et al. Relationship between sleep-related erections and testosterone levels in men. J Androl 1997;18(5):522–7.

68. Aversa A, Isidori AM, De Martino MU, et al. Androgens and penile erection: evidence for a direct relationship between free testosterone and cavernous vasodilation in men with erectile dysfunction. Clin Endocrinol 2000;53(4):517–22.

69. Stoleru SG, Ennaji A, Cournot A, et al. LH pulsatile secretion and testosterone blood levels are influenced by sexual arousal in human males. Psychoneuroendocrinology 1993;18(3):205–18.

70. Becker AJ, Uckert S, Stief CG, et al. Cavernous and systemic testosterone levels in different phases of human penile erection. Urol 2000;56(1):125–9.

71. Giuliano F, Rampin O, Schirar A, et al. Autonomic control of penile erection: modulation by testosterone in the rat. J Neuroendocrinol 1993;5(6): 677–83.

72. Lugg JA, Rajfer J, González-Cadavid NF. Dihydrotestosterone is the active androgen in the maintenance of nitric oxide-mediated penile erection in the rat. Endocrinol 1995;136(4):1495–501.

73. Dai YT, Stopper V, Lewis R, et al. Effects of castration and testosterone replacement on veno-occlusion during penile erection in the rat. Asian J Androl 1999;1(1–2):53–9.

74. Schirar A, Bonnefond C, Meusnier C, et al. Androgens modulate nitric oxide synthase messenger ribonucleic acid expression in neurons of the major pelvic ganglion in the rat. Endocrinol 1997;138(8): 3093–102.

75. Van den Broeck T, Soebadi MA, Falter A, et al. Testosterone Induces Relaxation of Human Corpus Cavernosum Tissue of Patients With Erectile Dysfunction. Sex Med 2020;8(1):114–9.

76. Maggi M, Buvat J, Corona G, et al. Hormonal causes of male sexual dysfunctions and their management

(hyperprolactinemia, thyroid disorders, GH disorders, and DHEA). J Sex Med 2013;10(3):661–77.

77. Leonard MP, Nickel CJ, Morales A. Hyperprolactinemia and impotence: why, when and how to investigate. J Urol 1989;142(4):992–4.

78. Krassas GE, Tziomalos K, Papadopoulou F, et al. Erectile dysfunction in patients with hyper- and hypothyroidism: how common and should we treat? J Clin Endocrinol Metab 2008;93(5):1815–9.

79. Nikoobakht MR, Aloosh M, Nikoobakht N, et al. The role of hypothyroidism in male infertility and erectile dysfunction. Urol J 2012;9(1):405–9.

80. Ma WL, Wang X, Mao JF, et al. [Changes of sex hormones and sex hormone-binding globulin levels in male adults with hyperthyroidism before and after antithyroid drug treatment]. Zhonghua yi xue za zhi 2019;99(24):1875–80.

81. Zheng TS, Ye LX, Wu ZY. [The observation of serum sexual hormone levels before and after treatment in male hyperthyroidisms]. Natl J Androl 2005;11(12):936–8.

82. Carosa E, Di Sante S, Rossi S, et al. Ontogenetic profile of the expression of thyroid hormone receptors in rat and human corpora cavernosa of the penis. J Sex Med 2010;7(4 Pt 1):1381–90.

83. Ozdemirci S, Yildiz F, Utkan T, et al. Impaired neurogenic and endothelium-dependent relaxant responses of corpus cavernosum smooth muscle from hyperthyroid rabbits. Eur J Pharmacol 2001; 428(1):105–11.

84. Hu CL, Wu YD, Liu HT, et al. [Effect of thyroid hormone on the contents of NOS and CO in the penile corpus cavernosum of rats]. Natl J Androl 2009; 15(1):37–40.

85. Karadeniz T, Topsakal M, Aydogmus A, et al. Erectile dysfunction under age 40: etiology and role of contributing factors. TheScientificWorldJournal 2004;4(Suppl 1):171–4.

86. Donatucci CF, Lue TF. Erectile dysfunction in men under 40: etiology and treatment choice. Int J Impot Res 1993;5(2):97–103.

87. Caskurlu T, Tasci AI, Resim S, et al. The etiology of erectile dysfunction and contributing factors in different age groups in Turkey. Int J Urol 2004; 11(7):525–9.

88. Cera N, Delli Pizzi S, Di Pierro ED, et al. Macrostructural alterations of subcortical grey matter in psychogenic erectile dysfunction. PLoS one 2012;7(6): e39118.

Optimizing Outcomes in Penile Implant Surgery

Raul E. Fernandez-Crespo, MD[a,*], Kristina Buscaino, DO[a,1], Rafael Carrion, MD[b,1]

KEYWORDS

- Inflatable penile prosthesis • Penile implant • Erectile dysfunction • Surgical technique
- Intraoperative complications

KEY POINTS

- Since their introduction in the 1970s, penile prostheses have undergone multiple modifications to increase their mechanical reliability, prevent infection, and improve patient satisfaction.
- Selection of implant and surgical approach should be based on patient's anatomy, expectations, and capacity to manipulate the device.
- Intraoperative complications should be recognized and corrected immediately; this is critical for satisfactory outcomes.
- Several techniques, preoperative and intraoperative, can be used to maximize patient satisfaction with respect to penile length and other outcomes.

 Video content accompanies this article at http://www.urologic.theclinics.com.

INTRODUCTION

Penile prosthesis (PP) placement can be considered a first-line option against erectile dysfunction (ED) but is most often used after a patient has failed, has contraindications, or is otherwise not interested in nonsurgical treatment modalities.[1] PP surgery was revolutionized in the early 1970s when groups from the University of Miami and Baylor College introduced semirigid and inflatable devices that could be safely inserted into the penis to create penile turgidity sufficient for intercourse.[2] The soft semirigid penile implant introduced by Drs Small, Carrion, and Gordon served as a pioneer for the current malleable and mechanical semirigid PP.[3] While Drs Scott, Bradley, and Timm from Baylor College introduced the first inflatable penile prosthesis (IPP).[4]

IPP is a mainstay of ED management. A notable advantage of the IPP compared with on-demand modalities and the malleable implant is that it allows the patient to control when he wishes to have an erection while closely mimicking the natural flaccidity and tumescence of the penis.[5] Among the patients with ED who underwent PP surgery, the self-reported satisfaction for three-piece IPP is very high, exceeding 90% in many published series.[6–8]

TYPES OF INFLATABLE PENILE PROSTHESIS

The North American PP market is dominated by two companies: Boston Scientific (BS) and Coloplast (previously American Medical System [AMS] and Mentor, respectively). **Table 1** depicts an update on the long-term outcomes and lifetime survival with the contemporary PP.[9]

[a] Sexual Medicine-Department of Urology, Morsani College of Medicine, University of South Florida, 12901 Bruce B Downs Boulevard, Tampa, FL 33612, USA; [b] Department of Urology, Morsani College of Medicine, University of South Florida, 12901 Bruce B Downs Boulevard, Tampa, FL 33612, USA
[1] Present address: 2 Tampa General Circle, STC 6 Tampa, FL 33606.
* Corresponding author. 2 Tampa General Circle, STC 6, Tampa, FL 33606.
E-mail address: raulf@usf.edu
Twitter: @drrauli (R.E.F.-C.); @drxtinabuscaino (K.B.); @urol11 (R.C.)

Urol Clin N Am 48 (2021) 527–542
https://doi.org/10.1016/j.ucl.2021.06.010
0094-0143/21/Published by Elsevier Inc.

Table 1
Update on the long-term outcomes and lifetime survival combining the existing data for the contemporary penile prosthesis

	5y	8y	10y	15 y
Overall survival rate	90.4%	-	86.6%	-
Mechanical survival rate	94.7%	-	79.4%	71%
Infection rate	-	1.5%	1.8%	-

Data from Dick, B., et al., An update on: long-term outcomes of penile prostheses for the treatment of erectile dysfunction. Expert Rev Med Devices, 2019. **16**(4): p. 281-286.

All contemporary IPPs manufactured by BS are composed of paired, triple-layered cylinders consisting of an inner and outer silicone layer surrounding a middle-woven Dacron and Lyrca layer.[10] The latter is responsible for girth-only expansion or girth and length expansion, with a unidirectional or bidirectional weave configuration of the Dacron and Lycra, respectively.[10] Current models available are the "CX" controlled expansion, "CXR" controlled expansion restricted (useful for scarred or smaller corpora), and the "LGX" length girth expansion.[10] This latter model permits up to a 25% increase in its longitudinal dimension.[11] All of these models are attached to a reservoir via a scrotal pump. The Ambicor inflatable prosthesis omits the reservoir, with fluid stored in the proximal aspect of the cylinders and is transferred to the distal aspect of the cylinders (located in the pendulous phallus) via the operation and activation of a small scrotal pump.[12]

Coloplast's three-piece IPP reservoir and cylinders are made with biocompatible polyurethane material, Bioflex.[13] Current models available are the Titan and Titan narrow-based cylinders.

The scrotal pump is an essential element of any inflatable devices. Older generation pumps were occasionally subject to autoinflation, the phenomenon in which fluid would shunt from the reservoir into the cylinders due to inadequate coaptation. Both the AMS Momentary Squeeze and the Coloplast Touch pumps have a lock-out valve to prevent autoinflation.[14]

PATIENT SELECTION AND SATISFACTION

IPPs have a high satisfaction rate for both the patients and their partners, with greater than 95% for both groups in a large series, regardless of the brand of the implant used.[8] Placement of a PP is associated with a normalization of erectile function in men with severe ED as assessed by the International Index of Erectile Function – Erectile Function

scores (IIEF-EF) domain (mean IIEF-EF 10.1 ± 4.5 vs 23.4 ± 1.5 preoperatively and postoperatively, respectively).[15] Although satisfaction rates are high, an IPP is not necessarily the optimal option for every patient. The famed penile implant surgeon Dr Steve Wilson articulated the importance of patient selection in penile implant surgery, stating "the first thing I wish I had known earlier about prosthetic urology is that just because the patient wants an implant does not mean he is a good candidate."[16] With this in mind, the surgeon's decision to proceed with surgery should not be solely determined by the patient's ED or perceived motivation. Other factors must be considered before moving forward with the procedure from the surgeon's standpoint. These include the patient's past medical and surgical history, overall health status, reasons for their surgical decision, and most importantly, their expectations. The prosthetic surgeon must ensure that the patient's expectations are attainable and realistic, as these are associated with their postoperative satisfaction. Interventions to improve patient's ultimate satisfaction with PP placement must therefore being at the preoperative consultation.

During that initial preoperative consultation, it is also important to identify the "difficult patient." A review of the urologic and cosmetic literature was performed by Trost and colleagues[17] to identify some of the characteristics of these patients. He introduced and described the "CURSED patient," which stands for Compulsive, Unrealistic, Revision, Surgeon shopping, Entitled, Denial, and Psychiatric. These patients are not only psychologically challenging but are also at higher risk for postoperative dissatisfaction. It is imperative to identify these patients in a timely fashion, to properly establish a healthy relationship with them with the ultimate goal of increasing the patient's satisfaction, or to simply avoid operating on them and referring them to another provider.

IMPLANT SELECTION

Implant selection is determined and selected by the surgeon and the patient. There is no high-quality evidence indicating that one manufacturer or model is universally superior to any other.[8] Surgeon preference and experience, as well as patient factors (eg, history, anatomy, expectations), may make a certain PP model superior to others in specific circumstances. In patients whose main concern is penile length maximization, the AMS LGX implant can be considered, as this model will expand more longitudinally rather than circumferentially.[18]

An ex vivo study directly compared AMS 700 LGX and Coloplast Titan in terms of axial and horizontal rigidity, with the Titan implant demonstrating greater rigidity in both variables, and not being as sensitive to the filling pressures as was noted with the LGX cylinders.[18] These results were later confirmed in cadavers as the biomechanical properties of three of the current IPP (ie, AMS CX, AMS LGX, and Coloplast Titan) were evaluated and compared.[19] Both these aforementioned studies can be used as a generalized guide for implant selection in patients scheduled to undergo implantation of an IPP, taking into consideration certain patient's characteristics and expectations/needs; these are summarized in **Table 2**.[18,19] Ultimately, surgical experience is the most critical component in optimizing penile length and axial rigidity so these recommendations should not be seen as absolute.

PREOPERATIVE DETAILS

Most men undergoing PP surgery have multiple comorbid conditions. Appropriate medical and cardiac optimization should be instituted before surgery. Most anticoagulation therapy should be stopped or bridged 3 to 7 days before surgery,[20,21] dependent on the advice of the patient's primary physician or cardiologist. Perioperative aspirin may be safely continued if medically necessary.[22]

Prevention of Infections

Any type of foreign material implanted in the body has the inherent risk of becoming infected. Improvement in materials and surgical techniques

have decreased but not eliminated infection as a complication of PP surgery. Tobacco use is associated with a higher risk of infection and/or need for revision surgery; smoking cessation should thus be recommended to patients who are tobacco users.[23,24]

Most PP infections are caused by skin flora, and it is unlikely that they are necessarily influenced by the sterility of the preoperative urine culture.[25] Nevertheless, a urine culture should be part of the patient's preoperative evaluation and when possible, should be negative. Patient's prone to urinary tract infections are placed on antibiotic therapy several days before the procedure to ensure the urine sterility on the day of surgery.[26]

Some surgeons recommend that patients shower with chlorhexidine several days before surgery to decrease the risk of surgical site infection. A Cochrane review[27] did not demonstrate any benefit of preoperative bathing with chlorhexidine over placebo or a bar of soap. However, the rate of surgical site infection is lower when the skin is prepped with chlorhexidine-alcohol scrub compared with povidone iodine scrub.[28] Skin cultures taken after prep with the above solutions and before implantation of a genitourinary prosthetic device demonstrated that chlorhexidine was superior in the eradication of skin flora.[29]

Data from the general surgery literature have indicated that the use of razors for shaving is associated with an increased risk of surgical site infection when compared with other modalities including clippers and chemical depilation.[30,31]

Table 2
Recommendations for the selection of inflatable penile prosthesis by model and patient's characteristic

	AMS CX®	AMS LGX®	Coloplast Titan®
Penile size	-	Allows for longitudinal expansion	-
Rigidity	Best rigidity in short phalluses	-	Overall best rigidity, and best rigidity in longer phalluses
Intromission force	-	-	Better suited for those patients whose partners require more force for intromission
Corporal fibrosis Peyronie's disease	-	-	Overall best implant
Difficulty compressing the pump	-	On LTMI, unable to withstand the force needed for vaginal penetration	Best implant, since on LTMI, provides the best rigidity

Abbreviation: LTMI, less than maximum inflation.
 Data from Scovell, J.M., et al., Longitudinal and Horizontal Load Testing of Inflatable Penile Implant Cylinders of Two Manufacturers: An Ex Vivo Demonstration of Inflated Rigidity. J Sex Med, 2016. **13**(11): p. 1750-1757; and Wallen, J.J., et al., Biomechanical Comparison of Inflatable Penile Implants: A Cadaveric Pilot Study. J Sex Med, 2018. **15**(7): p. 1034-1040.

Although this may be true in smooth skin areas, the scrotal skin is elastic with irregular folds, making it unsuitable in many cases for trimming with clippers.[32] Moreover, the use of a razor for hair removal of the male genitalia results in less skin trauma and a better prepped surgical field without an increased risk for surgical site infection, when directly compared with clippers.[32] The Sexual Medicine Society of North America (SMSNA) recommends that the surgeon uses the hair removal strategy that he/she prefers,[33] not necessarily what hospital policy might dictate. Shaving before the day of surgery is not recommended because if any nicks or cuts occur, bacteria may colonize these areas.[26]

Antibiotic prophylaxis is used to prevent postprocedural infections.[34] These should be administered 1 to 2 hours before the surgical incision.[12,34] The current antibiotic recommendations by the American Urological Association for patients undergoing PP placement are depicted in **Table 3**.[34] Fluconazole or other antifungal medication may be indicated in diabetic patients and in those with a history of fungal rashes in the groin area.[22,35]

A groundbreaking advancement in PP infection prevention was the introduction of antibiotic cylinder coatings. AMS introduced the Inhibizone antibiotic coating in 2001, which is present in all the components of the implant, with the exception of the rear tip extenders.[36,37] The external surface of the silicone cylinder is impregnated with two antibiotics, Rifampin and Minocycline, dispersing to the surrounding tissue creating a zone of bacterial growth inhibition.[36] When both antibiotic-impregnated and nonantibiotic impregnated devices from AMS are directly compared, the use of Inhibizone coated devices is associated with a lower revision rate for infection-related complications (2.5% in noncoated vs 1.1% in coated devices at a mean follow-up of 7.7 years).[38]

Mentor introduced, in 2002, the Titan implant coated with a hydrophilic substance, polyvinylpyrrolidone (PVP), which is covalently bonded to surface of the prosthesis. PVP inhibits bacterial adherence to the implant. This PVP coating also absorbs antibiotics when the device is immersed in antibiotic solution; this feature allows the surgeon to coat the implant in antibiotics of their preference, which are subsequently eluted into tissue postplacement.[36,39] A trimethropim/sulfamethoxazole solution "dip" for Coloplast's implant has been demonstrated very effective in preventing infection when compared with other antibiotic dips, exhibiting effectiveness against *Staphylococcus epidermidis*, *Staphylococcus lidgunensis*, *Staphylococcus aureus*, *Pseudomonas*, and *Enterococcus*.[39] However, the choice of antibiotic can be customized to local antibiograms.

Intraoperative irrigation of the surgical field with antibiotic solution during primary implantation is commonly practiced although evidence bases for this practice are weak.[40] The most common solution is aminoglycoside-based irrigation alone or with a combination of either vancomycin or a cephalosporin.[41] When a prosthesis is already coated with an antibiotic solution, copious irrigation may actually cause elution of these antibiotics before insertion and should be avoided.[40]

Diabetic patients

Diabetic patients have an increased risk of infection requiring surgery after initial implantation; the reason for this is likely multifactorial.[42] Chronic hyperglycemic environments are known to blunt the body's immune response, generate poor circulation subsequently delaying and causing poor wound healing, leading to end-organ damage; thus creating an ideal environment for bacterial growth.[42,43]

Serum hemoglobin A1C (HbA1C) is a measure of average glucose control over the past 3 to 4 months. Many implanting surgeons use this metric to screen patients before surgery.[43] Although this is commonly used as a screening tool by numerous implanters, the published data are very contradictory and inconsistent.

It is noteworthy to highlight that using this measurement to evaluate the susceptibility of diabetic

---

Table 3
Antibiotic prophylaxis recommendations for prosthetic urologic surgery as per the American Urological Association

Antimicrobial of Choice	Antimicrobial Alternative
• Aminoglycoside and • 1st/2nd generation Cephalosporin 　or Vancomycin	• Aminopenicillin 　○ Ampicillin/Sulbactam 　○ Ticarcillin/Clavulanate 　○ Piperacillin/Tazobactam

Data from Wolf, J.S., Jr., et al., Best practice policy statement on urologic surgery antimicrobial prophylaxis. J Urol, 2008. **179**(4): p. 1379-90.

patients to develop an infection after a PP placement, an assumption is indirectly being made in which the risk of infection is only associated with the glycemic control of the past 3 months; completely ignoring the end-organ damage associated with chronic hyperglycemia.

In a prospective multicenter study, Habous and colleagues[44] established that a threshold HbA1c of 8.5% could be used to identify diabetic patients who are at higher risk to develop a penile implant infection. Having the procedure performed by a low volume surgeon as well as a diagnosis of Peyronie's disease was also identified as predictors of infections. The data presented by Canguven and colleagues,[45] as well as the data presented by Osman and colleagues,[46] did not find any association between postoperative infection rates after penile implantation in diabetic patients with the serum HbA1c. In both these studies, high-volume implanters performed the procedures, but both were retrospective in nature. The mean HbA1c in all three studies were 8%, 7.6%, and 7.5%, respectively.

All 3 studies have multiple limitations. Although Habous study[44] is the only one prospective in nature, the infection rate presented was almost 9%. It is noteworthy to mention that around one-third of the implants placed were in patients with PD, in which increased operative time secondary to additional procedures were undertaken. Also "high volume surgeons" were those who performed more than 5 procedures per year. Both Canguven's[45] and Osman's[46] data are retrospective in nature; therefore, an inherent bias is present. Also, the infected group in Canguven's[45] data is very small, therefore drawing conclusions from it can be problematic, despite their results suggest that indeed there is no associated risk of infection with serum HbA1c.

Although controversy exists as to whether preoperative HbA1c or blood glucose is predictive of infection risk, diabetic patients, in general, are known to be at increased risk for infection, and optimization of glycemic control is recommended before PP placement.[20,23] Serum HbA1C can be used as an objective measure of medical compliance and need for perioperative glucose control.[22]

Pain Management

Appropriate pain management is crucial for postoperative success.[47] Currently, postoperative pain control is focused on minimizing opioid usage.[48] Multimodal analgesia (MMA), consisting of local nerve block and medications acting on different pathways, are being incorporated into the PP surgery field.[48,49] Preemptive analgesia is

based on this principle, preventing the sensitization of the central and the peripheral nervous system nociceptors.[50] The use of cyclooxygenase-2 inhibitors, gabapentin and acetaminophen, provided 1 to 2 hours before the incision, have been demonstrated to be effective in the prevention of inflammatory chemicals, and thus improving postoperative pain control.[50] Local nerve blocks will help with pain relief immediately and after the procedure, preventing pain signal propagation from the surgical site.[51] A dorsal penile nerve block before IPP placement demonstrated less pain immediately and 4 hours in the postoperative period in men who received the block compared with those who did not receive it.[51] **Table 4** depicts the MMA published by Lucas and colleagues.[49]

SURGICAL TECHNIQUES
Approach and Incision

Placement of the IPP can be done through several approaches, with the penoscrotal (PS) and the infrapubic (IP) most commonly used in North America. Satisfaction and infection rates are not conclusively influenced by the surgical approach so neither approach appears intrinsically superior.[52]

The subcoronal (SC) approach has also been described for placement of multicomponent PP, although it is more traditionally used for semirigid penile implantation. Weiberg and colleagues[53] described their technique for placement of a three-piece IPP through a SC incision accompanied by a modified no-touch technique. In their publication, they cite that one of the main advantages of this approach—in addition to its excellent cosmetic results—is the exposure provided to the corporas allowing additional reconstructive procedures to be performed (ie, penile plication, incision/excision of plaque with/without patch grafting), which are of critical importance, especially in patients with Peyronie's disease.

With the PS approach, an indwelling Foley catheter is typically placed before starting the procedure to drain the bladder for reservoir placement if the space of Retzius is used, and to assist identification of the urethra during initial dissection.[54] The initial incision may be performed vertically or transversely.[13] A vertical incision may be extended proximally or distally if needed, the latter can aid in more corporal exposure. A frog-leg position can be used to this approach, allowing easier distal dilation.

The tunica albuginea of the corpora can be exposed using the Henry Finger Sweep Technique[55] preventing the use of sharp dissection, further minimizing any potential injury to the corpus spongiosum/urethra, and bleeding.

Table 4
Multimodal analgesia pathway

Preoperative	Intraoperative	Postoperative	Discharge
Acetaminophen 975 mg Gabapentin 300–600 mg Meloxicam 7.5–15 mg or Celecoxib 200 mg	Pudendal nerve block Dorsal penile nerve block	Acetaminophen 975 mg q 6h Gabapentin 300 mg TID Meloxicam 7.5–15 mg or Celecoxib 200 mg daily Oxycodone 5 mg q 4h PRN for moderate pain Morphine 2 mg q 2h or Hydromorphone 1 mg q 3h for severe pain	Acetaminophen 975 mg q 6h Gabapentin 300 mg TID Meloxicam 7.5–15 mg or Celecoxib 200 mg daily Oxycodone 5 mg q 4h PRN for moderate pain
All meds given x1 dose	Consisting of 10 mL of 0.5% Marcaine and 10 mL of 1% Lidocaine		30-d supply of MMA and 3-d supply or opioid-based medication

Data from [Lucas, J., et al., A Multi-institutional Assessment of Multimodal Analgesia in Penile Implant Recipients Demonstrates Dramatic Reduction in Pain Scores and Narcotic Usage. J Sex Med, 2020. **17**(3): p. 518-525].

The scrotal septum should be separated from the urethral attachment for better proximal corporal exposure,[56] with sutures preplaced as proximally as exposure allows. A 1.5 to 2 cm corporotomy is then performed on both corporal bodies. Proximal placement of corporotomies is crucial to assure tubing exits into the scrotum and not into the penile skin, which can create a "tail-pipe" appearance and poor cosmetic result.[56] If the corporotomies need to be extended, this should be done proximally if possible.[56]

The PS approach is well-suited for obese patients.[57] It allows for easier distal dilation and the ability to directly fix the scrotal pump to prevent its migration, and also avoids the possibility of injuring the neurovascular bundle (NVB).[56] Blind placement of the reservoir and increased postoperative scrotal swelling are the main disadvantages of the PS approach.[56]

The IP approach was initially popularized by Dr William Furlow.[13] The incision is performed between the pubis and the penis, either vertically or horizontally.[5] The former can be specifically considered in patients with bilateral hernia repairs with mesh. Patients are positioned in the dorsal recumbent position and the table should be hyperextended, creating a flat surface in the area of the mons pubis, allowing easier and more accurate distal dilation and measurement.[58]

The IP approach is associated with shorter operative times and allows direct visualization for reservoir placement.[52,59] Anecdotally, less scrotal edema is noted and the training for inflation of the prosthesis can be started earlier, when compared with the PS approach.[52] To avoid injuring the NVB, the corporotomies should be made dorsally using a blade (not electrocautery) at 10 and 2-o'clock.[26] In revision surgeries with abundant scar tissue, electrocautery may be needed for dissection and for performing the corporotomies.[5]

The principle disadvantages of the IP approach include difficulty placing and fixing the pump within the scrotum, limited corporeal exposure, greater odds of tubing being palpable postoperatively, and the inherent risk of injury to the dorsal nerve of the penis.[5] Patients are encouraged to gently pull on the pump in the immediate postoperative period to reduce the risk of cephalad pump migration.[60] Shah and colleagues[60] developed and published a technique to reduce bother from palpable tubing by creating a subphallic window to pass the contralateral cylinder's tubing to the side where the pump will be located.

Dilation

During the dilation process, crossover and/or perforation of the corpora can occur either proximally or distally. To avoid this, the dilating instrument should be pointed slightly laterally to the axis of the penis and advanced with gradual and gentle pressure.[54] When dilating distally, the tip of the instrument used should be slightly visible under the skin as dilation progresses.[61] Crossover should be suspected when the measurements of the corporas are different, if symmetry is not noted on placing dilators bilaterally in each corporal cavity, when the second cylinder is not easily threaded or when the erection looks lopsided, tilted, or unusual.[61] See **Fig. 1** and Video 1.

When crossover is encountered, a dilator should be placed in the common cavity and the contralateral space developed, ensuring that dilation is directed laterally to avoid entering the common cavity.[61] Careful use of Metzembaum scissors and the subsequent use of dilators can aid in the development of this new space. On developing this space properly, with the contralateral dilator in place, the ipsilateral cylinder is threaded and placed in the new cavity.[61] Only then can the dilator be removed and the second cylinder placed.[61] This troubleshooting maneuver can be used for both proximal and distal crossover.

Proximal perforation should be suspected when there is a sudden loss of resistance to dilation and the dilator is not noted in its expected resting area along the ischial tuberosity.[20,61] This can be confirmed performing the "classic field goal test" (**Fig. 2**). If a narrow dilator was initially used, a larger dilator should be used to see if it rests on the bone avoiding further dilation of the false passage.[57,61] Proximal migration of inflatable cylinders is not common, mainly because of the presence of the input tubing exiting the cylinders and the corpora.[61] Risk of migration is higher in malleable implants. Tightly closing the corpora at the point of tubing exits may prevent adverse outcomes from proximal perforation, especially in the setting of small proximal perforations.[62] A suture sling should be considered in all cases, especially in the setting of a large proximal perforation.[62] A suture sling consists of a nonabsorbable suture passed through the tunica on one side of the corporotomy, then through the proximal end of the implant cylinder, and finally through the tunica of the contralateral corporotomy edge. This suture should be cut at least 1 cm in length so it can be easily located in the future if a revision surgery is warranted/performed.[61] When a proximal perforation occurs, the length of the unaffected corpora should be used to size the implant.[20] Formal repair of a proximal crural perforation is of minimal benefit and carries substantial risk.[63]

Distal urethral and corporal perforation can be identified by grossly noticing the dilator through the meatus/corporal defect, or by a positive "distal fluid challenge test" (Video 2); where fluid is present shooting out of the meatus/corporal defect when the ipsilateral corpora is irrigated.[62] In the setting of distal perforation, the safest course of

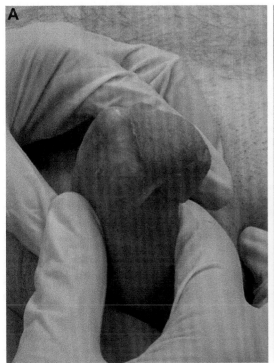
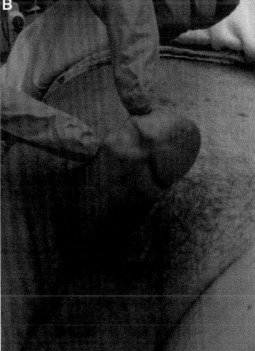

Fig. 1. (*A, B*) Two different patients with a left to right distal crossover, both noted postoperatively.

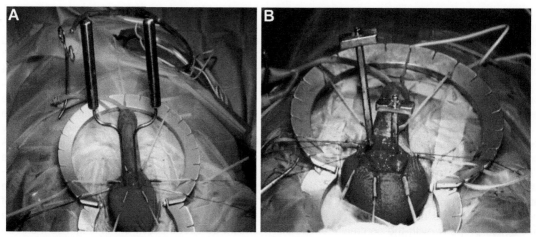

Fig. 2. (*A*) A negative "field goal test". (*B*) Positive "field goal test" with a left-sided proximal perforation.

action is to abort the procedure and return at a later date.[62] As this injury heals, corporal fibrosis will inevitably occur. For this reason, some surgeons advocate the placement of a single cylinder in the contralateral side if it has been successfully dilated before the distal perforation.[62] If the penile urethra is injured during the initial corporal/scrotal exposure, the injury should be repaired in 2 nonoverlapping layers and the procedure could be continued.[20] In this setting, an indwelling Foley catheter should be left in place only for a few days. However, if the laceration is only limited to the corpus spongiosum, it should also be repaired, without the need to leave the catheter in place.

Corporal Measurement

A more aggressive form of corporal measurement (new measurement length technique) has been promulgated to address penile shortening, the most common complaint among men undergoing IPP placement.[64] With this approach, 1 cm is added to the total length measurement so long as the dilator does not reach midglans or ischial bone when dilating distally and proximally, respectively.

The length for each corpora is measured individually and the "classic field goal test" can be used to assess the presence of crossover or perforation. This is especially useful in the setting of any length discrepancy. If none are present and the length discrepancy is less than 2 cm, then the larger measurement should be the one used.[54,64] If the measurement discrepancy is more than 2 cm, a careful reassessment should be done, as this may represent a technical error.[54,64]

Cylinder Placement

After both cylinders are completely seated inside the corpora, they should be test inflated to ensure

that the distal tips are symmetric and in the midglans area. Persistent bulging through the corporotomy, significant buckling of the cylinders inside the corporas, or the presence of a new-onset severe curvature should raise the suspicion for oversizing (**Fig. 3**, Video 3). Undersizing or improper distal dilation may present with glans bowing also known as "floppy glans" (**Fig. 4**).[12] When this is noted intraoperatively and distal dilation was properly performed, a rear-tip extender should be placed to increase the total length of the cylinder and assessing if the issue was corrected or not.[12] If distal dilation has not been properly performed, this should be repeated with the subsequent addition of rear-tip extenders as indicated to permit the cylinders to reach the midglans.

The surgeon should avoid having the input tubing run intracorporally secondary to possible decreased length for the pump to reach the most dependent aspect of the scrotum and because this can hinder the cycling process of the inflatable penile implant.[26] If the corporas are tight or severely fibrotic, narrow cylinders (ie, CXR or Titan narrow base) should be placed.[20]

The AMS 700 series implants have a polytetrafluoroethylene sleeve surrounding the tubing adjacent to the cylinders. These were introduced in 1983 to prevent friction damage of the single-layered silicone cylinder on contact with input tubing. It is our practice to remove these before placement, particularly when using an IP approach, as the potential scar these sleeves may form in the vicinity of the NVB may complicate revision or replacement surgery.[62]

Reservoir Placement

Reservoir placement is one of the most critical aspects of PP placement. Life-threatening

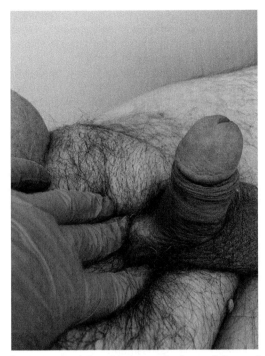

Fig. 3. Proximal dorsal bulge at the base of the penis secondary to oversizing the cylinders.

complications (ie, bowel or bladder perforation, major vascular injury) may occur with blind placement of a reservoir. Some surgeons advise against the placement of three-piece PP in patients with extensive retroperitoneal scarring that may make reservoir placement difficult or dangerous.[54]

Traditionally, the PP reservoir is placed in the Space of Retzius (SOR). Patients with a history of pelvic surgery or radiation may have extensive scarring, making placement of the reservoir in this space inadvisable.[61] Placement of the reservoir in a tightly scarred space adjacent to the bladder can cause urinary urgency/frequency and may even predispose the patient to bladder erosion.[61]

Placement of the reservoir in the space of Retzius

Regardless of the approach used to place the implant, the bladder must be emptied before placing the reservoir in the SOR with placement of a Foley catheter. If there is difficulty placing a catheter, the surgeon must consider addressing any urethral issues immediately and postponing the prosthetic surgery.[62] To ensure an uneventful catheter placement, some surgeons perform a cystoscopy as part of their preoperative workup.[62]

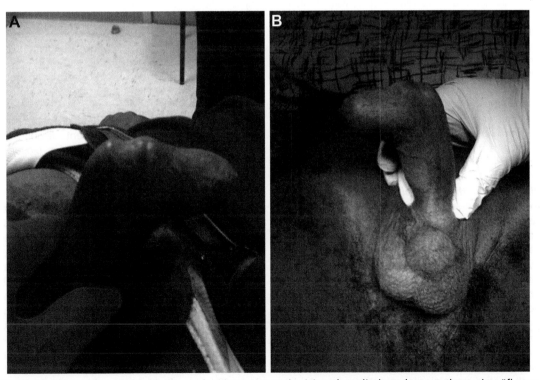

Fig. 4. (*A*, *B*) Improper distal dilation with subsequent undersizing the cylinder subsequently causing "floppy glans."

After the bladder is emptied, the patient should be reclined in Trendelenburg position to increase safety.[54] Gravitational force causes the bladder, bowel, and abdominal fat to move cephalad, away from the inguinal ring. This also decompresses the external iliac vein, decreasing the chances of a vascular injury. The reservoir's lockout valve should not be placed against a hard structure (ie, pubic bone) because constant pressure may indent the valve, causing it to malfunction and autoinflate.[26]

Despite all these maneuvers for safe reservoir placement, immediate intraoperative complications can occur. If gross hematuria is noted, a cystoscopy with or without a cystogram should be performed.[20] Alternatively, the surgical assistant can distend the bladder with a mixture of normal saline and methylene blue[21] to assess the integrity of the bladder. If an injury is encountered, the procedure should be halted and attention turned to the repair of the bladder.

A vascular injury can occur when placing or removing the reservoir. If copious blood is noted in the surgical field during this step, the surgeon should place pressure and the incision extended for better exposure. An intraoperative consultation from a vascular surgeon is strongly recommended.[61] The procedure must be aborted and general surgery service consulted if the bowel is injured.[20]

Herniation of the reservoir is rare, with an incidence of less than 1%, almost exclusively seen with the PS approach.[12] This may be secondary to vigorous coughing in the postoperative period, or more commonly due to an initial failure of proper reservoir placement.[12] When this is noted in the immediate postoperative period, the reservoir can be replaced through the same PS incision.[12] Alternatively, a small ipsilateral inguinal counter-incision can be performed and the reservoir placed in the perivesical space, while the defect is closed from above.[12]

Placement of the reservoir in alternate locations

As previously described, life-threatening injuries can arise when placing the reservoir in the SOR. Alternative locations have been sought out and evaluated to promote patient safety. With the introduction of the lockout valve within the reservoir/pump, autoinflation is no longer a major concern.

Before development of the "poplet" valve, all reservoirs allowed water to flow freely within the system with changes in abdominal pressure, increasing the risk of autoinflation.[36] The concept of alternative reservoir placement was introduced and first published by Wilson and colleagues[65] in 2002. Eventually, further modifications regarding reservoir construction and development allowed these to be placed in ectopic/alternative locations, while being more easily concealed.[16]

Through the IP and PS approaches, as well as through a counter incision, Perito[66,67] has provided and described detailed anatomic landmarks with placement of the reservoir anterior or posterior to transversalis fascia. Hakky and colleagues[68] published their technique for placement of the reservoir in the submuscular space. Morey and colleagues[69] presented their technique for safely placing the reservoir in a high submuscular space through a PS approach, without the need for a counter incision with the aid of a Foerster lung clamp.[69] Placement of the reservoir in the subcutaneous space can be considered in significantly obese patients; the potential for a palpable pump remains an important consideration and subcutaneous placement should be avoided if at all possible..[23] These strategies have provided options to surgeons in terms of reservoir placement; however, the final locations can be different from the intraoperative assessment.

Hemostasis and Drains

Adequate intraoperative hemostasis is key during any surgical procedure, especially with penile implant surgery. Watertight corporotomies and careful hemostasis of the subdartos pouch must be performed. Closure is typically performed in multiple layers, with 2 layers of absorbable suture before closure of the skin. At the end of the procedure, the cylinders can be left partially inflated to aid with hemostasis by compression of the corporal edges.

Inadequate hemostasis may lead to postoperative hematomas, increasing patient discomfort and risk of infection.[70,71] The use of a closed-suction drain after PP placement is controversial. Some experts argue that a drain represents a risk for infection through retrograde bacterial migration.[72] Proponents of drain placement tout decreased rates of hematoma formation and increased patient comfort in the postoperative period.[72] The incidence of hematoma formation, ecchymosis, and scrotal swelling is less if a closed-suction drain is used. In regards to scrotal hematomas, Wilson and colleagues[73] reported an incidence of 0.9% and almost 3% in patients with and without a drain, respectively. A Jackson-Pratt drain left in place after uncomplicated IPP placement can drain between 75 and 100 mL[74] within the first 24 hours. Drains are typically removed 24 to 48 hours after surgery, when output is less than 50 mL in 8 hours.[56]

MAXIMIZING PENILE LENGTH (PERCEPTION)

Stretched penile length (SPL, the distance from the pubic bone to the tip of the glans of the penis) should be measured and documented before surgery.[75] Using the same points of reference, erect length can be measured after a pharmacologically induced erection. Both measurements provide excellent predictors of postoperative inflated penile length.[75] Decreased penile size is the main cause of disappointment after penile implant surgery.[61] Most men will have an objective decrease in length postimplantation.[75,76] Perception is of critical import, because patients who have not been counseled may expect to recover the penile length they recall having (which may not necessarily be their factual length) before onset of ED.[77] Lack of glans engorgement occurs after IPP placement, may play a role in the perception of lost penile length.[76] Aside from issues of perception, one cause for "penile shortening" after PP relates to tissue healing, which may lead to the formation of a pseudocapsule. This capsule may eliminate the elastic properties of the tunica albuginea surrounding the corpora cavernosa.[61] Generalized patient issues such as weight gain and increased pubic fat can lead to the perception of a shorter penile length.[77]

Some surgeons recommend that patients use a vacuum erection device (VED) without penile constriction rings to stimulate daily penile engorgement starting at least 1 to 2 months before the surgery.[78,79] This technique is intended to reduce length loss implantation, not to actually increase penis size.[79] Patient compliance is critical for this protocol; close engagement may help set up realistic postoperative expectations and improved satisfaction with final penile length.[79] Subjectively, Sellers and colleagues[79] reported that the use of the VED helps improve the compliance of the corpora, decreasing the postoperative pain on cylinder inflation, as well as easier pump cycling. However, any evidence of objective measurements to support these claims were not reported.

Penile traction devices are touted as an alternative to VED and are recommended by some experts. Levine and colleagues[80] reported their experience on 10 patients administering external traction therapy with the FastSize penile extender (Aliso Viejo, CA, USA). In their protocol, this device was used daily for a minimum of 2 hours for 2 to 4 months before PP placement. Before and after SPL were measured; and an average increase of 1.5 cm was noted in all men after the use of the device, before the PP implantation. After PP implantation, only 70% of them demonstrated an increase in length post-traction but none reported loss of length. As with the use of a VED, using traction therapy directly involves the patient in their care and helps to understand the limitations of increasing penile length.[80]

Several adjuvant procedures may be performed at the time of PP placement to maximize the perception of penile length, without increasing actual measurement.[81] The suspensory ligamentous system of the penis is composed of the fundiform ligament, the suspensory ligament, and the arcuate subpubic ligament.[82] These ligaments are responsible for fixing, supporting, and stabilizing the penis to the pubis, while maintaining it toward the front.[82] The net effect of these ligaments is to aid penile penetration.[83]

Releasing this ligament surgically may permit the penis to slightly lay more dependently, giving it an apparent increase in length at the expense of some degree of penile stability.[83] After adequate exposure, the ligament is divided close to the pubic bone while the penis is held on stretch, ensuring all the midline attachments have been freed.[83] Typically, this will allow for a lengthening of 1 to 2 cm of the flaccid penis. Intraoperative and postoperative strategies have been described to optimize outcome with this technique.[83] Patients should be advised that the slight increase in length might be offset by penile instability, making intercourse more difficult.

Release of the PS web can provide the perception of increased penile length. The use of a Z-plasty, either single or double, skin closure has been extensively described for the correction of the PS web with excellent cosmetic results.[84]

Miranda-Sousa and colleagues[85] described two ventral phalloplasty techniques for excising the PS web during implantation of an IPP. One using a V-shape incision and another using a checkmark-shaped incision to excise the web, with the latter preferred as it avoids any residual "dog-ears." Attention to the closure is emphasized using interrupted sutures, both in the deep layers as well as in the skin, to avoid superficial wound separation. This is a safe and easy technique that improves patient satisfaction, is easily reproducible and only adds an average of 12 minutes intraoperatively.[85]

In another series, Gupta and colleagues[86] reported the use of a high longitudinal PS incision with a V-Y-plasty closure to reduce the PS webbing at the time of initial IPP placement. Patients who underwent correction of the PS web with this technique and those who were diabetic were more likely to experience wound dehiscence complications. With the latter still being a risk factor for wound dehiscence even when the scrotoplasty technique was changed to the one described by Miranda-Sousa and colleagues.[85]

In obese patients, the suprapubic fat pad can contribute to an apparent decreased phallic length due to burying of the penis under the panniculus.[81,87] Baumgarten and colleagues[87] presented their experience, which consisted of 8 patients with an average body mass index of 36.6 kg/m^2, who underwent suprapubic fat pad excision with concomitant IP IPP placement. The technique used is thoroughly detailed in their publication, emphasizing the key elements of patient positioning and marking. In their limited pilot series, only one patient required explantation due to prosthetic infection, whose postoperative course was remarkable for inadvertent removal of both subcutaneous drains during postoperative day zero.

POSTOPERATIVE CARE

Close postsurgical follow-up has to be provided to maximize patient satisfaction, assess for any complications that may arise, and to ensure that the device has been adequately placed and is functioning correctly.[77] Patients are instructed to use supportive underwear for at least the first month. During this time, the patient is encouraged to keep the penis in the cephalad position (ie, against the abdomen).[54] Strenuous and sexual activity should be avoided during the first 6 weeks after the procedure.

A recent retrospective study compared patients with and without risk factors who did not receive antibiotic therapy, and those with risk factors who did receive antibiotics.[88] It showed no difference among the 3 groups in regard to device explantation due to infection or for any cause, nor for nonoperative infectious complications. Another retrospective study demonstrated that despite two-thirds of patients receiving oral antibiotics after IPP placement, explantation rates did not differ when compared with those who did not receive them.[89] Despite lack of evidence supporting the value and use of oral antibiotics more than 24 hours postoperatively, many prosthetic surgeons do so; a survey among members of the Sexual Medicine Society of North America (SMSNA) demonstrated that 94% prescribed them.[41]

Scrotal ecchymosis and edema are commonly encountered after placement of a PP, especially when using the PS approach. Ice packs can be used for the first 48 hours.[21] If a scrotal hematoma occurs, it typically resolves conservatively without the need for surgical intervention, as long as the incision is closed.[71,77] However, if the incision is open and/or has bloody drainage, surgical exploration, hematoma evacuation, and placement of a new closed-suction drained are recommended, as established by an algorithm described by Garber and Bickell.[71] Anticoagulation should be held (when possible) for at least 5 days and preferably 10 to 14 to decrease the risk of delayed hematoma formation.[21,71]

Patients are typically taught how to cycle their devices 2 to 4 weeks postoperatively; pain is the most common limiting factor for early device cycling. After IPP placement, the cylinders are often left partially inflated and should not remain this way for a prolonged period because of the potential for capsule formation around the reservoir. A capsule around the reservoir may restrict the expansion of the reservoir, limiting the cylinders to fully deflate.[77] After being taught how to cycle their device, patients are instructed to start cycling their device and maintaining it inflated initially for 15 minutes (or as tolerated) every day, with each day increasing the time that they are able to maintain/tolerate it inflated up to a maximum of 1 hour. This is typically used during the first 6 to 8 weeks postoperatively. Afterward, they are instructed to cycle the device on a daily basis.

Henry and colleagues[90] published an aggressive postoperative rehabilitation (coupled with NLMT) with maximum inflation of the device for 1 to 2 hours daily for 1-year postimplantation. Penile measurements in the immediate postoperative period were compared to the measurements obtained after the postoperative inflation rehabilitation was performed for 1 year. The measurements obtained from pubic bone to meatus demonstrated an increase by 1.14 cm ($P = .003$), 0.99 cm ($P = .002$), and 1.04 cm ($P = .006$) for erect, flaccid, and stretched penis. The circumference as well as the width of the penis also increased significantly during this period ($1.08 + 0.82$, $P = .001$ and $.47 + 0.32$, $P = .001$, respectively). All these increased measurements were demonstrated to be statistically significant.

SUMMARY

In patients undergoing initial PP placement, the best chance for a successful end result rests within this initial attempt.[77] It is extremely important that the prosthetic surgeon adheres to the evidence-based guidelines and recommendations to ensure uneventful placement with the best outcomes.

CLINICS CARE POINTS

- The patient's and the partner's expectations should be met; during the preoperative evaluation, proper counseling should be performed to ensure that these expectations are realistic and attainable.

- Decreased penile length is the main reason for the patient's lack of satisfaction after the surgery. Patient satisfaction may be enhanced with the aid of adjuvant procedures including the use of VED and traction devices as well as release of suspensory ligament, ventral phalloplasty, and suprapubic fat pad excision.

- AMS' LGX implant can be recommended in patients with short penises, as it will allow for some longitudinal expansion, and avoided in patients with significant fibrosis and Peyronie's disease.

- Intraoperative irrigation with antibiotic solution during first-time implants is commonly practiced despite no actual evidence suggests any actual benefit.

- Preoperative showering with chlorhexidine does not decrease the risk of infections but the use of a chlorhexidine-alcohol scrub for skin prep does decrease the risk of infection.

- The American Urological Association has guidelines regarding preoperative antibiotics in patients who are going to be undergoing prosthetic placement. There is no high-grade evidence that perioperative antibiotics beyond 24 hours of surgery decrease the risk of infection or repeat surgery.

- No definitive value for HbA1C in diabetic patients has been established as associated with markedly increased risk of infection; diabetes control should nevertheless be optimized before PP placement.

- A multimodal analgesia protocol should be used for pain management to decrease the need for postoperative opioids.

- The use of a closed-suction drain prevents hematoma formation and scrotal edema; there is no evidence that drain placement increases the risk of infection.

DISCLOSURE

R.E. Fernandez-Crespo and K. Buscaino have nothing to disclose. R. Carrion is a consultant for Coloplast and Endo Pharmaceutical.

SUPPLEMENTARY DATA

Supplementary data related to this article can be found online at https://doi.org/10.1016/j.ucl.2021.06.010.

REFERENCES

1. Nose BD, Grimberg DCD, Lentz AC. Update on Intraoperative Cultures, Biofilms, and Modifiable Factors During Revision of Clinically Non-Infected Penile Implants. Sex Med Rev 2021;9(1):160–8.

2. Carrion H, Martinez D, Parker J, et al. A History of the Penile Implant to 1974. Sex Med Rev 2016;4(3):285–93.

3. Small MP, Carrion HM, Gordon JA. Small-Carrion penile prosthesis. New implant for management of impotence. Urology 1975;5(4):479–86.

4. Scott FB, Bradley WE, Timm GW. Management of erectile impotence. Use of implantable inflatable prosthesis. Urology 1973;2(1):80–2.

5. Montague DK, Angermeier KW. Inflatable penile prosthesis: The American Medical Systems' Experience. In: Carson CC, editor. Urologic prosthesis: the complete guide to devices, their implantation, and patient follow up. Totowa (NJ): Humana Press Inc.; 2002. p. 179–90.

6. Wilson SK, Delk JR, Salem EA, et al. Long-term survival of inflatable penile prostheses: single surgical group experience with 2,384 first-time implants spanning two decades. J Sex Med 2007;4(4 Pt 1):1074–9.

7. Habous M, Tal R, Tealab A, et al. Predictors of Satisfaction in Men After Penile Implant Surgery. J Sex Med 2018;15(8):1180–6.

8. Cayan S, Aşcı R, Efesoy O, et al. Comparison of Long-Term Results and Couples' Satisfaction with Penile Implant Types and Brands: Lessons Learned From 883 Patients With Erectile Dysfunction Who Underwent Penile Prosthesis Implantation. J Sex Med 2019;16(7):1092–9.

9. Dick B, Tsambarlis P, Reddy A, et al. An update on: long-term outcomes of penile prostheses for the treatment of erectile dysfunction. Expert Rev Med Devices 2019;16(4):281–6.

10. Mulcahy JJ. The Development of Modern Penile Implants. Sex Med Rev 2016;4(2):177–89.

11. Pastuszak AW, Lentz AC, Farooq A, et al. Technological Improvements in Three-Piece Inflatable Penile Prosthesis Design over the Past 40 Years. J Sex Med 2015;12(Suppl 7):415–21.

12. Sadeghi-Nejad H. Penile prosthesis surgery: a review of prosthetic devices and associated complications. J Sex Med 2007;4(2):296–309.

13. Wilson SK, Delk JR 2nd. Historical advances in penile prostheses. Int J Impot Res. 2000 Oct;12 Suppl 4:S101-7. doi: 10.1038/sj.ijir.3900586.

14. Fernandez-Crespo RE, Buscaino K, Carrion R. "Pumpology": the Realistic Issues Associated with Pump Placement in Prosthetic Surgery. Curr Urol Rep 2021;22(2):10.

15. Bozkurt IH, Arslan B, Yonguc T, et al. Patient and partner outcome of inflatable and semi-rigid penile prosthesis in a single institution. Int Braz J Urol 2015;41(3):535–41.

16. Wilson S. The Top 5 Surgical Things That I Wish I had Known Earlier in My Career: Lessons Learned From a Career of Prosthetic Urology. J Sex Med 2018;15(6):809–12.

17. Trost LW, Baum N, Hellstrom WJ. Managing the difficult penile prosthesis patient. J Sex Med 2013;10(4): 893–907 [quiz: 907].

18. Scovell JM, Ge L, Barrera EV, et al. Longitudinal and Horizontal Load Testing of Inflatable Penile Implant Cylinders of Two Manufacturers: An Ex Vivo Demonstration of Inflated Rigidity. J Sex Med 2016;13(11):1750–7.

19. Wallen JJ, Barrera EV, Ge L, et al. Biomechanical Comparison of Inflatable Penile Implants: A Cadaveric Pilot Study. J Sex Med 2018;15(7):1034–40.

20. Scherzer ND, Dick B, Gabrielson AT, et al. Penile Prosthesis Complications: Planning, Prevention, and Decision Making. Sex Med Rev 2019;7(2):349–59.

21. Pathak RA, Broderick GA. Inflatable penile prosthesis implantation. In: Smith JA, Howards SS, Preminger GM, Dmochowski RR, editors. Hinman's Atlas of Urologic Surgery. Philadelphia (PA): Elsevier; 2018. p. 878–87.

22. Gross MS. Penile Prosthesis Infection. AUA Update Series: Lesson 11, Volumen 37; April 2018.

23. Osmonov D, Christopher AN, Blecher GA, et al. Clinical Recommendations From the European Society for Sexual Medicine Exploring Partner Expectations, Satisfaction in Male and Phalloplasty Cohorts, the Impact of Penile Length, Girth and Implant Type, Reservoir Placement, and the Influence of Comorbidities and Social Circumstances. J Sex Med 2020;17(2):210–37.

24. Lacy JM, Walker J, Gupta S, et al. Risk Factors for Removal or Revision of Penile Prostheses in the Veteran Population. Urology 2016;98:189–94.

25. Kavoussi NL, Siegel JA, Viers BR, et al. Preoperative urine culture results correlate poorly with bacteriology of urologic prosthetic device infections. J Sex Med 2017;14(1):163–8.

26. Mulcahy JJ, Austoni E, Barada JH, et al. The penile implant for erectile dysfunction. J Sex Med 2004; 1(1):98–109.

27. Webster J, Osborne S. Preoperative bathing or showering with skin antiseptics to prevent surgical site infection. Cochrane Database Syst Rev 2015;(2):CD004985.

28. Darouiche RO, Wall MJ, Itani KMF, et al. Chlorhexidine–Alcohol versus Povidone–Iodine for Surgical-Site Antisepsis. N Engl J Med 2010;362(1):18–26.

29. Yeung LL, Grewal S, Bullock A, et al. A comparison of chlorhexidine-alcohol versus povidone-iodine for eliminating skin flora before genitourinary prosthetic surgery: a randomized controlled trial. J Urol 2013; 189(1):136–40.

30. Kjønniksen I, Andersen BM, Søndenaa VG, et al. Preoperative hair removal-a systematic literature review. AORN J 2002;75(5):928–40.

31. Lefebvre A, Saliou P, Lucet JC, et al. Preoperative hair removal and surgical site infections: network meta-analysis of randomized controlled trials. J Hosp Infect 2015;91(2):100–8.

32. Grober ED, Domes T, Fanipour M, et al. Preoperative Hair Removal on the Male Genitalia: Clippers vs. Razors. J Sex Med 2013;10(2):589–94.

33. Razor and Preoperative Preparation of the Male Genitalia. January 2020.

34. Wolf JS Jr, Bennett CJ, Dmochowski RR, et al. Best practice policy statement on urologic surgery antimicrobial prophylaxis. J Urol 2008;179(4):1379–90.

35. Gross MS, Phillips EA, Carrasquillo RJ, et al. Multicenter Investigation of the Micro-Organisms Involved in Penile Prosthesis Infection: An Analysis of the Efficacy of the AUA and EAU Guidelines for Penile Prosthesis Prophylaxis. J Sex Med 2017; 14(3):455–63.

36. Henry GD. Historical review of penile prosthesis design and surgical techniques: part 1 of a three-part review series on penile prosthetic surgery. J Sex Med 2009;6(3):675–81.

37. Corporation, B.S., AMS 700TM with MS PumpTM Penile Prosthesis: Operating Room Manual. 2018.

38. Carson CC 3rd, Mulcahy JJ, Harsch MR. Long-term infection outcomes after original antibiotic impregnated inflatable penile prosthesis implants: up to 7.7 years of followup. J Urol 2011;185(2): 614–8.

39. Wilson SK, Salem EA, Costerton W. Anti-infection dip suggestions for the Coloplast Titan Inflatable Penile Prosthesis in the era of the infection retardant coated implant. J Sex Med 2011;8(9):2647–54.

40. Selph JP, Carson CC 3rd. Penile prosthesis infection: approaches to prevention and treatment. Urol Clin North Am 2011;38(2):227–35.

41. Wosnitzer MS, Greenfield JM. Antibiotic patterns with inflatable penile prosthesis insertion. J Sex Med 2011;8(5):1521–8.

42. Lipsky MJ, Onyeji I, Golan R, et al. Diabetes Is a Risk Factor for Inflatable Penile Prosthesis Infection: Analysis of a Large Statewide Database. Sex Med 2019;7(1):35–40.

43. Dick BP, Yousif A, Raheem O, et al. Does Lowering Hemoglobin A1c Reduce Penile Prosthesis Infection: A Systematic Review. Sex Med Rev 2020. https://doi.org/10.1016/j.sxmr.2020.06.004.

44. Habous M, Tal R, Tealab A, et al. Defining a glycated haemoglobin (HbA1c) level that predicts increased risk of penile implant infection. BJU Int 2018; 121(2):293–300.

45. Canguven O, Talib R, El Ansari W, Khalafalla K, Al Ansari A. Is Hba1c level of diabetic patients associated with penile prosthesis implantation infections? Aging Male 2018;9:1–6. https://doi.org/10.1080/13685538.2018.1448059.

47. Reinstatler L, Shee K, Gross MS. Pain Management in Penile Prosthetic Surgery: A Review of the Literature. Sex Med Rev 2018;6(1):162–9.

48. Tong CMC, Lucas J, Shah A, et al. Novel Multi-Modal Analgesia Protocol Significantly Decreases Opioid

Requirements in Inflatable Penile Prosthesis Patients. J Sex Med 2018;15(8):1187–94.

49. Lucas J, Gross M, Yafi F, et al. A Multi-institutional Assessment of Multimodal Analgesia in Penile Implant Recipients Demonstrates Dramatic Reduction in Pain Scores and Narcotic Usage. J Sex Med 2020;17(3):518–25.

50. Moucha CS, Weiser MC, Levin EJ. Current strategies in anesthesia and analgesia for total knee arthroplasty. J Am Acad Orthop Surg 2016;24(2):60–73.

51. Raynor MC, Smith A, Vyas SN, et al. Dorsal penile nerve block prior to inflatable penile prosthesis placement: a randomized, placebo-controlled trial. J Sex Med 2012;9(11):2975–9.

52. Palmisano F, Boeri L, Cristini C, et al. Comparison of Infrapubic vs Penoscrotal Approaches for 3-Piece Inflatable Penile Prosthesis Placement: Do We Have a Winner? Sex Med Rev 2018;6(4):631–9.

53. Weinberg AC, Pagano MJ, Deibert CM, et al. Sub-Coronal Inflatable Penile Prosthesis Placement With Modified No-Touch Technique: A Step-by-Step Approach With Outcomes. J Sex Med 2016;13(2):270–6.

54. Henry GD, Mahle P, Caso J, et al. Surgical Techniques in Penoscrotal Implantation of an Inflatable Penile Prosthesis: A Guide to Increasing Patient Satisfaction and Surgeon Ease. Sex Med Rev 2015;3(1):36–47.

55. Henry GD. The Henry mummy wrap and the Henry finger sweep surgical techniques. J Sex Med 2009;6(3):619–22.

56. Gupta NK, Ring J, Trost L, et al. The penoscrotal surgical approach for inflatable penile prosthesis placement. Transl Androl Urol 2017;6(4):628–38.

57. Hellstrom WJ, Montague DK, Moncada I, et al. Implants, mechanical devices, and vascular surgery for erectile dysfunction. J Sex Med 2010;7(1 Pt 2):501–23.

58. Vollstedt A, Gross MS, Antonini G, et al. The infrapubic surgical approach for inflatable penile prosthesis placement. Transl Androl Urol 2017;6(4):620–7.

59. Simon R, Hakky TS, Henry G, et al. Tips and tricks of inflatable penile prosthesis reservoir placement: a case presentation and discussion. J Sex Med 2014;11(5):1325–33.

60. Shah BB, Baumgarten AS, Morgan K, et al. V-Neck Technique: A Novel Improvement to the Infra-Pubic Placement of an Inflatable Penile Implant. J Sex Med 2017;14(7):870–5.

61. Mulcahy JJ. The Prevention and Management of Noninfectious Complications of Penile Implants. Sex Med Rev 2015;3(3):203–13.

62. Henry G, Macedo G, Bella A, Mutter M, et al. Intraoperative management I. In: Moncada I, Martinez-Salamanca JI, LLedo-Garcia E, Mulcahy JJ, et al, editors. Textbook of urogenital prosthetic surgery: erectile restoration & urinary incontinence. Madrid, España: Editorial Medica Panamericana; 2021. p. 101–19.

63. Mulcahy JJ. Crural perforation during penile prosthetic surgery. J Sex Med 2006;3(1):177–80.

64. Henry G, Houghton L, Culkin D, et al. Comparison of a new length measurement technique for inflatable penile prosthesis implantation to standard techniques: outcomes and patient satisfaction. J Sex Med 2011;8(9):2640–6.

65. Wilson SK, Henry GD, Delk JR, et al. The mentor Alpha 1 penile prosthesis with reservoir lock-out valve: effective prevention of auto-inflation with improved capability for ectopic reservoir placement. J Urol 2002;168(4 Pt 1):1475–8.

66. Perito PE. Ectopic reservoir placement–no longer in the space of Retzius. J Sex Med 2011;8(9):2395–8.

67. Perito PE, Wilson SK. Traditional (retroperitoneal) and abdominal wall (ectopic) reservoir placement. J Sex Med 2011;8(3):656–9.

68. Hakky TS, Kohn TP, Ramasamy R. Submuscular Abdominal Wall Placement of IPP Reservoir. J Sex Med 2016;13(10):1573–7.

69. Morey AF, Cefalu CA, Hudak SJ. High submuscular placement of urologic prosthetic balloons and reservoirs via transscrotal approach. J Sex Med 2013;10(2):603–10.

70. Kramer A, Goldmark E, Greenfield J. Is a closed-suction drain advantageous for penile implant surgery? The debate continues. J Sex Med 2011;8(2):601–6.

71. Garber BB, Bickell M. Delayed postoperative hematoma formation after inflatable penile prosthesis implantation. J Sex Med 2015;12(1):265–9.

72. Sadeghi-Nejad H, Ilbeigi P, Wilson SK, et al. Multi-institutional outcome study on the efficacy of closed-suction drainage of the scrotum in three-piece inflatable penile prosthesis surgery. Int J Impot Res 2005;17(6):535–8.

73. Wilson S CM, Delk JI. Hematoma formation following penile prosthesis implantation: to drain or not to drain. J Urol 1996;634A.

74. Perito PE. Minimally invasive infrapubic inflatable penile implant. J Sex Med 2008;5(1):27–30.

75. Osterberg EC, Maganty A, Ramasamy R, et al. Pharmacologically induced erect penile length and stretched penile length are both good predictors of post-inflatable prosthesis penile length. Int J Impot Res 2014;26(4):128–31.

76. Wang R, Howard GE, Hoang A, et al. Prospective and long-term evaluation of erect penile length obtained with inflatable penile prosthesis to that induced by intracavernosal injection. Asian J Androl 2009;11(4):411–5.

77. Levine LA, Becher EF, Bella AJ, et al. Penile Prosthesis Surgery: Current Recommendations From the International Consultation on Sexual Medicine. J Sex Med 2016;13(4):489–518.

78. Canguven O, Talib RA, Campbell J, et al. Is the daily use of vacuum erection device for a month before penile prosthesis implantation beneficial? a randomized controlled trial. Andrology 2017;5(1):103–6.

79. Sellers T, Dineen M, Salem EA, et al. Vacuum preparation, optimization of cylinder length and postoperative daily inflation reduces complaints of shortened penile length following implantation of inflatable penile prosthesis. Asm 2013;03(01):14–8.

80. Levine LA, Rybak J. Traction therapy for men with shortened penis prior to penile prosthesis implantation: a pilot study. J Sex Med 2011;8(7):2112–7.

81. Hakky TS, Suber J, Henry G, et al. Penile enhancement procedures with simultaneous penile prosthesis placement. Adv Urol 2012;2012:314612.

82. Hoznek A, Rahmouni A, Abbou C, et al. The suspensory ligament of the penis: an anatomic and radiologic description. Surg Radiol Anat 1998;20(6): 413–7.

83. Li CY, Kayes O, Kell PD, et al. Penile suspensory ligament division for penile augmentation: indications and results. Eur Urol 2006;49(4):729–33.

84. Alter GJ. Correction of penoscrotal web. J Sex Med 2007;4(4 Pt 1):844–7.

85. Miranda-Sousa A, Keating M, Moreira S, et al. Concomitant ventral phalloplasty during penile implant surgery: a novel procedure that optimizes patient satisfaction and their perception of phallic length after penile implant surgery. J Sex Med 2007;4(5):1494–9.

86. Gupta NK, Sulaver R, Welliver C, et al. Scrotoplasty at Time of Penile Implant is at High Risk for Dehiscence in Diabetics. J Sex Med 2019;16(4):602–8.

87. Baumgarten AS, Beilan JA, Shah BB, et al. Suprapubic Fat Pad Excision with Simultaneous Placement of Inflatable Penile Prosthesis. J Sex Med 2019; 16(2):333–7.

88. Dropkin BM, Chisholm LP, Dallmer JD, et al. Penile Prosthesis Insertion in the Era of Antibiotic Stewardship-Are Postoperative Antibiotics Necessary? J Urol 2020;203(3):611–4.

89. Adamsky MA, Boysen WR, Cohen AJ, et al. Evaluating the Role of Postoperative Oral Antibiotic Administration in Artificial Urinary Sphincter and Inflatable Penile Prosthesis Explantation: A Nationwide Analysis. Urology 2018;111:92–8.

90. Henry GD, Carrion R, Jennermann C, et al. Prospective evaluation of postoperative penile rehabilitation: penile length/girth maintenance 1 year following Coloplast Titan inflatable penile prosthesis. J Sex Med 2015;12(5):1298–304.

Is There a Role for Vascular Surgery in the Contemporary Management of Erectile Dysfunction?

Ricardo Munarriz, MD[a],*, Nannan Thirumavalavan, MD[b],
Martin S. Gross, MD[c]

KEYWORDS

- ED • Bypass • Impotence • Penis • Vascular

KEY POINTS

- Young men with focal vascular disease are thought to benefit most from vascular surgery for erectile dysfunction, although exact criteria have not been agreed upon.
- Current microvascular artery bypass techniques for penile revascularization consist of an anastomosis between the inferior epigastric artery and the dorsal artery or the deep dorsal vein of the penis.
- Venous vascular surgery or embolization procedures for the treatment of veno-occulsive erectile dysfunction are not recommended.

INTRODUCTION

Michal and colleagues[1] reported the first penile microvascular artery bypass surgery (MABS) for erectile dysfunction (ED) in 1973. He and his collaborators directly anastomosed the inferior epigastric artery (IEA) to the corpus cavernosum (Michal I), which resulted in intraoperative erections and excellent flow rates (>100 mL/min). This approach was also associated with close to 100% anastomotic stenosis/thrombosis, and thus the results were not durable. Subsequently, Michal's team anastomosed the IEA with the dorsal penile artery using an end-to-side anastomosis technique in an attempt to improve patency rates. The documented success rate using nonvalidated instruments of this Michal II procedure was 56%.[2]

Eight years later, Virag and colleagues[3] reported 92 cases with 54 MABS using an IEA to deep dorsal vein technique. The goal was to increase penile perfusion in a retrograde fashion. The reported success rate was 49% with an additional 20% of men reporting improvement in ED.[3] This artery-to-vein technique unfortunately also resulted in glans hyperemia in most patients, which was minimized by ligation of the circumflex branches. Furlow and Fisher[4] reported a 62% success rate using an artery-to-vein technique with ligation of the circumflex branches. Hauri[5] continued to modify the penile arterial bypass technique by performing a complicated side-to-side anastomosis between the dorsal artery (DA) and vein covered by a spatulated IEA in an attempt to improve outcomes and satisfaction rates.

In the modern era, penile revascularization procedures are rarely performed for a variety of reasons, principle among them being the availability of safe and efficacious oral therapy for ED. However, in select young, healthy men with vasculogenic ED secondary to arterial insufficiency, MABS has

[a] Department of Urology, Boston Medical Center, One Boston Medical Center Place, Boston, MA 02118, USA;
[b] Urology Institute, University Hospitals Cleveland Medical Center, Case Western Reserve University School of Medicine, 11100 Euclid Ave, Cleveland, OH 44106, USA; [c] Section of Urology, Dartmouth-Hitchcock Medical Center, Geisel School of Medicine at Dartmouth College, Lebanon, NH 03756, USA
* Corresponding author.
E-mail address: munarriz@bu.edu

Urol Clin N Am 48 (2021) 543–555
https://doi.org/10.1016/j.ucl.2021.07.002
0094-0143/21/© 2021 Elsevier Inc. All rights reserved.

the potential to reverse the pathophysiology of ED and restore normal erectile function.

Venous vascular surgery was a common procedure for ED in the 1980s and 1990s. Current guidelines on ED recommend against these procedures owing to poor long-term surgical outcomes. In select patients, venous ligation surgery by an experienced surgeon may be an option.[6]

MICROARTERIAL BYPASS SURGERY
Ideal Surgical Candidate

Patient selection is crucial for optimal outcomes after vascular interventions for ED. In general, young healthy men with focal vascular disease are thought to benefit the most from vascular surgery. In the 2015 International Consultation on Sexual Medicine Report, the authors recommend considering vascular interventions for men younger than 55 years old, with "recently acquired ED from focal arterial occlusive disease in the absence of other risk factors."[7] Although exact criteria have not been agreed upon, we have expanded the patient criteria based on the limited available literature and our institutional experience.[7–10]

1. Age: Trost and colleagues [7]reported that age less than 55 may be a predictor of better outcomes, but also that "data was insufficient to define a specific cut-off point" (Evidence Grade C). However, we believe the ideal candidate should be less than 50 years of age or even younger (<40 years old).
2. Absence of vascular risk factors (diabetes, hypertension, tobacco use, hypercholesterolemia, etc).
3. Absence of neurologic ED (eg, multiple sclerosis, pelvic surgery, lumbosacral radiculopathies).
4. Absence of untreated hormonal abnormalities.
5. Absence of active or significant psychiatric disorders (severe depression, bipolar disease, or schizophrenia) or the use of psychotropic drugs owing to their documented sexual side effects.
6. Absence of Peyronie's disease.
7. Absence of untreated premature ejaculation.
8. Absence of acute or chronic perineal or pelvic trauma.
9. Absence of corporo-occlusive dysfunction by duplex Doppler ultrasound examination and cavernosometry.
10. Focal occlusive disease of the common penile or cavernosal arteries documented by penile duplex Doppler ultrasound examination with

or without cavernosometry and confirmed by selective internal pudendal arteriography.

Vascular Anatomy

The blood supply to the penis is derived mainly from the internal pudendal artery and enters the perineum at the level of Alcock's canal. The internal pudendal artery's 3 terminal branches are the bulbourethral, the scrotal, and the common penile artery, which in turn divides into the dorsal and cavernosal arteries (**Fig. 1**A). The accessory pudendal arteries frequently provide additional blood to the corpora cavernosa and may play a critical role in men who undergo pelvic surgery.

The IEA is a branch of the external iliac artery and travels cephalad underneath the rectus muscle above the peritoneum ending near the umbilicus (**Fig. 2**A). It gives several small branches that feed the rectus muscle, which have to be carefully clipped or cauterized using bipolar electrocautery during IEA harvesting. Occasionally, the IEA and the obturator artery have a common trunk. If so, it is advisable to harvest the contralateral IEA if there is no common trunk to avoid a penile artery shunt syndrome in which blood flow preferentially flows to the obturator artery rather than the penile artery (see **Fig. 2**B).[11]

Hemodynamic Evaluation

Penile duplex Doppler ultrasound examination and dynamic infusion cavernosometry

We recommend a screening penile duplex Doppler ultrasound examination with redosing erectogenic agent if necessary.[12] Peak systolic velocities (PSV) of less than 25 cm/s are considered diagnostic for arterial insufficiency, with velocities between 25 and 30 cm/s considered borderline.[13] Chung and colleagues have reported that PSV are age dependent.[14] Thus, in young patients with a PSV of greater than 25 cm/s, cavernosometry documenting arterial gradients of greater than 20 mm of Hg between the brachial and cavernosal arteries may be helpful to confirm the diagnosis of arterial insufficiency. Ultimately, a pudendal arteriogram may be needed to document focal arterial occlusion.

The penile duplex Doppler ultrasound examination should reveal end-diastolic velocities and resistive index consistent with normal corporo-occlusive function. Teloken and colleagues[15] reported that penile duplex Doppler ultrasound examination has the propensity to inaccurately diagnose venous leak. Thus, in cases of borderline PSV in young men or unclear veno-occlusive function, cavernosometry may be a more accurate assessment for veno-occlusive ED.[15,16] We

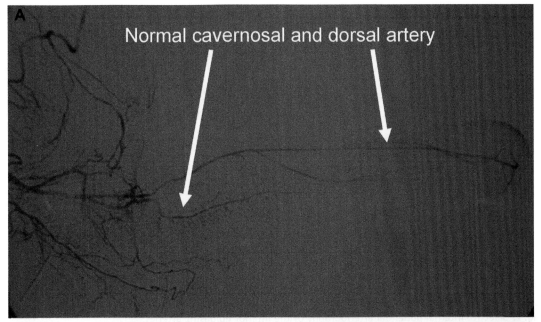

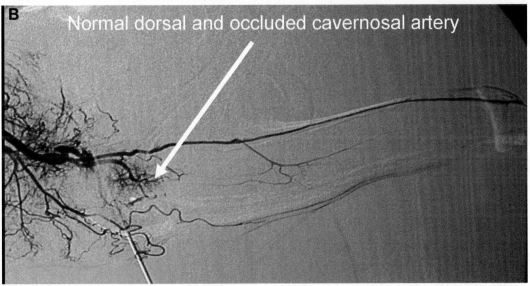

Fig. 1. Selective internal pudendal arteriography documenting patent dorsal artery with perforating cavernosal branch (*A*) and occluded cavernosal artery (*B*).

routinely perform dynamic infusion cavernosometry to further document arterial occlusive disease and normal corporo-occlusive function. Flows to maintain of less than 5 mL/min and pressure decays of less than 45 mm of Hg over 30 seconds effectively rules out the possibility of venous leak.[10]

Selective internal pudendal arteriography
Digital subtraction angiography is the gold standard for diagnosing arterial insufficiency. Digital subtraction angiography confirms the presence

and location of focal occlusions (see **Fig. 1**B). Digital subtraction angiography also provides vascular anatomic information on the donor (IEA; see **Fig. 2**) and recipient vessels (DA; see **Fig. 2**) (eg, size, length, branches) that is critical for surgical planning.[9,10]

Surgical Technique

Current MABS techniques consist of an anastomosis between the IEA to the DA or the deep dorsal vein of the penis. Although an IEA to deep

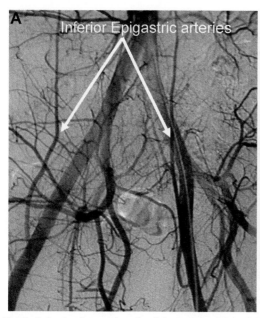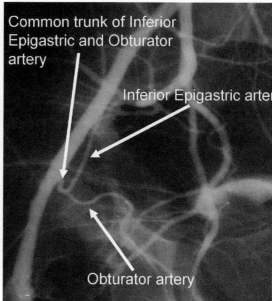

Fig. 2. Selective internal pudendal arteriography of the inferior epigastric arteries.

dorsal vein anastomosis is technically easier than IEA to DA, we favor IEA to DA MABS for several reasons. The use of a valvulotome to facilitate flow through the valves of the dorsal vein may cause endothelial injury, which may activate the intrinsic pathway of the clotting system and lead to thrombosis of the anastomosis. An IEA to DA MABS anastomosis also eliminates the possibility of glans hyperemia, a devastating complication.[17–19] Although there are no definitive data regarding the best technique, IEA to DA studies by Munarriz and colleagues[20] (the largest series to date) and Jarow and DeFranzo[21] show superior outcomes to those reported using artery-to-vein techniques.

Dorsal artery dissection
A 4- to 5-cm semilunar scrotal incision 2 finger-breadths below the penoscrotal junction on the opposite side from the planned abdominal incision for IEA harvesting provides excellent surgical exposure. Finger blunt dissection along Buck's fascia toward the glans is carried out and the penis is then inverted. The fundiform ligament is mobilized and preserved to minimize penile shortening. At this point, the selected DA is isolated and mobilized while avoiding injury to the dorsal nerves. The neurovascular bundle is irrigated with papaverine to prevent vasospasm. The scrotal wound is temporarily closed with staples (Fig. 3).

Harvesting of the inferior epigastric artery
Traditionally, open abdominal incisions are used to harvest the IEA. Robot-assisted laparoscopic harvesting of the IEA has been described and may result in shorter hospitalization times and faster recoveries.[22] If an open procedure is chosen, a 5- to 7-cm transverse incision three-quarters of the distance between the umbilicus and pubis is created with a scalpel (Fig. 4). Dissection is carried down through Scarpa's fascia and the rectus fascia is divided vertically. The rectus muscle is mobilized medially to allow exposure of the IEA, which is mobilized from its origin (the common external iliac artery) to the umbilicus. Papaverine is used to prevent vasospasm during the mobilization of the IEA. The distal end of the IEA is clipped and divided as high as possible.

Inferior epigastric artery transfer
The scrotal staples are removed and blunt dissection between the fundiform ligament and the neurovascular bundle is carried out until the lateral aspect of the pubic tubercle is palpated. At this point, the abdominal fascia is perforated bluntly using a technique similar to that used for the insertion of a penile prosthesis reservoir into the retroperitoneal space. A Schnitt clamp is advanced from the penis into the preperitoneal space where the IEA lies. The distal clip of the IEA is grasped with the clamp and the IEA is transferred to the dorsal aspect of the penis by pulling out the clamp(see Fig. 4). The abdomen is closed in a multilayer fashion using a running technique with 0 polyglycolic acid suture for the rectus fascia, a 2-0 polyglycolic acid suture for Scarpa's fascia, and a 4-0 poliglecaprone suture for the skin.

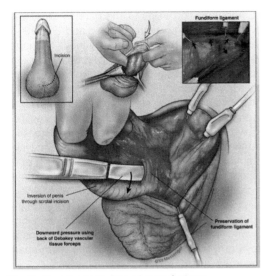

Fig. 3. Dorsal artery dissection technique.

Microvascular anastomosis

The penis is inverted again and a retractor with surgical hooks is used to accommodate the penis for microsurgery. The operating microscope is brought to the surgical field and the DA is mobilized proximally and divided. The proximal end is cauterized using bipolar electrocautery and aneurysmal clips are placed on the DA and IEA. The adventitia of the distal end of the IEA and proximal end of the DA are sharply excised with microscissors to prevent thrombosis of the anastomosis (see **Fig. 4**). A microsurgical anastomosis is performed using a simple interrupted technique with 10-0 nylon suture (**Figs. 5** and **6**). The aneurysmal clips are removed and blood flow is observed,

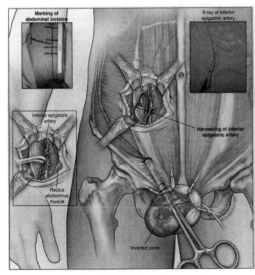

Fig. 4. IEA transfer technique.

documenting anastomotic patency. The penis is placed back on its normal anatomic position and the dartos and skin are reapproximated with 2-0 polyglactin and 4-0 poliglecaprone sutures, respectively. The patency of the anastomosis is confirmed again by Doppler ultrasound examination.

VENOUS VASCULAR SURGERY

The 2018 American Urological Association guideline on ED states that "for men with ED, penile venous surgery is not recommended." This recommendation is derived from poor long-term surgical outcomes.[8] However, in select cases, venous ligation surgery may be beneficial.

Ideal Surgical Candidate

1. Normal cavernous arteries on color duplex Doppler studies and/or cavernosometry. However, there are no definitive data.[10]
2. Abnormal, but limited veno-occlusion dysfunction demonstrated by penile Duplex Doppler ultrasound examination and/or cavernosometry.
3. Localization of the site of venous leakage on pharmacocavernosography to a discrete area of the corporal crura.
4. No medical contraindication to surgery.
5. No vascular risk factors.
6. Highly motivated patient who understands that venous ligation surgery has poor long-term outcomes, but may be effective in select cases.

Surgical Technique

Positioning and surgical approach

Penile degloving using a subcoronal or an inversion technique (**Fig. 6**) are excellent approaches for venous dissection and ligation surgery because they provide access to all important venous channels along the shaft of the penis. The dorsal lithotomy position is preferred if crural banding or ligation is necessary. A combination of blunt and sharp dissection is used to expose the venous system from the glans to the pubic area. Some surgeons dissect and divide the fundiform and suspensory ligaments to maximize vascular exposure to the more proximal deep dorsal penile vein and the cavernosal veins. There are concerns, however, that these maneuvers may result in penile shortening and instability.[20] As a result, we recommend mobilization of the fundiform ligament and reconstruction of the suspensory ligament if divided. In addition, we recommend loupe magnification and the use of bipolar electrocautery to avoid mechanical or thermal injury to the dorsal arteries and nerves.

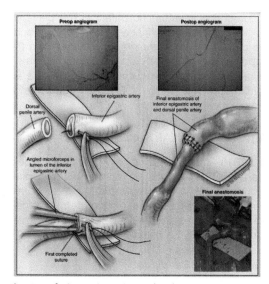

Fig. 5. Inferior epigastric to doral artery anstomosis technique.

Venous vascular ligation

A nonretractable butterfly needle is placed into one of the corpora cavernosa and fixed in place with a purse-string ligature in the tunical albuginea. Indigo carmine or methylene blue is administered to demarcate the vascular system.

Distally, the deep dorsal vein is mobilized and ligated as closed to the glanular sulcus as possible. Along the penile shaft, communicating circumflex veins near the corpora cavernosa and the spongiosum are identified, exposed under Buck's fascia, and ligated.

Communicating veins to the perineal side wall and the pubic regions are isolated and divided to maximize exposure to the deeper venous drainage system. The deep dorsal and cavernosal veins are dissected proximally under the pubic bone and ligated. Communicating veins between the deep and the superficial system are also ligated. We recommend the use of absorbable sutures (2-0 polyglactin) to avoid the patient or partner feeling permanent suture material during sexual activity. Other surgeons have promulgated the use of permanent sutures to ligate the deep dorsal and cavernosal veins under the pubis.

If crural ligation is elected, the crura are identified and carefully isolated from the corpus spongiosum. A right-angle clamp can be used to pass two 5-mm-wide cotton tape ligatures 1 cm apart around the crus (**Fig. 7**).

A closed suction drain is placed in the infrapubic region and withdrawn through a separate stab wound where it is affixed to the skin. The drain is usually removed in 24 to 48 hours if drainage is minimal. The skin is approximated with reabsorbable suture (chromic 3-0 or 3-0 poliglecaprone) and a loose circumferential elastic dressing is placed to decrease postoperative edema and swelling.

DISCUSSION
MABS Surgical Outcomes

Assessing outcomes after vascular interventions is challenging. Although vascular interventions for ED have been described as early as the 1970s,

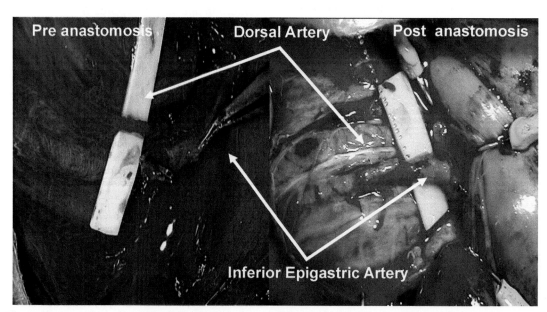

Fig. 6. Photography before and after the anastomosis between the inferior epigastric and dorsal arteries.

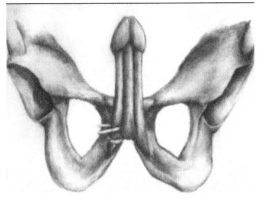

Fig. 7. A right-angle clamp can be used to pass two 5-mm-wide cotton tape ligatures 1 cm apart around the crus.

standardized validated questionnaires such as the International Index of Erectile Function (IIEF) were not developed until 1997.[23] Much of the available literature used subjective outcomes like nonvalidated questionnaires, imaging assessments (penile Doppler ultrasound examination, angiogram, nocturnal penile tumescence) or need for phosphodiesterase type 5 inhibitors. These nonstandard measures add to the heterogeneity of the literature, making it difficult to draw conclusions regarding therapeutic efficacy. **Table 1** summarizes most of the available publications and clearly shows a tremendous variation in treatment outcomes.

The American Urologic Association Erectile Dysfunction Guideline Panel attempted to analyze available literature regarding arterial insufficiency by using a defined "index patient"—a healthy man no older than 55 years with recently acquired ED from focal arterial occlusive disease and without other vascular risk factors such as smoking or diabetes. In trying to achieve homogeneity in their approach, the authors found that, at the time of their evaluation, only 4 articles met this definition.[8] The total studied population was 50 men with reported successful outcomes of 36% to 80% for IEA to dorsal vein and 91% for IEA-to-DA MABS, respectively.[21,24–26] **Table 2** summarizes the available studies that met the Erectile Dysfunction Update panel criteria.

Munarriz and colleagues[20] published the largest long-term outcome MABS study to date using validated questionnaires (71 men; aged 30.5 ± 9.2 years; mean follow-up of 34.5 ± 18 months). The mean preoperative and postoperative penile rigidity using analog scale (with and without phosphodiesterase type 5 inhibitors), total IIEF score (35.5 ± 14.8 and 56.2 ± 16.6), and Center for Epidemiologic Studies Depression Scale score (42.0 ± 10.0 33.7 ± 6.1) improved significantly. Treatment satisfaction according to the Erectile Dysfunction Inventory of Treatment Satisfaction scale was high; 62 of the 71 patients (87.3%) stated they would recommend the surgery to someone else[20] (**Table 3**).

The 2015 International Consultation for Sexual Medicine suggested that age less than 55 years may be a predictor of better outcomes, but also that "data was insufficient to define a specific cut-off point (Evidence Grade C)."[6] In our experience, the optimal patient should be 50 years of age or younger.

Munarriz and colleagues[20] evaluated MABS effectiveness by age using IIEF data and divided patients into 4 age groups (18–29, 30–39, 40–49, and 50–59 years) and found statistically significant improvements for all age groups except for the 50- to 59-year-old group, which had only 1 patient Interestingly, 77.46% of patients were younger than 40 years of age.[20]

Other work focusing on older men (>50 years old; mean age, 59.7 years old) has found an approximately 60.5% success rate in men undergoing deep dorsal vein arterialization. This series included carefully selected men without a history of major trauma, diabetes, nicotine use, hyperlipidemia, coronary artery disease, or hypertension. The mean follow-up was 22.1 months and the mean IIEF 15 improved from 19.2 to 25.5 (P<.05).[27]

Microvascular Artery Bypass Surgery Complications

There are few data regarding complications of penile MABS. With few exceptions, most complications (infection, bleeding, fevers, nausea, penile pain, anesthesia problems, etc) are rare (0%–3%) and short term.[20] The exception to this is penile hyperemia, a devastating complication associated with dorsal vein arterialization characterized by severe penile pain, glans vascular congestion, and ulcerations.[17–19]

Complications that are particularly bothersome to patients include decreased penile sensation, loss of penile length, and hernias. Munarriz and colleagues[20] reported that 3 (4%), 17 (24%), and 20 (28%) of 71 patients reported incisional hernias, loss of penile sensation and loss of penile length, respectively. The mean postoperative IIEF Orgasmic Function domain scores documented an improvement in orgasmic function (preoperative 5.71 ± 3.04 and postoperative 7.97 ± 2.58), suggesting that sensation is generally at least partially preserved. Despite these reports, the overall postoperative satisfaction was high and

Table 1
Microarterial bypass surgery outcomes

Study	Year	No. of Patients	Result
Virag	1981	36	41.6% good, 33.3% fair
Michal et al	1986	73	60% success
Balko et al	1986	11	73% significantly improved
Society for Study of Impotence (Belker and Bennett)	1988	50	78% success
Lizza and Zorgniotti	1988	13	77% success
Sharlip	1990	30	20% success, 27% improved
Virag and Bennett	1991	100	38% good, 30% improved
Furlow et al	1990	95	78%
Sohn	1992	65	31% success, 54% good or improved
Bock and Lewis	1992	36	53% success, 28% improved
Löbelenz et al	1992	19	58% success, 40% improved
Schramek et al	1992	35	60% success, 23% improved 54% excellent postoperative Doppler 23% good postoperative Doppler
Melman and Riccardi	1993	18	33% success
Janssen et al	1994	21	62% success, 5% improved
Lizza and Zorgiotti	1994	36 32 26	53% success, 31% improved 41% success, 34% improved 54% success, 19% improved
Jarow and DeFranzo	1996	11	64% success, 27% improved
Benet et al	1997	36	46% success, 14% improved
Mannine et al	1998	62	34% success, 20% improved
Munarriz et al 2009	2009	71	EF domains of IIEF significantly improved Question 3 IIEF significantly improved Question 4 IIEF significantly improved SDS significantly improved CES-D significantly improved Treatment satisfaction significantly improved

Abbreviations: CES-D, Center for Epidemiologic Studies Depression Scale and Treatment Satisfaction; IIEF, International Index of Erectile Function; SDS, Sexual Distress Scale.

Data from Ronald Lewis and Ricardo Munarriz. Vascular Surgery for Erectile dysfunction. Campbell's Urology. Walsh, Retik, Vaughan& Wein. Nine Edition, Chapter 24, 802-817.

87.7% of patients reported they would recommend or undergo surgery again.

Venous vascular surgery outcomes

Venous ligation surgery for ED was very popular in the 1980s and 1990s, but poor long-term success rates resulted in discontinuation of these procedures (**Table 4**).[28–33] The 2018 American Urological Association Guideline on Erectile Dysfunction recommends against penile venous surgery.[8]

Despite the American Urological Association recommendation, a number of studies have suggested that venous vascular surgery may be helpful in very carefully selected patients.[34–36] Rahman and colleagues[34] reported statistically significant improvements in mean IIEF scores (8.9 ± 4.5 and 17.5 ± 5.0) in 11 men who underwent crural ligation for ED and congenital venous leakage. Cayan[35] also reported significant improvement in mean IIEF scores at 1 year postoperatively in patients undergoing resection of the deep and superficial dorsal and the cavernous veins. Flores and colleagues[36] also documented statistically significant improvements in mean IIEF scores (6.7 ± 3.61–16.3 ± 6.4) in men undergoing crural ligation surgery for isolated crural venous leak.

A variety of endovascular procedures to manage veno-occlusive ED have been reported;

Table 2
Microarterial bypass surgery outcomes that met the criteria for the arterial occlusive disease index patient[8]

Investigators	Year	Patients	Outcome (%)	Success Criteria
Grasso et al[26]	1992	22	68	NPT
			36	Doppler
DePalma et al[25]	1995	11	60	Doppler
Jarow and DeFranzo[21]	1996	11	91	Doppler
Ang and Lim.[24]	1997	6	66	NPT, Doppler
Munarriz et al.[20]	2009	71	Preoperative: 40.03 ± 20.19 and 18.70 ± 12.99 Postoperative: 64.15 ± 23.35 and 32.06 ± 16.48	IIEF overall IIEF EF domain

Abbreviations: Doppler, penile duplex Doppler ultrasound examination; IIEF EF domain, erectile function domain of the IIEF; IIEF, International Index of Erectile Function; NPT, nocturnal tumescence testing.
  Data from Ronald Lewis and Ricardo Munarriz. Vascular Surgery for Erectile dysfunction. Campbell's Urology. Walsh, Retik, Vaughan & Wein. Nine Edition, Chapter 24, 802-817.

outcomes seem to be generally similar to surgical series, although there are no head-to-head comparison studies.[37–43]

Venous vascular surgery complications
There are limited data on the frequency of venous vascular complications and how they were

Table 3
Microarterial bypass surgery outcomes using validated questionnaires.[20]

	Preoperatively	Postoperatively
IIEF		
Total score	35.5 ± 14.8	56.2 ± 16.6
EF of IIEF	13.7 ± 6.7	23.8 ± 6.6
Question 3	2.2 ± 1.4	4.1 ± 1.4
Question 4	2.1 ± 1.3	3.9 ± 1.5
SDS	37.7 ± 11.1	17.5 ± 12.5
CES-D	42.0 ± 10.0	33.7 ± 7.1
Edits		72%–81%
Penile rigidity (%)		
Without PDE % inhibitors	41	71
With PDE 5 inhibitors	77	90

Abbreviations: CES, Center for Epidemiologic Studies Depression Scale and Treatment Satisfaction; IIEF EF domain, erectile function domain of the IIEF; IIEF, International Index of Erectile Function; Rigidity, Penile rigidity using analog scale; SDS, Sexual Distress Scale.
  Data from Munarriz, R., Uberoi, J., Fantini, G., Martinez, D., and Lee, C. (2009) Microvascular arterial bypass surgery: long-term outcomes using validated instruments. J. Urol. 182(2), 643–648.

managed. The most commonly reported complications include penile pain and numbness, skin necrosis, painful erections, penile curvature, and wound and tape infections[28–33] (**Table 5**).

LIMITATIONS IN STUDIES OF VASCULAR INTERVENTIONS

Although there are data showing a potential benefit of penile arterial revascularization or venous vascular surgery for select patient with vasculogenic ED, the procedures are not mainstream for a number of reasons. The lack of standardization in patient selection, hemodynamic evaluation, surgical technique, and limited long-term outcome data using validated instruments has marginalized these surgical procedures.

With the incidence of obesity, metabolic syndrome, and cardiovascular disease increasing over the past few decades, especially in younger patients, the index patient is becoming rarer.[43] Most men who present with ED are found to have concomitant subclinical cardiovascular disease, of which ED is merely the initial presenting symptom.[44] As such, even young patients may have vascular risk factors such as high blood pressure, high cholesterol, or diabetes. In addition, MABS requires significant microsurgical expertise, a skill not possessed by the majority of those who treat ED. The learning curve would be significant for the surgeon who does not perform microsurgery routinely. The equipment costs associated with microsurgery may also be prohibitive. The procedure takes experienced surgeons approximately 4 hours to complete, and reimbursement does not accurately reflect the complexity of the procedure.

Table 4
Penile venous ligation surgery for veno-occulsive ED

Investigator	Mean Age (y)	Technique	Outcome
Sasso et al,[28] 1999 N = 23 Follow-up: 12 mo	41	Superficial DDV Circumflex Emissary	Spontaneous erections at 12 mo: 74% Long term: 55%
Popken et al,[29] 1999 N = 122 Follow-up: 70 mo	49	Superficial DDV Circumflex	Spontaneous erections 14% ICI 9%
Al Assal et al,[30] 1998 N = 325 Follow-up: 1–13 mo	45		Cured <40 years 76% > 40 years 58%
Lukkarinen et al,[31] 1998 N = 21 Follow-up: >12 mo			Good 29% ICI 52%
Basar[33] N = 26 Follow-up: 25 mo			Complete erection 15% Partial erection 23%

Schultheiss[32]
N = 147
Follow-up: 6–76 mo
	48 ± 11.7	DDV	Complete spontaneous
			  erection 11.2%
			Postop response to
			  pharmacotherapy 19.0%
			No satisfactory improvement
			  69.8%

Rahmal et al,[34] 2005 N = 12	28	Crural ligation	IIEF EF domain 8.9–15.5 9/11 reported significant improvement

Cayan,[35] 2008
N = 24
Follow-up: 1 y
	34.6	Superficial
		DDV Cavernous V
		Crural ligation
			IIEF EF domain 6.7 ± 3.61–
			  16.3 ± 6.4
			73% reported some degree of
			  improvement
			42.3% reported complete EF
			  improvement
			30.8% reported partial
			  improvement

Flores et al,[36] 2011
N = 14
Follow-up: 12 mo
	29 ± 7	Crural ligation	Statistical improvement in IIEF
			  EF scores
			No patients needed
			  intracavernosal therapy
			4 of 14 patients needed DE5s.

Abbreviations: Cavernous V, cavernous vein; DDV, deep dorsal vein; IIEF EF domain, erectile function domain of the IIEF; IIEF, International Index of Erectile Function.

From a patient perspective, MABS procedures are invasive and require both an abdominal and scrotal incision, with a recovery time of a few weeks. This time is in addition to complex testing for those pursuing this option, such as dynamic infusion cavernosometry and selective internal pudendal arteriography. For young men with mild ED, an oral medication that provides satisfactory results is obviously much less invasive and potentially more appealing. In the past, cost considerations for the chronic use of phosphodiesterase type 5 inhibitors may have been exorbitant, but cost reductions and the availability of generic and compounded medications have made this less of an issue.[45]

For men who are not responsive to oral therapies for ED, less invasive options like intracavernosal injections may have more appeal. To our knowledge, no formal cost-effectiveness analysis of vascular surgery compared with other treatment modalities for ED has been performed to date, although it has been performed for phosphodiesterase type 5 inhibitors, injections, and penile implants.[46] Despite these considerations, a therapy

Table 5
Venous embolization for veno-occulsive ED

	Age	Technique	Agent	Follow-up (mo)	Outcome (%)
Fernandez et al,[37] 2001 N = 23	63	Transfemoral	Balloon ETOH	22	Complete 26 Patient report
Miwa et al,[38] 2001 N = 10	67	Open DDV canalization	ETOH	32	Complete 50 Patient report
Peskircioglu et al,[39] 2000 N = 32	46	Open DDV canalization	N-Butyl cyanoacrylate	25	Complete 69 Patient report
Malossini et al,[40] 1998 N = 17	36	Open DDV canalization	Coils	34	Good 73% Patient report
Rebonato et al,[41] 2014 N = 18	51	US guided DDV canalization	N-butyl cyanoacrylate Coils	13.3 ± 7.5	IIEF End diastolic V

Abbreviations: DDV, deep dorsal vein; US, ultrasound examination.
   Data from Hellstrom JG, Montague DK, Moncada I, Carson C, Minhas S, Faria G, Krishnamurti S. J Sex Med 2010 Jan;7(1 Pt 2):501-23. Implants, mechanical devices, and vascular surgery for erectile dysfunction.

that can reverse ED is appealing for patients and surgeons alike and interest in vascular surgery options for ED is likely to continue.

SUMMARY

The current treatment of ED is aimed at managing the condition but none of the current treatments approved by the US Food and Drug Administration can cure or reverse the pathophysiology of vasculogenic ED. Penile MABS may be the only treatment capable of restoring erectile function without the need for the chronic use of vasoactive medications or placement of a penile prosthesis. Similarly, in select cases, penile venous ligation surgery may beneficial. However, current guidelines do not support penile venous surgery. The lack of standardization in patient selection, hemodynamic evaluation, surgical technique, and limited long-term outcome data using validated instruments has resulted in these surgeries being considered experimental and rarely performed.

CLINICS CARE POINTS

- Young healthy men presenting with suspected vasculogenic ED may benefit from hemodynamic testing (penile duplex Doppler

ultrasound examination, cavernosometry and confirmatory selective internal pudendal arteriography).

- Young healthy men with ED secondary to confirmed vascular insufficiency may be considered for penile revascularization procedures.

- Venous vascular surgery or embolization procedures for the treatment of veno-occulsive ED are not recommended. However, these surgeries or procedures may be performed in select cases or in the setting of research studies.

- The lack of standardization in patient selection, hemodynamic evaluation, surgical technique, and deficiency of long-term outcome data using validated instruments has limited the use of these surgeries.

DISCLOSURE

Dr R. Munarriz and M.S. Gross are consultants for Coloplast.

REFERENCES

1. Michal V, Kramar R, Pospichal J, et al. Direct arterial anastomosis to the cavernous body in the treatment of erectile impotence. Czech Rozhledy Chir 1973; 52:587–93.

2. Michal V, Kramer R, Hejhal L. Revascularization procedures of the cavernous bodies. In: Zorgniotti AW,

Ross G, editors. Vasculogenic Impotence: Proceedings of the first International Conference on corpus cavernosum revascularization. Springfield, IL: Charles C Thomas; 1980. p. 239–55.

3. Virag R, Zwang G, Dermange H, et al. Vasculogenic impotence: a review of 92 cases with 54 surgical operations. Vasc Surg 1981;15:9–16.

4. Furlow WL, Fisher J. Deep dorsal vein arterialization: clinical experience with a new technique for penile revascularization. J Urol 1988;139:298A. Abstr. 543.

5. Hauri D. Therapiemoglichkeitem bei der vascular bedingten erectilei n impotenz. Akt Urol 1984;15:350.

6. Burnett AL, Nehra A, Breau RH, et al. Erectile dysfunction: AUA guideline. J Urol 2018;200(3): 633–41.

7. Trost LW, Munarriz R, Wang R, et al. External mechanical devices and vascular surgery for erectile dysfunction. J Sex Med 2016;13(11):1579–617.

8. Montague DK, Jarow JP, Broderick GA, et al. The management of erectile dysfunction: an update. Baltimore: American Urological Association; 2007.

9. Munarriz R, Mulhall J, Goldstein I. Penile arterial reconstruction. In: Graham Jr SD, Keane TE, Glenn JF, editors. Glenn's urologic surgery. 6th edition. Philadelphia: Lippincott Williams & Wilkins; 2004. p. 573–81.

10. Lewis R, Munarriz R. Vascular surgery for erectile dysfunction. Campbell's urology. 9th edition. Saunders, Philadelphia PA: Walsh, Retik, Vaughan & Wein; 2007. p. 802–17. Chapter 24.

11. Pavlinec JG, Hakky TS, Yang C, et al. Penile artery shunt syndrome: a novel cause of erectile dysfunction after penile revascularization surgery. J Sex Med 2014;11(9):2338–41.

12. Mulhall JP, Abdel-Moneim A, Abobakr R, et al. Improving the accuracy of vascular testing in impotent men: correcting hemodynamic alterations using a vasoactive medication re-dosing schedule. J Urol 2001;166(3):923–6.

13. Quam JP, King BF, James EM, et al. Duplex or color Doppler sonographic evaluation of vasculogenic impotence. Am J Roentgenol 1989;153:1141–7.

14. Chung WS, Park YY, Kwon SW. The impact of aging on penile hemodynamics in normal responders to pharmacologic injection: a Doppler sonographic study. J Urol 1997;157:2129–31.

15. Teloken PE, Kelly P, Parker M, et al. The false diagnosis of venous leak: prevalence and predictors. J Sex Med 2011;8(8):2344–9.

16. Vardi Y, Glina S, Mulhall JP, et al. Cavernosometry: is it a dinosaur? J Sex Med 2008;5(4):760–4.

17. Eichmann A, Krähenbühl A, Hauri D. Postoperative hyperemia of the glans penis with ulcers following revascularization surgery for vascular impotence. Dermatology 1992;184(4):291–3.

18. Claes H, Van Poppel H, Baert L. Hypervascularization of the glans penis after a venous leakage and revascularisation procedure: a case report. Acta Urol Belg 1993;61(3):17–9.

19. Wilms G, Oyen R, Claes L, et al. Glans ischemia after penis revascularization: therapeutic embolization. Cardiovasc Intervent Radiol 1990;13(5):304–5.

20. Munarriz R, Uberoi J, Fantini G, et al. Microvascular arterial bypass surgery: long-term outcomes using validated instruments. J Urol 2009;182(2):643–8.

21. Jarow JP, DeFranzo AJ. Long-term results of arterial bypass surgery for impotence secondary to segmental vascular disease. J Urol 1996;156:982.

22. Raynor MC, Davis R, Hellstrom WJG. Robot-assisted vessel harvesting for penile revascularization. J Sex Med 2010;7(1 Pt 1):293–7.

23. Rosen RC, Riley A, Wagner G, et al. The International Index of Erectile Function (IIEF): a multidimensional scale for assessment of erectile dysfunction. Urology 1997;49(6):822–30.

24. Ang LP, Lim PH. Penile revascularisation for vascular impotence. Singapore Med J 1997;38:285.

25. DePalma RG, Olding M, Yu GW, et al. Vascular interventions for impotence: lessons learned. J Vasc Surg 1995;21:576.

26. Grasso M, Lania C, Castelli M, et al. Deep dorsal vein arterialization in vasculogenic impotence: our experience. Arch Ital Urol Nefrol Androl 1992;64:309.

27. Kayigil O, Agras K, Okulu E. Is deep dorsal vein arterialization effective in elderly patients? Int Urol Nephrol 2008;40(1):125–31.

28. Sasso F, Gulino G, Weir J, et al. Patient selection criteria in the surgical treatment of veno-occlusive dysfunction. J Urol 1999;161:1145–7.

29. Popken G, Katzenwadel A, Wetterauer U. Long-term results of dorsal penile vein ligation for symptomatic treatment of erectile dysfunction. Andrologia 1999; 31(Suppl. 1):77–82.

30. Al Assal F, Delgado A, Al Assal R. Venous surgery for veno-occlusive dysfunction. Long-term results. Int J Impot Res 1998;10S:31.

31. Lukkarinen O, Tonttila P, Hellstrom P, et al. Non-prosthetic surgery in the treatment of erectile dysfunction. A retrospective study of 45 impotent patients in the University of Oulu. Scand J Urol Nephrol 1998;32:42–6.

32. Basar MM, Atan A, Yildiz M. Long-term results of venous ligation in patients with veno-occlusive dysfunction. Int J Impot Res 1998;10S:21.

33. Schultheiss D, Truss MC, Becker AJ, et al. Long-term results following dorsal penile vein ligation in 126 patients with veno-occlusive dysfunction. Int J Impot Res 1997;9:205–9.

34. Rahman NU, Dean RC, Carrion R, et al. Crural ligation for primary erectile dysfunction: a case series. J Urol 2005;173(6):2064–6.

35. Cayan S. Primary penile venous leakage surgery with crural ligation in men with erectile dysfunction. J Urol 2008;180(3):1056–9.

36. Flores S, Tal R, O'Brien K, et al. Outcomes of crural ligation surgery for isolated crural venous leak. J Sex Med 2011;8:3495–9.

37. Fernández Arjona M, Oteros R, Zarca M, et al. Percutaneous embolization for erectile dysfunction due to venous leakage: prognostic factors for a good therapeutic result. Eur Urol 2001;39:15–9.

38. Miwa Y, Shioyama R, Itou Y, et al. Pelvic venoablation with ethanol for the treatment of erectile dysfunction due to veno-occlusive dysfunction. Urology 2001;58:76–9.

39. Peskircioglu L, Tekin I, Boyvat F, et al. Embolization of the deep dorsal vein for the treatment of erectile impotence due to veno-occlusive dysfunction. J Urol 2000;163:472–5.

40. Malossini G, Ficarra V, Cavalleri S, et al. Long-term results of the veno-occlusive percutaneous treatment of erectile disorders of venous origin. Arch Ital Androl 1998;70:203–9.

41. Rebonato A, Auci A, Sanguinetti F, et al. Embolization of the periprostatic venous plexus for erectile dysfunction resulting from venous leakage. J Vasc Interv Radiol 2014;25(6):866–72.

42. Hellstrom JG, Montague DK, Moncada I, et al. Implants, mechanical devices, and vascular surgery for erectile dysfunction. J Sex Med 2010;7(1 Pt 2): 501–23.

43. Andersson C. Vasan RS. Epidemiology of cardiovascular disease in young individuals. Nat Rev Cardiol 2018;15(4):230–40.

44. Osundu CU, Vo B, Oni ET, et al. The relationship of erectile dysfunction and subclinical cardiovascular disease: a systematic review and meta-analysis. Vasc Med 2018;23(1):9–20.

45. Mishra K, Bukavina L, Mahran A, et al. Variability in prices for erectile dysfunction medications-are all pharmacies the same? J Sex Med 2018;15(12): 1785–91.

46. Rezaee ME, Ward CE, Brandes ER, et al. A review of economic evaluations of erectile dysfunction therapies. Sex Med Rev 2020;8(3):497–503.

Penile Fractures
Evaluation and Management

Allen Simms, MD, Nima Baradaran, MD, Tom F. Lue, MD, ScD (Hon), FACS,
Benjamin N. Breyer, MD*

KEYWORDS

- Penile fracture • Penile rupture • Penile trauma • Urethral injury • Corpus cavernosum
- Collagenase clostridium histolyticum

KEY POINTS

- Penile fracture is a urologic injury with unique etiologies depending on geography and culture.
- Diagnosis of penile fractures can be made based on history and physical examination alone, but ultrasound or MRI can be helpful adjuncts.
- Patients should be evaluated with retrograde urethrogram or cystoscopy when urethral injury is suspected.
- Surgical management is favored over conservative measures to improve outcomes.

INTRODUCTION

Penile fracture is a urologic injury defined as the disruption of the tunica albuginea with rupture of the corpus cavernosum, usually occurring as blunt trauma to the erect penis during intercourse.[1] Although penile fracture is a clinical diagnosis using history and physical examination, imaging is evolving as a helpful adjunct. Immediate surgical management is the standard of care per AUA and EUA guidelines.[2,3]

EPIDEMIOLOGY

The incidence and etiology of penile fractures is highly variable based on geography. The incidence of penile fractures in the United States is reported at 1.02 per 100,000 men per year,[4] although a rate as high as 10.48 per 100,000 men has been reported in a specific area of Iran.[5] The most common etiology of penile fracture in the United States is sexual intercourse,[6,7] representing 46% of cases in a recent meta-analysis.[8] Other causes include forced flexion of the penis (21%), masturbation (18%), and rolling over on the erect penis (8.2%).[8] The incidence of fracture occurring during sexual intercourse has been reported as up to 94% of cases,[9] whereas it was the reported cause in just 7.9% of cases in an Iranian series.[10] In Middle Eastern and Northern African countries, up to three-quarters of fractures are due to the practice of Taqaandan, the manual bending of the erect penis to achieve detumescence.[5,10] In Japan, masturbation was found to be the most common cause, with sexual intercourse representing only 19.9%.[11]

Penile fracture during intercourse is a result of the erect penis forcefully striking the perineum or pubic bone.[1] During heterosexual intercourse, the "woman on top" and rear-entry "doggy style" positions are associated with the highest risk of penile fracture, with the latter associated with more severe injuries.[3,7,12] Penile fractures may occur more commonly in stressful situations, such as illicit or extramarital sexual intercourse.[13]

A rising contributor to penile fractures is the use of Collagenase Clostridium Histolyticum (CCH) injections for the treatment of Peyronie's disease. In a safety analysis of patients receiving CCH injections, 0.5% of patients had surgically confirmed fractures,[14] an approximate 500-fold increase from reported incidence in the general population.

Department of Urology, University of California San Francisco, San Francisco, CA, USA
* Corresponding author. University of California San Francisco, 400 Parnassus Ave., 6th Fl, San Francisco, CA 94143-0330.
E-mail address: Benjamin.breyer@ucsf.edu

Urol Clin N Am 48 (2021) 557–563
https://doi.org/10.1016/j.ucl.2021.06.011

An additional study suggests the rate of fracture after CCH injection may be even higher at 4.9%, with majority (80%) occurring between 15 and 19 days.[14,15] Penile fractures after CCH injections can occur without any intercourse/manipulation, as up to 31% result from nocturnal erections alone.[16] The severity of these fractures tends to be lower and management is more likely to involve a nonoperative approach.

PRESENTATION

The tunica albuginea is a strong fascial layer, which envelopes the corpora cavernosa and helps maintain erections. The normal tunica albuginea is 2 mm thick,[17] but thins to 0.25 to 0.5 mm during an erection, losing elasticity.[18,19] During normal erection and intercourse, intracorporal pressures increase to several hundred mm Hg. The tunica can withstand pressures up to 1500 mm Hg before rupture.[19,20] The ventrolateral tunica has less collagen deposition and thus is thinner[21]; almost all penile fractures occur on the ventral or lateral aspect of the penis.[10] The vast majority of penile fractures occur in the proximal or midshaft, and nearly all occur distal to the suspensory ligament.[6–8,18] Rupture of the albuginea is usually unilateral (86%–96%), and more commonly right-sided (up to 74%).[19,22,23]

Rupture of the tunica albuginea usually occurs with an audible "pop" (69%); other presenting symptoms include pain, swelling, and rapid detumescence[1,6,18,23,24] (**Fig. 1**). On physical examination, hematoma is the most common finding, present in nearly all cases.[23] If Buck's fascia remains intact, a localized clot may form over the site of injury, which can be felt as an immobile lump when rolling a finger over the area ("rolling sign").[19,25–27] The "rolling sign" may be more appreciable in delayed presentations when edema and swelling have improved.[28] Likewise, when

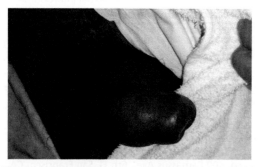

Fig. 1. A 50-year-old man presenting after penis hit tailbone during sex, causing acute pain, loud snap, and rapid detumescence; voiding small amount of bloody urine.

Buck's fascia remains intact, the classic "eggplant deformity" may develop, in which the swollen and bruised phallus deviates away from the injury due to mass effect.[1,19] Conversely, in penile fractures with concomitant disruption of Buck's fascia, hematoma can expand to scrotum, perineum, and suprapubic region, creating the "butterfly sign".[1,18,23] Gross or microscopic hematuria, blood at urethral meatus, and/or inability to urinate should raise concern for urethral injury, which occurs in 5.6% of cases.[8,29]

DIAGNOSIS

The diagnosis of a penile fracture can be made with a careful history and physical examination.[1,8] Patients presenting with audible "pop" followed by detumescence, swelling, and positive "rolling" signs have an underlying penile fracture in virtually all cases. "False" fractures are penile vascular injuries (superficial dorsal vein, deep dorsal vessels, or nonspecific bleeding from dartos) usually occurring during intercourse and can mimic penile fractures.[30,31] Key clinical differences include absence of rapid detumescence, ability to achieve an erection after injury, and absence of palpable tunical defect.[30–32] Although snapping sound can be heard with false fractures, it is less common, occurring in only 22% of patients.[33] Another uncommon mimicker is suspensory ligament rupture, which can be differentiated by lack of detumescence, minimal bruising/pain, penile hypermobility, and palpable gap between base of penis and pubic bone.[19,34]

Imaging for suspected fracture can be considered per AUA and EUA guidelines (**Fig. 2**), when diagnosis is unclear and may provide reassurance that tunica is intact.[1–3] Imaging can also be useful in the localization of injury. Ultrasonography has become the preferred imaging modality to evaluate penile fractures, as it is fast, readily available, and inexpensive.[1] Although highly operator dependent, ultrasound has proven to be quite accurate with sensitivity up to 88% and specificity up to 100%.[22,25,35] Ultrasound findings include disruption of the tunica (hypoechoic line or area) and/or intracavernosal or extracavernosal hematomas.[35–37] The "Turkish Eye" sign describes the appearance of an intracavernosal hematoma as a hypoechoic region surrounded by the echodense corpora, which can reliably diagnose penile fractures.[37] Urethral evaluation is difficult with ultrasound, but evidence of a distended proximal urethra or air within the corpora should raise suspicion for urethral rupture.[38,39]

Magnetic resonance imaging (MRI) is another accurate means for detecting penile fractures,[35,40–42] but its use is limited by cost and

	Imaging Findings	Reliability	Strengths	Weaknesses
Ultrasound	Disruption of the hyperechoic line around the corporal bodies, intra- or extra-cavernosal hematomas ("Turkish Eye" sign)	Sensitivity up to 88% Specificity up to 100%	• Fast • Inexpensive • Readily available	• Operator dependency • Poor urethral evaluation
MRI	Disruption of the tunica albuginea (low-signal intensity layer).	Sensitivity and negative predictive value of 100%	• Operator independent • Accuracy • May also detect corpus spongiosum disruption	• Availability • Cost • Time-consuming
Cavernosography	Injection of dye under live fluoro reveals extravasation	False negative rate of 28%	Useful when fracture suspected but not found intra-operatively	• Operator dependency • Time-consuming • Invasive • Risk of complications
RUG and/or cystoscopy	Urethral disruption; extravasation of contrast		Ability to detect urethral injury	• Time-consuming

Fig. 2. Diagnosis of penile fractures can be made with a careful history and physical examination. However, imaging can be useful in certain clinical scenarios.

availability. The tunica albuginea appears as a low-signal intensity layer on MRI, and its disruption can easily be detected.[40] MRI is operator-independent and has been proven to be superior to ultrasound with regard to accuracy. Both the sensitivity and negative predictive value of MRI in the diagnosis of penile fractures is 100%,[40,42,43] and localization accuracy is 97%.[35] This high rate of localizing the disruption may allow surgeons to make an incision directly over the defect.[41] Although MRI can also detect disruptions of corpora spongiosum, its accuracy is lower with sensitivity of 60% and specificity of 78%.[43]

EUA guidelines cite cavernosography as an additional option,[3] although its use in the initial evaluation of penile fractures is limited because of its time-consuming nature and unfamiliarity among most urologists and radiologists.[1,44] Cavernosography involves the injection of an erectogenic agent to facilitate tumescence; after a degree of tumescence is obtained, contras is injected into the corpora under live fluoroscopy.[18,23] Cavernosography has a high false-negative rate of up to 28%.[45,46] Cavernosography also carries the risks of pain, infection, corporal fibrosis, and priapism.[23,44,47,48] This technology may be useful in intraoperative settings when a fracture is suspected but not discovered.[19]

Because the aforementioned imaging studies have relatively poor accuracy with regards to urethral injuries, AUA and EUA guidelines recommend either retrograde urethrogram (RUG) or

cystoscopy at the time of surgical intervention if urethral injury is suspected[2,3] (**Fig. 3**). Urethral injury should be suspected in patients with gross or microscopic hematuria, difficulty voiding, or blood at meatus.[8,29] In addition, RUG or cystoscopy should be performed in the setting of bilateral rupture, as concomitant urethral injury is near ubiquitous in this circumstance.[7,22,27,29]

MANAGEMENT AND OUTCOMES

Conservative management of penile fractures includes application of hot or cold compresses, pressure dressings, suppression of erections, and anti-inflammatory drugs.[18] Conservative

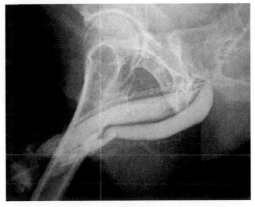

Fig. 3. Retrograde urethrogram concerning for concomitant penile urethral injury.

management has fallen out of favor because of higher complication rates and inferior erectile preservation outcomes compared with surgical management.[8,49–52] Specifically, conservative management is associated with a greater risk of penile curvature, erectile dysfunction, painful erections, arteriovenous fistulas, and infections.[8,51,52] Conservative management is also associated with prolonged hospitalizations.[8,49,51]

Urgent (not necessarily emergent) surgical repair is considered the standard of care for penile fractures.[28] In absence of urethral injury, delay of surgery does not seem to be overly detrimental with regards to outcomes. Kozacıoğlu and colleagues[53] found no difference in erectile dysfunction, penile curvature, or painful erections when comparing surgery within 6 hours, 6 to 12 hours, and 12 to 24 hours of injury. Some advocate for even longer delay of 7 to 12 days so that edema may resolve and the site of injury can be better appreciated.[28,54] In a study of 24 patients with unilateral penile fractures without urethral involvement, a 7 to 12 day delay with an incision directly over injury was not associated with any long-term complications.[54] In a systematic review of immediate (<24 hours) and delayed (>24 hours) surgical repair, there was no difference in erectile dysfunction, nor scar formation. There was a statistically significant increase in the rate of penile curvature in the delayed group, but in most cases, this was mild and exerted no negative effects on sexual function.[55] In a large retrospective study, Bozzini and colleagues[56] did note a statistically significant correlation between erectile dysfunction and undergoing surgery beyond 8.23 hours;

this may not yield clinical significance given only mild erectile dysfunction noted.

Multiple surgical approaches to fracture repair have been described including circumferential degloving, inguinoscrotal, midline ventral penoscrotal, and lateral. There is no data suggesting any approach is universally superior.[57] The main advantage of the subcoronal circumferential incision is maximum exposure, allowing examination of all 3 corporal bodies and reducing the risk of missing a bilateral injury or urethral injury.[1,18,23,57] The disadvantage of the circumferential degloving approach is the extensive dissection, which can lead to decreased sensation and rarely, skin necrosis.[23,54,58] This incision also makes exploration of the proximal penis difficult, especially when there is a large amount of hematoma or tissue edema. The ventral midline penoscrotal incision allows excellent exposure of the site of most penile fractures (proximal, ventral, and lateral) and the urethra[1,59] (**Fig. 4**). A direct longitudinal incision directly over the fracture site may be beneficial when location of the fracture is known and there is no concern for bilateral or urethral involvement.[1,28,54,60] This approach may be performed under local anesthesia and allows for less dissection; it has generated satisfactory outcomes in immediate and delayed settings.[28,54,60,61]

Regardless of the incision of choice, the key principles in surgical repair of penile fractures are exposure, evacuation of hematoma, identification of the site of injury, wound toilet and debridement, suturing of tears in tunica albuginea, and urethral repair as needed.[19] Closure of the tunical defect should be performed with 2-0 or 3-0 absorbable

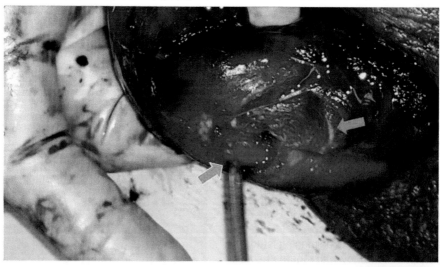

Fig. 4. Ventral midline penoscrotal incision provides excellent exposure, allowing the penile fracture (*blue arrow*) and concomitant urethral injury (*green arrow*) to be identified.

sutures in an interrupted or running fashion.[1,8,26,41] Palpable suture can be avoided by inverting the knots.[10,27] After tunica closure, some experts recommend artificial erection with saline or methylene blue to assess for leak in the repair and separate injuries.[1,19,27,46,57] Urethral defects should be repaired over a catheter with fine (4-0 or 5-0) absorbable suture[1,19,29,57,62,63] **(Fig. 5)**. The catheter should remain in place for at least 7 to 10 days.[57] Postoperatively, patients should be advised to abstain from sexual intercourse for 4 to 6 weeks, as early erections may lead to dehiscence of the corporal repair.[1,9,41,48,62]

Although surgical repair is superior to conservative management, postoperative complications occur at a rate of approximately 20%.[8] The most common complications are palpable penile nodule (13.1%), penile curvature (2.8%), erectile dysfunction (1.9%), painful erections (1.4%), and wound infections (0.2%).[8] Despite erectile dysfunction being uncommon after surgical repair, many patients suffer from performance anxiety and fear of recurrence, which may affect sexual function.[58,64] Surgical repair of urethral disruption in the setting of penile fractures does not seem to predispose to urethral stricture disease.[65]

Of note, the management of post-CCH fractures remains controversial. A survey of clinicians (specifically, members of the Sexual Medicine Society of North America [SMSNA]) who administer CCH and had experience managing postinjection fracture indicated that the vast majority (85%) of post-CCH fractures occurred at the location of Collagenase injection. Most participants (62%) reported that the tunica tissue at the time of surgical repair was of worse quality than what is typical in penile fracture. Of the 44 cases reported in the survey, 33% were managed nonoperatively; SMSNA members reported no significant difference between surveillance and surgery with regards to sexual function, curvature, and patient satisfaction.[16] Larger data sets and long-term data are required, but initial experience appears to indicate that conservative management may be appropriate in some cases of post-CCH penile fractures.

SUMMARY

Penile fracture is a urologic injury with an etiology that varies based on the cultural milieu. Diagnosis can be made based on history and physical examination alone. Patients should be evaluated with RUG or cystoscopy when urethral injury is suspected. Ultrasound or MRI is a helpful adjunct when the diagnosis is unclear, and can assist in identifying the location of the rupture. Surgical management is favored over conservative measures to improve outcomes. Delayed surgical repair may not be inferior to immediate intervention.

CLINICS CARE POINTS

- Penile fractures require urgent urologic evaluation.
- Diagnosis should be promptly made with careful history and physical exam.
- Imaging to aid in the diagnosis can be considered when diagnosis is unclear.
- Immediate surgical exploration remains the standard of care.

DISCLOSURE

The authors have nothing to disclose.

REFERENCES

1. Morey AF, Zhao LC. Genital and lower urinary tract trauma. In: Wein A, Kavoussi L, Partin A, et al, editors. Campbell-walsh urology, Vol 4, Ed. 11. Philadelphia: Elsevier; 2016. p. 2379–92. chap 101.
2. Morey AF, Brandes S, Dugi DD 3rd, et al. Urotrauma: AUA guideline. J Urol 2014;192(2):327–35.
3. Summerton DJ, Djakovic N, Kitrey ND, et al. Guidelines on urological trauma. 2018. Available at: http://uroweb.org/guideline/urological-trauma/. Accessed October 2019.
4. Rodriguez D, Li K, Apoj M, et al. Epidemiology of penile fractures in United States emergency departments: access to care disparities may lead to suboptimal outcomes. J Sex Med 2019;16(2):248–56.
5. Mirzazadeh M, Fallahkarkan M, Hosseini J. Penile fracture epidemiology, diagnosis and management in Iran: a narrative review. Transl Androl Urol 2017; 6(2):158–66.

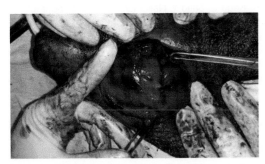

Fig. 5. Repair of the tunical defect, and closure of urethral defect over catheter.

6. Eke N. Fracture of the penis. Br J Surg 2002;89(5): 555–65.

7. Barros R, Schilze L, Ornellas AA, et al. Relationship between sexual position and severity of penile fracture. Int J Impot Res 2017;29(5):207–9.

8. Amer T, Wilson R, Chlosta P, et al. Penile Fracture: a meta-analysis. Urol Int 2016;96:315–29.

9. Mydlo JH. Surgeon experience with penile fracture. J Urol 2001;166(2):526–9.

10. Zargooshi J. Sexual function and tunica albuginea wound healing following penile fracture: An 18-year follow-up study of 352 patients from Kermanshah, Iran. J Sex Med 2009;6(4):1141–50.

11. Ishikawa T, Fujisawa M, Tamada H, et al. Fracture of the penis: nine cases with evaluation of reported cases in Japan. Int J Urol 2003;10(5):257–60.

12. Reis LO, Cartapatti M, Marmiroli R, et al. Mechanisms predisposing penile fracture and long-term outcomes on erectile and voiding functions. Adv Urol 2014;2014:768158.

13. Kramer AC. Penile fracture seems more likely during sex under stressful situations. J Sex Med 2011;8: 3414–7.

14. Carson CC 3rd, Sadeghi-Nejad H, Tursi JP, et al. Analysis of the clinical safety of intralesional injection of collagenase Clostridium histolyticum (CCH) for adults with Peyronie's disease (PD). BJU Int 2015; 116(5):815–22.

15. Beilan JA, Wallen JJ, Baumgarten AS, et al. Intralesional injection of collagenase clostridium histolyticum may increase the risk of late-onset penile fracture. Sex Med Rev 2018;6(2):272–8.

16. Yafi FA, Anaissie J, Zurawin J, et al. Results of SMSNA survey regarding complications following intralesional injection therapy with collagenase clostridium histolyticum for peyronie's disease. J Sex Med 2016;13(4):684–9.

17. Bitsch M, Kromann-Andersen B, Schou J, et al. The elasticity and the tensile strength of tunica albuginea of the corpora cavernosa. J Urol 1990;143(3):642–5.

18. Miller S, McAninch JW. Penile fracture and soft tissue injury. In: McAninch JW, editor. Traumatic and reconstructive urology. 1st ed. Philadelphia, PA: W. B. Saunders; 1996. p. 693–8.

19. Al-Shaiji TF, Amann J, Brock GB. Fractured penis: Diagnosis and management. J Sex Med 2009; 6(12):3231–40.

20. De Rose AF, Giglio M, Carmignani G. Traumatic rupture of the corpora cavernosa: New physiopathologic acquisitions. Urology 2001;57(2):319–22.

21. Hsu GL, Brock G, Martínez-Piñeiro L, et al. Anatomy and strength of the tunica albuginea: its relevance to penile prosthesis extrusion. J Urol 1994;151(5): 1205–8.

22. Koifman L, Barros R, Junior RAS, et al. Penile fracture: Diagnosis, treatment and outcomes of 150 patients. Urology 2010;76(6):1488–92.

23. Jack GS, Garraway I, Reznichek R, et al. Current treatment options for penile fractures. Rev Urol 2004;6:114–20.

24. Falcone M, Garaffa G, Castidlione F, et al. Current management of penile fracture: an up-to-date systematic review. Sex Med Rev 2018;6(2):253–60.

25. Agarwal MM, Singh SK, Sharma DK, et al. Fracture of the penis: a radiological or clinical diagnosis? A case series and literature review. Can J Urol 2009; 16(2):4568–75.

26. Naraynsingh V, Raju GC. Fracture of the penis. Br J Surg 1985;72(4):305–6.

27. Nawaz H, Khan M, Tareen FM, et al. Penile fracture: presentation and management. J Coll Physicians Surg Pak 2010;20(5):331–4.

28. Naraynsingh V, Hariharan S, Goetz L, et al. Late delayed repair of fractured penis. J Androl 2010;31: 231–3.

29. Amit A, Arun K, Bharat B, et al. Penile fracture and associated urethral injury: Experience at a tertiary care hospital. J Can Urol Assoc 2013;7(3–4): E168–70.

30. Kurkar A, Elderwy AA, Orabi H. False fracture of the penis: Different pathology but similar clinical presentation and management. Urol Ann 2014;6(1):23–6.

31. El-Assmy A, El-Tholoth HS, Abou-El-Ghar ME, et al. False penile fracture: value of different diagnostic approaches and long-term outcome of conservative and surgical management. Urology 2010;75(6):1353–6.

32. Feki W, Derouiche A, Belhaj K, et al. False penile fracture: report of 16 cases. Int J Impot Res 2007; 19(5):471–3.

33. Dias-Filho AC, Fregonesi A, Martinez CAT, et al. Can the snapping sound discriminate true from false penile fractures? Bayesian analysis of a case series of consecutively treated penile fracture patients. Int J Impot Res. 2020;32(4):446–54.

34. Kropman RF, Venema PL, Pelger RC. Traumatic rupture of the suspensory ligament of the penis. Case report. Scand J Urol Nephrol 1993;27(1):123–4.

35. Zare Mehrjardi M, Darabi M, Bagheri SM, et al. The role of ultrasound (US) and magnetic resonance imaging (MRI) in penile fracture mapping for modified surgical repair. Int Urol Nephrol 2017;49(6):937–45.

36. Koga S, Saito Y, Nakamura N, et al. Sonography in fracture of the penis. Br J Urol 1993;72(2):228–9.

37. Metzler IS, Reed-Maldonado AB, Lue TF. Suspected penile fracture: to operate or not to operate? Transl Androl Urol 2017;6(5):981–6.

38. Avery LL, Scheinfeld MH. Imaging of penile and scrotal emergencies. Radiographics 2013;33(3): 721–40.

39. Napier D. The role of ultrasound in the diagnosis of penile fracture. Sonography 2019;6:15–23.

40. Guler I, Ödev K, Kalkan H, et al. The value of magnetic resonance imaging in the diagnosis of penile fracture. Int Braz J Urol 2015;41(2):325–8.

41. Abolyosr A, Abdel Moneim AE, Abdelatif AM, et al. The management of penile fracture based on clinical and magnetic resonance imaging findings. BJU Int 2005;96(3):373–7.

42. Saglam E, Tarhan F, Hamarat MB, et al. Efficacy of magnetic resonance imaging for diagnosis of penile fracture: A controlled study. Investig Clin Urol 2017; 58(4):255–60.

43. Sokolakis I, Schubert T, Oelschlaeger M, et al. The role of magnetic resonance imaging in the diagnosis of penile fracture in real-life emergency settings: comparative analysis with intraoperative findings. J Urol 2019;202(3):552–7.

44. Morey AF, Metro MJ, Carney KJ, et al. Consensus on genitourinary trauma: external genitalia. BJU Int 2004;94(4):507–15.

45. Beysel M, Tekin A, Gurdal M, et al. Evaluation and treatment of penile fractures: accuracy and clinical diagnosis and the value of corpus cavernosography. Urology 2002;60(3):492–6.

46. Mydlo JH, Hayyeri M, Macchia RJ. Urethrography and cavernosography imaging in a small series of penile fractures: a comparison with surgical findings. Urology 1998;51(4):616–9.

47. Pliskow RJ, Ohme RK. Corpus cavernosography in acute "fracture" of the penis. AJR Am J Roentgenol 1979;133(2):331–2.

48. Sawh SL, O'Leary MP, Berry AM, et al. Fractured penis: A review. Int J Impot Res 2008;20(4):366–9.

49. Yapanoglu T, Aksoy Y, Adanur S, et al. Seventeen years' experience of penile fracture: conservative vs. surgical treatment. J Sex Med 2009;6(7): 2058–63.

50. Yamaçake KG, Tavares A, Padovani GP, et al. Long-term treatment outcomes between surgical correction and conservative management for penile fracture: retrospective analysis. Korean J Urol 2013;54(7): 472–6.

51. Nicolaisen GS, Melamud A, Williams RD, et al. Rupture of the corpus cavernosum: Surgical management. J Urol 1983;130(5):917–9.

52. Muentener M, Suter S, Hauri D, et al. Long-term experience with surgical and conservative treatment of penile fracture. J Urol 2004;172(2):576–9.

53. Kozacıoğlu Z, Ceylan Y, Aydoğdu Ö, et al. An update of penile fractures: long-term significance of the number of hours elapsed till surgical repair on long-term outcomes. Turk J Urol 2017;43(1):25–9.

54. Nasser TA, Mostafa T. Delayed surgical repair of penile fracture under local anesthesia. J Sex Med 2008;5(10):2464–9.

55. Wong NC, Dason S, Bansal RK, et al. Can it wait? A systematic review of immediate vs. delayed surgical repair of penile fractures. Can Urol Assoc J 2017; 11(1–2):53–60.

56. Bozzini G, Albersen M, Otero JR, et al. Delaying surgical treatment of penile fracture results in poor functional outcomes: Results from a large retrospective multicenter European study. Eur Urol Focus 2018;4(1):106–10.

57. Kamdar C, Mooppan UMM, Kim H, et al. Penile fracture: Preoperative evaluation and surgical technique for optimal patient outcome. BJU Int 2008;102(11): 1640–4.

58. Barros R, Schul A, Ornellas P, et al. Impact of surgical treatment of penile fracture on sexual function. Urology 2019;126:128–33.

59. Mazaris EM, Livadas K, Chalikopoulos D, et al. Penile fractures: immediate surgical approach with a midline ventral incision. BJU Int 2009;104(4): 520–3.

60. Naraynsingh V, Maharaj D, Kuruvilla T, et al. Simple repair of fractured penis. J R Coll Surg Edinb 1998;43(2):97–8.

61. Mansi MK, Emran M, el-Mahrouky A, et al. Experience with penile fractures in Egypt: Long-term results of immediate surgical repair. J Trauma 1993; 35(1):67–70.

62. Barros R, Silva M, Antonucci V, et al. Primary urethral reconstruction results in penile fracture. Ann R Coll Surg Engl 2018;100(1):21–5.

63. Maharaj D, Naraynsingh V. Fracture of the penis with urethral rupture. Injury 1998;29(6):48.

64. Bolat MS, Özen M, Önem K, et al. Effects of penile fracture and its surgical treatment on psychosocial and sexual function. Int J Impot Res 2017;29(6): 244–9.

65. Derouiche A, et al. Management of penile fractures complicated by urethral rupture. Int J Impot Res 2008;20(1):111–4.

Management of Priapism
2021 Update

Christian Ericson, MD, Bryce Baird, MD, Gregory A. Broderick, MD*

KEYWORDS

- Priapism • Management • Shunt • Guidelines • Penile prosthesis

KEY POINTS

- Priapism management, Intracavernosal shunting, Penile prosthesis
- Ischemic priapism, Non ischemic priapism, Stuttering priapism, Priapism management, Shunting

INTRODUCTION

Priapism is defined as a penile erection that lasts longer than 4 hours after completion of sexual activity or that is unrelated to sexual activity.[1] Priapism is a disorder of the hemodynamic systems that control erection and detumescence of the penis. Priapism is relatively rare, with an incidence of 1.5 per 100,000 person-years.[2] Contemporary management of priapism is directed toward 3 goals: resolution of the acute event, preservation of the erectile function, and preventing recurrence.[3]

There are 2 pathophysiologic variants that are essential to distinguish in the emergent setting: ischemic (low-flow) and nonischemic (high-flow).[4] Each variant has specific etiologies, diagnostic criteria, and management. Ischemic priapism may be conceptualized as a compartment syndrome of the penis. Emergent categorization of ischemic versus nonischemic versus recurrent ischemic priapism (RIP) (stuttering priapism) is essential because ischemic priapism may result in penile fibrosis and erectile dysfunction (ED).[1] Although the priapic erection provokes anxiety in both patient and provider, nonischemic priapism does not mandate emergent intervention.[5]

Patients with suspected priapism should be evaluated by an emergency medicine physician and ideally a urologist. A complete medical and sexual history should be documented. Points to discuss with the patient include the erection onset, duration, presence or absence of penile pain, antecedent genital or perineal trauma (straddle injury),

prior episodes of prolonged erection, and general erectile quality.[4] Medical history should be directed at risk factors for priapism, especially prescribed of intracavernosal injectables, hematologic diseases (eg, sickle cell disease [SCD], glucose-5-phosphate dehydrogenase deficiency, hereditary spherocytosis, and leukemia), medications (eg, psychotropic medications, especially trazodone), use of oral phosphodiesterase type 5 (PDE5) inhibitors, over-the-counter medications/supplements for ED, and recreational drugs (cocaine).[4,6] A focused physical examination should be performed. The physical examination is important to determine the degree of penile rigidity and any evidence of perineal trauma.[1] Patients with ischemic priapism present with rigid corporal bodies, the tips of which often are palpable through the typically soft glans penis; the degree of tenderness is a function of the duration of ischemic priapism. In nonischemic priapism, the corporal bodies are partially erect and generally not tender to palpation.[4]

In both ischemic priapism and nonischemic priapism, the precipitating event may be a nocturnal erection that fails to subside. The physiology of ischemic priapism begins with a normal erection; the pathology is related to time-dependent changes in corporal oxygenation, hypercarbia, and acidosis as the erection persists beyond 4 hours to 10 hours.[4]

Nonischemic priapism almost universally is associated with prior pelvic or penile trauma. Straddle injuries may cause disruption of the

Department of Urology, Mayo Clinic Florida, 4500 San Pablo Road, Jacksonville, FL 32224, USA
* Corresponding author.
E-mail address: broderick.gregory@mayo.edu

Urol Clin N Am 48 (2021) 565–576
https://doi.org/10.1016/j.ucl.2021.07.003

cavernous artery or cavernous sinusoids resulting in arteriolar-sinusoidal fistula. The onset of nonischemic priapism may not be evident for hours to days following the initial trauma. A partial persistent erection typically becomes evident following a nocturnal erection some days to weeks later. Nonischemic priapism is not a compartment syndrome and may not be associated with discomfort other than at the site of a prior injury.[7]

This commentary discusses the current literature and practices surrounding the diagnosis and management of ischemic and nonischemic priapism. Few randomized controlled trials of priapism management exist due to the emergent nature of the condition. There are many published society guidelines, surgical case reports, and basic science investigations. A general understanding of this pathophysiology and penile hemodynamics allows the urologist to safely and effectively triage patients to the appropriate medical and surgical interventions.

ISCHEMIC PRIAPISM ETIOLOGY AND PATHOPHYSIOLOGY

Ischemic priapism is the most common subtype of priapism and accounts for more than 95% of all reported priapism episodes.[7,8] Ischemic priapism is a medical emergency. Failure to achieve prompt and complete detumescence typically results in cavernous thrombosis and smooth muscle necrosis. The natural history of ischemic priapism is days to weeks of penile erection and pain, which progresses to fibrosis and ED.[9] Extraneous factors, such as busy emergency departments, delayed transportation, patient embarrassment, and intoxication, can delay diagnosis. A study of US emergency room visits between 2006 and 2009 identified 32,462 diagnostic codes for priapism (a national incidence of 5.4 per 100,000 men per year). Priapism incidence was 30% higher in summer months, and 13% of visits resulted in hospitalizations.[10]

Ischemic priapism is defined by rigid corpora, minimal or no cavernous nonischemic inflow, and complete occlusion of venous outflow. The result of this hematologic stasis is a progressively acidotic environment within the corpora, secondary to hypoxia and hypercarbia. Aspirated blood from the corpora is dark red due to the absence of bound oxygen. The progressive acidity within the closed compartment activates corporal nociceptors; hence, pain is a key factor in differentiating ischemic priapism from nonischemic priapism.[11]

The hallmark physical finding of ischemic priapism is fully erect, rigid, and tender corporal bodies. The glans and corpus spongiosum may be flaccid or partially engorged but are not rigid. History and physical examination alone may be sufficient for the experienced provider to diagnose ischemic priapism, but corporal aspiration and penile blood gas are confirmatory and warranted when possible. Inquiries into previous episodes of priapism and interventions for such are important and may help diagnose and direct evaluation and treatment.

Intracavernous injection (ICI) therapy with vasodilator agents is a common treatment of men with ED refractory to oral PDE5 inhibitors. The incidence of prolonged erection or ischemic priapism following diagnostic penile injection (prostaglandin E1, papaverine, papaverine/phentolamine, or combination of all 3, Trimix) in the office is reported to vary between 1.3% and 5.3%.[12] The likelihood of prolonged erection or priapism following diagnostic alprostadil injection varies with the etiology of ED and may be considerably higher in younger men, and in patients with neurogenic or psychogenic ED.[12] Urologists should be aware that recreational use of ICIs has been reported as the primary etiology of priapism in specific community settings. A retrospective of cases from a major Los Angeles medical center identified 169 events of ischemic priapism over 8 years; 49% of events were related to recreational use of ICIs; 50% of patients using recreational ICIs also were human immunodeficiency virus positive. Only 25% of patients had been prescribed ICI therapy; oral PDE5 inhibitors were reported in 5% of cases; SCD in 4%; and trazodone use in 5%.[7,13]

Multiple classes of medications are well known to cause priapism by themselves or in combination with erection potentiating medications. Although the package inserts for all PDE5 inhibitors commercially available in the United States (ie, avanafil, sildenafil, tadalafil, and vardenafil) warn of prolonged erections, ischemic priapism following PDE5 inhibitor therapy is rare in the average patient with ED. A query of the FDA Adverse Event Reporting System (FAERS) Public Dashboard found 411 cases of PDE5 inhibitor–related priapism since 1998. Drug-induced priapism was 2-times to 2.6-times more likely with antipsychotics or trazodone than PDE5 inhibitors.[14,15]

Another important etiology for ischemic priapism is hematological abnormalities. Blood dyscrasias have been proposed to cause vascular stasis, leading to decreased venous outflow, which prevents detumescence.[7] The blood dyscrasia most often associated with ischemic priapism is SCD.[16] SCD is the result of a mutation in the gene coding for hemoglobin. Boys and men who are homozygous for the hemoglobin S gene are likely to manifest SCD.

The incidence of priapism in patients with SCD under 18 is 3.6% versus 42% in patients over the age of 18 years. Other hematologic pathologies (eg leukemia) have been associated with ischemic priapism in up to 5% of cases.[17]

The pathophysiology of ischemic priapism from SCD is complex. Historically ischemic priapism was attributed to sludging of sickled red cells in the penile sinusoids.[7] Although the primary event in the sickling of red cells is polymerization of abnormal hemoglobin, there are downstream pathophysiologic events related to chronic hemolysis and oxidant damage that may be germane to the pathogenesis of ischemic priapism in SCD. It has been proposed that nitric oxide synthase deficiency (down-regulation cyclic guanosine monophosphate [cGMP] protein kinase 1 and Rho-kinase pathways) in SCD patients leads to an impaired negative feedback loop in the cGMP and PDE5 pathway. The results are erections that are unchecked. This hypothesis has been demonstrated in a rodent model: cGMP is left in an uninhibited state due to a lack of enough PDE5 to allow cGMP breakdown. Oxidative stress, also known to occur in sickle cell anemia, further alters the balance of the nitric oxide/cGMP (NO/cGMP) pathway. These pathways have been proposed as therapeutic targets for stuttering priapism (**Table 1**).[18]

The urologist and emergency provider should be familiar with SCD-associated RIP and with general recommendations for oral or intravenous hydration and pain control in SCD patients. To screen for SCD in the patient presenting with ischemic priapism, current American Urological Association (AUA) guidelines recommend complete blood cell count, reticulocyte count, and hemoglobin electrophoresis.[1] Consultation with a hematologist is recommended before transfusing for anemia or if other complications of vaso-occlusive crisis (VOC) are suspected. Priapism in SCD patients is not necessarily accompanied by acute VOC. VOC generally is thought to result from ischemia induced by vaso-occlusion in the bones and bone marrow. VOC requires the attention of a hematologist because associated complications include fever/infection, acute kidney injury, acute anemia, hepatobiliary complications, acute chest syndrome, and stroke.[7]

Advanced pelvic malignancies may lead to priapism; this commonly is referred to as "malignant priapism." The pathophysiology of malignant priapism may be direct infiltration of tumor implants or occlusion of venous outflow. Magnetic resonance imaging may be most helpful in distinguishing a patient with penile induration due to malignant infiltration of corporal bodies. A recent study of 412 men with idiopathic ischemic priapism found a 3.5% prevalence of a malignant cause.[9,19]

Other etiologies that should be noted but are not discussed further in this article include thalassemias, lymphomas, amyloidosis, scorpion stings, spider bites, spinal cord injury, and medications for attention-deficit/hyperactivity.

STUTTERING PRIAPISM ETIOLOGY AND PATHOPHYSIOLOGY

Stuttering priapism, or RIP, refers to multiple erection episodes, generally sleep-related, that often are painful, last up to 4 hours, and typically affect adolescents and adult men with SCD.[20] Patients often detail a history of stuttering, awakening with prolonged erections with increasing frequency leading up to an episode of true ischemic priapism.[21]

Sleep-related erections are a natural phenomenon in hormonally intact men. Nocturnal penile

---

Table 1
New molecular targets for treatment of stuttering priapism

Study	Molecular Target	Therapeutic Agent
Burnett and Pierorazio 2011[47]	Nitric oxide, cGMP system	PDE5 inhibitors
Musicki and Burnett 2020[48]	Oxidative stress	Apocynin (NADPH oxidase inhibitors)
Mi et al 2008[49]	Adenosine	ADA-PEG (supplemental enzyme therapy)
Kanika et al 2009[50]	Opiorphins	ODC inhibitor
Musicki, Karakus et al 2018[51]; Morrison, Madden et al 2015[52]; Rachid-Filho, Cavalcanti et al 2009[53]	Androgens	Testosterone replacement therapy; Finasteride
Olujohungbe and Burnett 2013[54]	Adrenergic system	Ephedrine; etilefrine

Abbreviations: ADA-PEG, polyethylene-glycol–modified adenosine deaminase; ODC, ornithine decarboxylase.

tumescence coincides with rapid eye movement sleep; 3 to 5 erections can occur in an 8-hour sleep cycle with erection of varying degrees (tumescence) lasting from 10 minutes to 20 minutes. Unfortunately for men with RIP, the erections can last up to 3 hours to 4 hours and may persist on awakening requiring interventions. RIP needs to be distinguished clinically from the psychological phenomenon, known as sleep-related painful erections (SRPEs). SRPEs are classified as rapid-eye-movement (REM) parasomnias; patients complain of awakening recurrently with painful erections. Awakening from SRPE results in natural detumescence unlike RIP. Nocturnal penile tumescence and rigidity testing in SRPE does not show prolonged erections, and these men have no history of priapism and erectile dysfunction. SRPEs typically are treated with baclofen and other neuroleptic agents.[7]

Treatment options for RIP aim to inhibit specific pathways and factors controlling sleep-related erections. Medications that have been proposed to this effect include ketoconazole, finasteride, antiandrogens (flutamide, bicalutamide, and chlormadinone), gonadotropin-releasing hormone agonists, and diethylstilbesterol. These agents have in common interruption of androgen synthesis and or blockage of androgen receptors resulting in inhibition of nocturnal erections.[22,23]

In vitro studies of antiandrogenic agents also show direct inhibitory effects at the molecular level. They inhibit corporal smooth muscle relaxation by altering cellular calcium transport. The potential side effects of GnRH agonists, antiandrogens, and DES are profound and include gynecomastia, hot flushes, loss of libido, osteoporosis, increased body fat, and insulin resistance. Additionally, DES is associated with risk of deep vein thrombosis.[24]

Ketoconazole is an orally bioavailable antifungal medication. Ketoconazole, at dosages of 200 mg, causes total and free testosterone to fall 60% within hours of dosing. To prevent adrenal insufficiency, patients should be coadministered a corticosteroid. Oral ketoconazole has been shown efficacious in suppressing RIP, with initial dosing of 200 mg, 3 times daily, plus 5 mg of prednisone, for 2 weeks, followed by 200 mg, nightly, without prednisone.[25]

Finasteride and dutasteride are 5α-reductase inhibitors, which block conversion of testosterone to dihydrotestosterone. Finasteride, in dosages from 1 mg to 5 mg daily, and dutasteride, at 0.5 mg daily, both have been shown to reduce frequency and duration of RIP episodes.[26,27]

Direct ICIs of α-adrenergic agents (phenylephrine, metaraminol, and etilefrine) reverse prolonged erections and can terminate an episode of RIP. Self-administration of phenylephrine 100 μg to 200 μg is an effective tool for reliable patients with RIP. Patients started self-administered therapy should be counseled about sympathomimetic side effects including hypertension, headache, and bradycardia.[28,29]

Oral nightly α-adrenergic drugs (pseudoephedrine and etilefrine) potentiate sympathetic pathways causing vasoconstriction of erectile tissues and have been investigated in nightly dosing.[29]

Oral terbutaline has been touted as a treatment of ischemic priapism.[30] Evidence for efficacy of oral terbutaline in management of priapism has not met efficacy standards for priapism according to both the AUA and the European Association of Urology guidelines. This treatment has few side effects but has no significant efficacy in reversing ischemic priapism or preventing RIP and may delay administration of more effective therapy.[1,5]

Finally, daily oral PDE5 inhibitor dosing in SCD patients with RIP has been investigated in a placebo-controlled study. PDE5 inhibitors dosing did not show increased efficacy over placebo during the 8-week trial but sildenafil dosing, at 50 mg, did show a reduction in RIP in the 8-week open-label phase.

Each of those therapies has significant side effects. Antiandrogens suppress testosterone and may have an impact on sexual drive and spermatogenesis. Antiandrogens are contraindicated in prepubescent children and adolescents who have not experienced closure of the epiphyseal plates because this stunts growth. Oral ketoconazole can interrupt androgen synthesis effectively but also interrupts steroidogenesis and combination therapy with prednisone is required.[25] Oral baclofen has shown some efficacy in patients with spinal cord injury or men with SRPE but has little or no impact in neurologically intact men with RIP.[1]

NONISCHEMIC PRIAPISM ETIOLOGY AND PATHOPHYSIOLOGY

Nonischemic priapism, also called high-flow priapism, is a much less common than ischemic priapism. This condition is the result of unregulated cavernous nonischemic inflow following formation of an arteriolar-sinusoidal fistula.[4] In contrast to ischemic priapism, there is appropriate flow of well oxygenated blood through the system, which maintains appropriate pH and oxygenation of the cavernous environment. Unregulated high corporal blood (arteriolar–sinusoidal fistula) does cause partial persistent erection. The etiology of nonischemic priapism most often is blunt perineal trauma, most often straddle injury related to bicycles, falls, or sports trauma. There are reports of nonischemic priapism after correction of ischemic priapism via T-shunt and corporal snake procedure.[31] Direct penetrating injury to the cavernous artery (most commonly needle laceration during treatment of ischemic priapism) also can cause a cavernous fistula. Sustained erection may begin within 24 hours of trauma but typically the sinusoid fistula takes several weeks to mature.[4]

EVALUATION OF PRIAPISM

Careful history and diligent physical examination, as described previously, are the preliminary keys to differentiating ischemic versus nonischemic priapism. A priapism checklist has been proposed to help urologists and emergency room providers (**Table 2**).[4] Laboratory testing with complete blood cell count (blood cell differential and platelet count) and coagulation panel is advised to evaluate for hematologic abnormalities. A penile blood gas effectively differentiates nonischemic from ischemic priapism.[5] Use of a drug screening panel is indicated if there is concern for psychotropic or recreational drug use. Alcohol intoxication and illicit drug use have been shown to be causative in up to 21% of cases of ischemic piapism.[4] If sickle cell anemia is suspected as the underlying cause, additional laboratory studies should be considered: hemoglobin electrophoresis, reticulocyte count, and lactate dehydrogenase. The AUA guidelines do not recommend directing priapism treatment solely at the underlying cause. Treatment of a sickle cell crisis without concomitant emergent management of ischemic priapism is likely to lead to substantial delay in resolution and higher risk of long-term ED. Hematological consultation and investigations of any abnormal laboratories can be pursued after emergent decompression of the priapism.[1]

Initial diagnostic and therapeutic management begins with corporal aspiration. Blood aspirate from ischemic priapism contains deoxygenated blood that appears dark, like motor oil, versus the oxygenated blood of nonischemic priapism, which is much lighter in color. Initial aspirates should be sent for blood gas analysis of P_{O_2}, P_{CO_2}, and pH. Normal nonischemic blood maintains a P_{O_2} of greater than 90 mm Hg with a P_{CO_2} of less than 40 mm Hg. The pH of normal blood is approximately 7.4. Values concerning for ischemic priapism (**Table 3**) are consistent with profound hypoxemic acidosis, often with a P_{O_2} of less than 30 and a P_{CO_2} of greater than 60. pH is acidotic, often less than 7.25. In line with the pathophysiology of nonischemic priapism, the blood gas values from penile aspirates mirror systemic oxygenated blood values.[4]

Color duplex Doppler ultrasonography (CDDU) of the penis is a diagnostic tool that is recommended as an option (where available) by AUA guidelines.[1] EAU guidelines go 1 step further and specify that CDDU of both the penis and perineum are recommended, can differentiate nonischemic from ischemic priapism, can identify fistula in 70% of cases, and may be used as an alternate to penile blood gas in the evaluation of priapism.[5] Ischemic priapism manifests as little to no blood flow in the cavernosal arteries on CDDU imaging. Nonischemic priapism manifests as normal to high blood flow velocities (numeral) within the arteries. It often may appear turbulent secondary to fistula blood flow. When nonischemic priapism is suspected, CDDU also may be used to look for anatomic abnormality, such as pseudoaneurysm. It is recommended that CDDU be performed

Table 2
Priapism checklist

Finding	Ischemic	Nonischemic
Fully rigid corpora	Common	Sometimes present
Penile pain	Common	Sometimes present
Penile blood gas: low PO_2, high CO_2	Common	Rare
Recent penile injection	Common	Sometimes present
Chronic erection without full rigidity	Rare	Common
Perineal trauma	Rare	Common

Table 3
Penile blood gas diagnostic values

Source	P_{O_2} (mm Hg)	P_{CO_2} (mm Hg)	pH
Normal nonischemic blood	>90	<40	7.4
Normal mixed venous blood	40	50	7.35
Ischemic blood from aspirate	<30	>60	<7.25

with the patient frog legged or in lithotomy, to permit scanning of the perineum as well as the penile shaft.[5]

INITIAL MANAGEMENT OF ISCHEMIC PRIAPISM

A variety of nonspecific home remedies, including exercise, ejaculation, ice packs, cold baths, and cold enemas, have been proposed for ischemic priapism; data on efficacy for these are scant and these are not recommended, particularly if they lead to delay in administration of more appropriate evidence-based therapies. Initial management of ischemic priapism should include administration of a dorsal nerve block with appropriate local anesthetic agent. After administration of local anesthetic, a large-bore needle (19 gauge or higher) is placed into the base of the pendulous shaft. Some centers recommend bilateral placement of 19-gauge needles to facilitate simultaneous irrigation and aspiration. The needles subsequently are used for diagnostic aspiration followed by therapeutic aspiration, aspiration/irrigation, and/or injection of a sympathomimetic drug (**Fig. 1**).[4,7] It is the authors'

practice to utilize a single butterfly needle or angiocatheter at the base of the pendulous shaft, leaving just enough room to manually compress the penis below at the penoscrotal junction. Alternatively, 19-gauge needles can be placed bilaterally at the 9-o'clock or 3-o'clock positions if aspiration/irrigation is to be used. The authors compress the penoscrotal junction and aspirate the pendulous penis until it is completely detumesced. Maintaining the butterfly needle, compression is released and the penis allowed to refill. After several rounds of aspiration, red oxygenated blood consistently is observed. Restoration of the corporal environment with oxygenated blood is required for effective smooth muscle contraction in response to sympathomimetic drugs (phenylephrine, ephedrine, epinephrine, norepinephrine, metraminol, and etilefrine). Phenylephrine is the agent of choice, given higher selectivity of α_1-adrenoreceptors with lower stimulation of β-mediated ionotropic and chronotropic effects on the heart, leading to a more favorable side-effect profile.[32] Resuming finger compression at the penoscrotal junction, the authors begin dosing with phenylephrine in 100-μg to 200-μg aliquots every 5 minutes. Smaller aliquots of phenylephrine

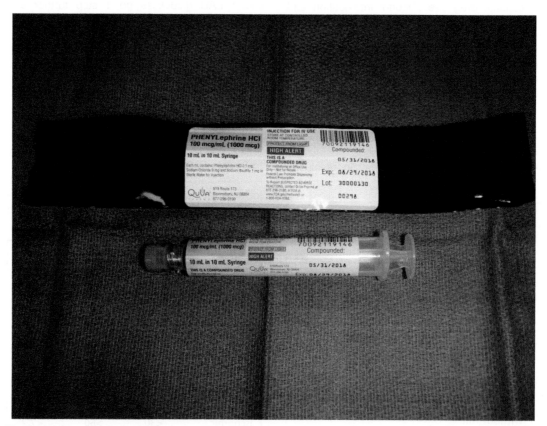

Fig. 1. At the author's institution, proprietary syringes of phenylephrine are available (10-mL syringe with 100 mcg/mL). This permits safe dosing. The authors typically use 2-mL aliquots with repeated aspirations followed by repeated injections. This avoids the dangers inherent with mixing solutions.

are recommended in children. This process of peno-scrotal compression, aspiration, and injection generally can be repeated up to 1000 μg of phenylephrine without significant hypertension/reflex bradycardia in a healthy normotensive adult. At the authors' institution, proprietary syringes of phenylephrine are used (10 mL syringe with 200 μg/mL saline), allowing easy dosing in 1-mL aliquots. This avoids the dangers of mixing and sorting out diluent volumes. Priapism related to in office erectile function testing with ICIs easily may be reversed in most cases, with a single injection of 200 μg of phenylephrine; it is the authors' practice to reverse diagnostic erections at 1 hour.[4,7]

Methodical aspiration and irrigation with 0.9% normal saline as first-line therapy by AUA guideline.[1] A combination of corporal blood aspiration and saline irrigation effectively terminates priapism in 66% of cases compared with aspiration alone (reported success rate of 24%–36%).[33] Aspiration and saline irrigation continued throughout administration of phenylephrine is associated with increase in successful resolution in 81% of cases. In comparison the efficacy of injecting phenylephrine alone is lower 58%. These studies are consistent with the known physiology of ischemic priapism; the corporal smooth muscle will not contract and the ischemic priapism will not reverse so long as the environment is hypoxemic and hypercarbic. Aspiration followed by phenylephrine injection or irrigation with a diluted phenylephrine solution are more effective.[17]

Patients should be apprised of potential adverse events from phenylephrine administration, including headache, palpitations, and dizziness. In most clinic settings, automated blood pressure cuffs and heart rate monitoring are readily available; it is prudent for patients undergoing repeated aspiration/sympathomimetic injections or irrigations to be on sequential monitoring. Oral systemic therapy for sympathomimetics is not indicated in the treatment of acute ischemic priapism but has shown some efficacy in preventing stuttering priapism.[8]

SHUNTING PROCEDURES

Should initial management fail, second-line therapy for ischemic priapism is a distal shunting procedure. A variety of corporo-glanuar distal shunting procedures have been described, each with relatively similar rates of priapism resolution. The AUA (2003 and 2010) reviewed priapism resolution rates with their associated rates of postoperative ED in 3 common distal shunt procedures: Ebbehoj, Winter, and Al-Ghorab. These are detailed in **Table 4** and **Fig. 2**.[1]

Table 4
Distal Penile Shunting - Resolution and Outcomes

Distal Shunt	Resolution (%)	Erectile Dysfunction (%)
Ebbehoj	73	14
Winter	66	25
Al-Ghorab	74	25

Two modifications of distal shunt have been reported within the past decade. The T-shaped shunt involves placement of a no. 10 blade through the glans, 4 mm lateral to the meatus, into the corpora unilaterally; rotating the blade 90° away from the meatus; and then removing the blade.[34,35] Deoxygenated blood is milked out of the incision until there is flow of bright red oxygenated blood. The procedure can be repeated on the contralateral side if there is no resolution of the erection; if bilateral shunt creation fails, corporal tunneling with a smooth-tipped dilator through the incision can be considered.

The corpora snake maneuver is another recent innovation, consisting of bilateral distal corporoglanular shunting (Al-Ghorab) followed by passage of a 7/8 Hegar dilator down the length of the penis to the crura. The initial report indicated success in 8 of 10 patients, with a mean duration of priapism 75 hours.[36]

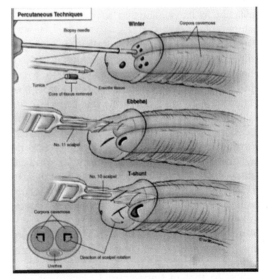

Fig. 2. Percutaneous shunting techniques. (*From* Tom F. Lue, Edoardo S. Pescatori,Surgical Techniques: Distal Cavernosum–Glans Shunts for Ischemic Priapism, The Journal of Sexual Medicine,Volume 3, Issue 4, 2006, Pages 749-752.)

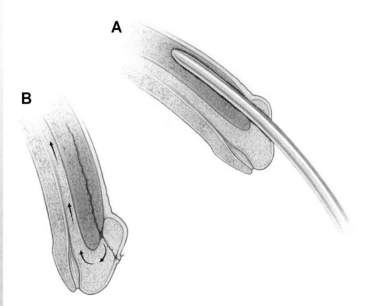

Fig. 3. (*A*) Corporal snake with Hegar dilator; (*B*) postdilation blood flow pathway. (*From* Burnett AL, Pierorazio PM. Corporal "snake" maneuver: corporoglanular shunt surgical modification for ischemic priapism. J Sex Med. 2009 Apr;6(4):1171-1176. doi: 10.1111/j.1743-6109.2008.01176.x. Epub 2009 Feb 4.)

As shown in **Figs. 3 and 4**A–D, Zacharakis and colleagues[37] describe 45 patients with priapism who underwent T-shunt with corporal snaking. For patients with priapism with duration less than 24 hours, 100% of patients had resolution of their erection. For erections of greater than 48 hours, only 30% had resolution. In the less than 24-hour duration group, approximately 50% of patients developed erectile dysfunction, whereas in the greater than 48-hour group, all patients had smooth muscle necrosis and long-term erectile dysfunction. Time to intervention was statically significant in its relationship to erectile function postoperatively.[37]

Despite high success rates of distal shunting to resolve ischemic priapism, approximately 50% of patients in 1 study became candidates for a penile implant.[38] Persistent ischemic priapism of greater than 36 hours uniformly results in erectile dysfunction. Informed consent prior to shunting procedures should clearly delineate for the patient that he will have some degree of ED; he may develop severe ED refractory to medical therapy. The goal of the successful shunt is to shorten the natural history of ischemic priapism, which is persistent painful erection of several weeks.

A recent novel surgical technique for refractory ischemic priapism is known as penoscrotal decompression (PSD). The surgical approach is identical to that of trans-scrotal placement of a penile prosthesis. One or both corporal bodies are isolated and opened sufficiently to permit advancing of a pediatric Yankauer suction distally and proximally to evacuate corporal thrombus.

The technique, as first described, was used in patients failing distal corporo-glanular shunting.[39] In a subsequent multi-institutional study, primary PSD was completely effective in 15 patients, with a mean ischemic duration of 71 hours.[40] The authors propose that primary PSD for ischemic priapism avoids trauma to the distal corpora and glans, which both is cosmetically deforming and makes the patient susceptible to future penile prosthetic erosion.

Conversion of ischemic to nonischemic hyperemic state may yield the appearance the day after surgery that ischemic erection persists. Before returning the patient to operating room for more interventions, it is prudent to perform penile blood gas and/or CDDU and determine whether cavernous flows have resumed.

Older literature described the creation of proximal shunts when distal shunting failed. Examples include shunts between the corpus cavernosum and corpus spongiosum (Quackles and Sacher). Proximal shunting of 1 or both corpora cavernosa directly to the saphenous or deep dorsal vein also has been described (known as Grayhack and Barry shunts, respectively). These procedures are associated with significant risks and unclear benefit; none appears in contemporary ischemic priapism management algorithms.

Early data suggest that there may be a role for antithrombotic therapy (ATT) in the management of ischemic priapism.[41] ATT may prevent thrombotic occlusion of shunts, which is thought to cause early recurrence of priapism.[41] One single-center study, in which 13 patients underwent shunting procedures without ATT therapy

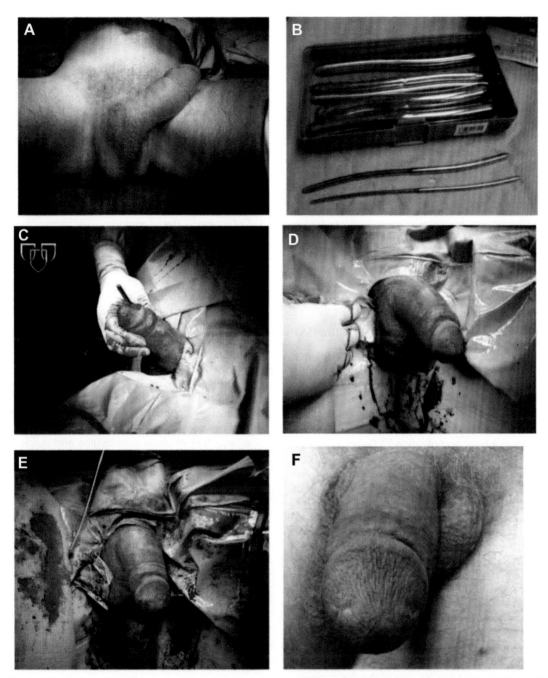

Fig. 4. (*A*) A 54-year-old white man with priapism following Trimix self-injection. He presented to outside hospital after 3 days of ischemic priapism. A Winter shunt failed to reverse priapism. (*B, C,* and *D*) On day 5, he was transferred and underwent bilateral T-shunts and corporal snake maneuver using Hegar dilators with successful detumescence. (*E*) Closed T-shunts. (*F*) Two-week postoperative wound check. (*Used with permission* of Mayo Foundation for Medical Education and Research, all rights reserved.)

compared with 9 patients who had both ATT and a shunting procedure, showed less recurrence of priapism, at rates of 11% versus 69%, respectively.[41] These preliminary findings from a single center should be investigated further, ideally in controlled and randomized studies.

EARLY VERSUS DELAYED PENILE PROSTHESIS PLACEMENT

Penile prosthesis placement is a useful management option for severe erectile dysfunction. In patients with a history of priapism, severe corporal fibrosis can make placement of a prosthesis challenging for even the experienced implanter. For this reason, some experts advocate immediate or early (within several weeks of shunting procedures) penile prosthesis implantation in patients with ischemic priapism likely to result in severe ED.[42] Techniques, including extended corporotomies, excision of corporal fibrosis, and sharp dilation, are requisite.[43] Specialized dilators with a cutting edge may be utilized.[44] The EAU guidelines recommend consideration of penile implant in cases of ischemic priapism of greater than 48 hours' duration.[5] Immediate placement theoretically avoids the risk of penile foreshortening and narrowing that is common in postpriapism penile fibrosis. Unfortunately, immediate or early placement of penile prosthesis is in the setting of priapism carries some risks, including distal erosion, cavernositis, prosthetic infection, and significantly higher rates of reoperation.[45]

MANAGEMENT OF NONISCHEMIC PRIAPISM

Unlike ischemic priapism, nonischemic priapism is not an emergency. Symptoms can persist for years without adverse effects to sexual function.[4] Spontaneous resolution or response to conservative therapy has been reported in up to 62% of published series.[11] The mainstay of treatment remains selective arterial embolization.[1,5] Selective pudendal arteriography is invasive and requires significant skill set of an interventional radiologist familiar with pelvic anatomy. Pudendal arteriography should be reserved for those situations when the patient and urologist have elected to embolize nonischemic priapism and the risks and benefits have been discussed in detail.[4] The most common side effect after embolization is ED. The success rates with selective pudendal artery catheterization followed by embolization are reported between 89% and 100%, with normal erectile function postembolization seen in 75% to 86% of patients.[4] Recurrence has been identified to occur in up to 30% of patients, and retreatment with repeat embolization is an option in that setting.[7]

In patients who are not candidates for angioembolization or who do not have access to a center with the correct personnel or technology, surgical ligation of the cavernosal fistula is an alternate treatment option.[4] Even in these cases, transfer to a center with angiography capabilities is preferred. The surgical approach for this is transcorporal with corporal exploration and often requires intraoperative doppler examination. Care must be taken to not ligate the cavernosal artery in lieu of the true fistula.[46] Patients often must wait 1 months to 2 months after onset of nonischemic priapism secondary to perineal trauma in order for the fistula to fully mature prior to surgical intervention.[4]

SUMMARY

Priapism is a common urologic emergency that the urologist should be comfortable managing. Resolution of the acute event, preservation of the erectile function, and preventing recurrence are the goals of diagnosis and management. Treatment of priapism is diagnosis specific. Key Clinical Care Points of Priapism are:

1. Run the Priapism Checklist (**Table 2**)
2. Determine the etiology: ischemic vs. nonischemic
3. For ischemic priapism:
   a. Consider toxicology screening for substance abuse
   b. Consider Sickle Cell Disease supportive care: oxygenation, hydration, pain control, Hematology Consult
   c. Treat the ischemic compartment with penile aspiration and alpha adrenergic injection (phenylephrine)
   d. Surgical interventions are required for failure of pharmacologic reversal.
4. Nonischemic priapism is typically associated with perineal trauma.
   a. Injection of alpha adrenergics and surgical shunting are not appropriate.
   b. Spontaneous resolution has been reported.
   c. Supportive care with ice and compression on the perineum are reasonable.
   d. Selective pudendal arteriography for imaging and embolization can be considered for persistence and patient bother.

This article is a compilation of the evidence-based recommendations published by the American Urological Association in 2003 and the European Association of Urology published in 2014. The authors have updated those guidelines with current literature to facilitate best practices in the diagnosis and managemet of priapism.

DISCLOSURE

The authors have no disclosures.

REFERENCES

1. Montague DK, Jarow J, Broderick GA, et al. American Urological Association guideline on the management of priapism. J Urol 2003;170:1318–24.
2. Eland IA, et al. Incidence of priapism in the general population. Urology 2001;57(5):970–2.

3. El-Bahnasawy MS, Dawood A, Farouk A. Low-flow priapism: risk factors for erectile dysfunction. BJU Int 2002;89(3):285–90.

4. Broderick, G.A. Priapism. Campbell - Walsh - Wein. Urology, 12th edition, pp. 1539-1563. Elsevier, copyright 2021.

5. Salonia A, Eardley I, Giuliano F, Hatzichristou D, et al, European Association of Urology. European Association of Urology guidelines on priapism. Eur Urol 2014;65(2):480–9. https://doi.org/10.1016/j.eururo.2013.11.008. Epub 2013 Nov 16. PMID: 24314827.

6. Prabhakaran K, Jacobs BL, Smaldone MC, et al. Stuttering priapism associated with hereditary spherocytosis. Can J Urol 2007;14(5):3702–4. PMID: 17949526.

7. Broderick GA, Kadioglu A, Bivalacqua TJ, et al. Priapism: pathogenesis, epidemiology, and management. J Sex Med 2010;7(1 Pt 2):476–500. https://doi.org/10.1111/j.1743-6109.2009.01625.x. PMID: 20092449.

8. Sidhu AS, Wayne GF, Kim BJ, et al. The Hemodynamic Effects of Intracavernosal Phenylephrine for the Treatment of Ischemic Priapism. J Sex Med 2018;15(7):990–6. https://doi.org/10.1016/j.jsxm.2018.05.012. PMID: 29960632.

9. Broderick GA, Harkaway R, et al. Pharmacologic erection: time-dependent changes in the corporal environment. Int J Impot Res 1994;6(1):9–16. PMID: 8019618.

10. Roghmann F, Becker A, Sammon JD, et al. Incidence of priapism in emergency departments in the United States. J Urol 2013;190(4):1275.

11. Muneer A, Ralph D. Guideline of guidelines: priapism. BJU Int 2017;119(2):204–8. https://doi.org/10.1111/bju.13717. Epub 2016 Dec 29. PMID: 27860090.

12. Linet OI, Neff LL. Intracavernous prostaglandin E1 in erectile dysfunction. Clin Investig 1994;72(2):139–49.

13. Zhao H, Berdahl C, Bresee C, et al. Priapism from recreational intracavernosal injections in a high-risk metropolitan community. J Sex Med 2019;16(10):1650–4.

14. Rezaee ME, Gross MS. Are we overstating the risk of priapism with oral phosphodiesterase type 5 inhibitors? J Sex Med 2020;17(8):1579–82. https://doi.org/10.1016/j.jsxm.2020.05.019. Epub 2020 Jul 2. PMID: 32622767.

15. Karayagmurlu A, Coskun M. Successful management of methylphenidate or atomoxetine-related priapism during attention-deficit hyperactivity disorder treatment. J Clin Psychopharmacol 2020;40(3):314–5.

16. Broderick GA. Priapism and sickle-cell anemia: diagnosis and nonsurgical therapy. J Sex Med 2012;9(1):88–103.

17. Broderick GA, Gordon D, Hypolite J, et al. Anoxia and corporal smooth muscle dysfunction: a model for ischemic priapism. J Urol 1994;151(1):259–62.

18. Burnett AL, Chang AG, Crone JK, et al. Noncholinergic penile erection in mice lacking the gene for endothelial nitric oxide synthase. J Androl 2002;23(1):92–7. https://doi.org/10.1002/j.1939-4640.2002.tb02601.x. PMID: 11780929.

19. James Johnson M, Hallerstrom M, Alnajjar HM, et al. Which patients with ischaemic priapism require further investigation for malignancy? Int J Impot Res 2020;32:195–200.

20. Morrison BF, Burnett AL. Stuttering priapism: insights into pathogenesis and management. Curr Urol Rep 2012;13(4):268–76.

21. Kheirandish P, Chinegwundoh F, Kulkarni S. Treating stuttering priapism. BJU Int 2011;108(7):1068–72.

22. Gbadoe AD, Assimadi JK, Segbena YA. Short period of administration of diethylstilbestrol in stuttering priapism in sickle cell anemia. Am J Hematol 2002;69(4):297–8.

23. Serjeant GR, de Ceulaer K, Maude GH. Stilboestrol and stuttering priapism in homozygous sickle-cell disease. Lancet 1985;2(8467):12.

24. Levine LA, Guss SP. Gonadotropin-releasing hormone analogues in the treatment of sickle cell anemia-associated priapism. J Urol 1993;150(2 Pt 1):475–7.

25. Abern MR, Levine LA. Ketoconazole and prednisone to prevent recurrent ischemic priapism. J Urol 2009;182(4):1401–6.

26. Baker RC, Bergeson RL, Yi YA, Ward EE, et al. Dutasteride in the long-term management of stuttering priapism. Transl Androl Urol 2020;9(1):87–92.

27. Dahm P, Rao DS, Donatucci CF. Antiandrogens in the treatment of priapism. Urology 2002;59(1):138.

28. Steinberg J, Eyre RC. Management of recurrent priapism with epinephrine self-injection and gonadotropin-releasing hormone analogue. J Urol 1995;153(1):152–3.

29. Virag R, Bachir D, Lee K, Galacteros F. Preventive treatment of priapism in sickle cell disease with oral and self-administered intracavernous injection of etilefrine. Urology 1996;47(5):777–81 [discussion 781].

30. Ahmed I, Shaikh NA. Treatment of intermittent idiopathic priapism with oral terbutaline. Br J Urol 1997;80(2):341.

31. Vagnoni V, Franceschelli A, Gentile G, et al. High-flow priapism after T-shunt and tunneling in a patient with ischemic priapism. Turk J Urol 2020;46(6):488–91.

32. Mishra K, Loeb A, Bukavina L, et al. Management of priapism: a contemporary review. Sex Med Rev 2020;8(1):131–9.

33. Ateyah A, et al. Intracavernosal irrigation by cold saline as a simple method of treating iatrogenic prolonged erection. J Sex Med 2005;2(2):248–53.

34. Brant WO, Garcia MM, Bella AJ, et al. T shaped shunt and intracavernous tunneling for prolonged priapism. J Urol 2009;181:1699–705.

35. Hoeh MP, Levine LA. Management of recurrent ischemic priapism 2014: a complex condition with devastating consequences. Sex Med Rev 2015; 3(1):24–35.

36. Burnett AL, Pierorazio PM. Corporal "snake" maneuver: corporoglanular shunt surgical modification for ischemic priapism. J Sex Med 2009;6(4):1171–6.

37. Zacharakis E, Raheem AA, Freeman A, Skolarikos A, Garaffa G, Christopher AN, Muneer A, Ralph DJ, et al. The efficacy of the T-shunt procedure and intracavernous tunneling (snake maneuver) for refractory ischemic priapism. J Urol 2014;191(1):164–8.

38. Ortaç M, Çevik G, Akdere H, et al. Anatomic and Functional Outcome Following Distal Shunt and Tunneling for Treatment Ischemic Priapism: A Single-Center Experience. J Sex Med 2019;16(8): 1290–6.

39. Fuchs JS, Shakir N, McKibben MJ, et al. Penoscrotal decompression-promising new treatment paradigm for refractory ischemic priapism. J Sex Med 2018; 15(5):797–802.

40. Baumgarten AS, VanDyke ME, Yi YA, et al. Favourable multi-institutional experience with penoscrotal decompression for prolonged ischaemic priapism. BJU Int 2020;126(4):441–6.

41. Ramstein JJ, Lee A, Cohen AJ, et al. Clinical outcomes of periprocedural antithrombotic therapy in ischemic priapism management. J Sex Med 2020; 17(11):2260–6.

42. Rees RW, Kalsi J, Minhas S, et al. The management of low-flow priapism with the immediate insertion of a penile prosthesis. BJU Int 2002;90(9):893–7.

43. Sadeghi-Nejad H. Penile prosthesis surgery: a review of prosthetic devices and associated complications. J Sex Med 2007;4(2):296–309.

44. Bettocchi C, et al. Penile prosthesis: what should we do about complications? Adv Urol 2008;573560.

45. Ralph DJ, Garaffa G, Muneer A, et al. The immediate insertion of a penile prosthesis for acute ischaemic priapism. Eur Urol 2009;56:1033–8.

46. Shapiro RH, Berger RE. Post-traumatic priapism treated with selective cavernosal artery ligation. Urology 1997;49(4):638–43.

47. Pierorazio PM, Bivalacqua TJ, Burnett AL. Daily phosphodiesterase type 5 inhibitor therapy as rescue for recurrent ischemic priapism after failed androgen ablation. J Androl 2011;32(4):371–4.

48. Musicki B, Burnett AL. Mechanisms underlying priapism in sickle cell disease: targeting and key innovations on the preclinical landscape. Expert Opin Ther Targets 2020;24(5):439–50.

49. Mi T, Abbasi S, Zhang H, Uray K, Chunn JL, Xia LW, Molina JG, Weisbrodt NW, Kellems RE, Blackburn MR, Xia Y. Excess adenosine in murine penile erectile tissues contributes to priapism via A2B adenosine receptor signaling. J Clin Invest 2008;118(4):1491–501.

50. Kanika ND, Tar M, Tong Y, Kuppam DS, Melman A, Davies KP. The mechanism of opiorphin-induced experimental priapism in rats involves activation of the polyamine synthetic pathway. Am J Physiol Cell Physiol 2009;297(4):C916–27.

51. Musicki B, Karakus S, Akakpo W, Silva FH, Liu J, Chen H, Zirkin BR, Burnett AL. Testosterone replacement in transgenic sickle cell mice controls priapic activity and upregulates PDE5 expression and eNOS activity in the penis. Andrology 2018;6(1): 184–91.

52. Morrison BF, Madden W, Clato-Day S, Gabay L. Testosterone Replacement Therapy in Adolescents With Sickle Cell Disease Reverses Hypogonadism Without Promoting Priapism: A Case Report. Urol Case Rep 2015;3(6):179–80.

53. Rachid-Filho D, Cavalcanti AG, Favorito LA, Costa WS, Sampaio FJ. Treatment of recurrent priapism in sickle cell anemia with finasteride: a new approach. Urology 2009;74(5):1054–7.

54. Olujohungbe A, Burnett AL. How I manage priapism due to sickle cell disease. Br J Haematol 2013; 160(6):754–65.

A Conceptual Approach to Understanding and Managing Men's Orgasmic Difficulties

David L. Rowland, PhD

KEYWORDS

- Orgasmic disorders • Ejaculatory disorders • Premature ejaculation • Inhibited ejaculation
- Delayed ejaculation • Sex therapy • Pharmacologic • Ejaculatory latency

KEY POINTS

- Premature ejaculation (PE) and delayed/inhibited ejaculation (DE) may result from a mix of biological and psychogenic factors.
- Medical issues should be investigated when the problem has recently been acquired.
- Addressing ejaculatory latency may be the immediate concern, but communication between sexual partners is important to mutual sexual satisfaction.
- Treatment success for PE based on an integrated approach is high. Treatment success for DE based on psychobehavioral strategies is moderate.

INTRODUCTION

This review discusses 2 ejaculation disorders that represent disturbances in psychosexual responding, *premature ejaculation (PE)* and *delayed/inhibited ejaculation (DE)*. Both disorders are related to the timing/occurrence of ejaculation (ie, ejaculation latency [EL]) during partnered sex, and men with either condition can often be treated successfully and achieve (or regain) a satisfying sex life.

These 2 conditions are discussed separately, touching briefly on definition, prevalence, cause/risk, diagnosis, and treatment. Although a holistic approach is taken for each problem—considering biological, psychological, relationship, and cultural issues—various therapeutic tools may be more suited to or preferred by some patients and practitioners than others. However, *efficacy* and *patient satisfaction*—outcomes that are clearly intertwined—remain the primary concerns of treatment.

Ejaculation/Orgasm as Part of the Sexual Response Cycle in Men

Within the framework of the sexual response, orgasm (and ejaculation) in men is both a biological (reproductive) and psychological (reward) endpoint. Sexual interest and arousal are essential precursors to ejaculation and indicate the man's "readiness" to respond within a perceived sexual situation. This readiness depends on both internal (hormonally "primed" diencephalic brain structures) and external (appropriate/desirable partner and situation) cues. During the sexual activity, levels of arousal gradually increase, eventually culminating in the 2 phases of ejaculatory response. The first phase is emission, represented by urethral distension and bladder neck closure, and is associated with the man's subjective experience of "ejaculatory inevitability," the feeling that impending ejaculation cannot be stopped. The second phase is semen expulsion via striate/smooth muscle contractions in the groin region

Department of Psychology, Valparaiso University, 1001 Campus Drive, Valparaiso, IN 46383, USA
E-mail address: david.rowland@valpo.edu

Urol Clin N Am 48 (2021) 577–590
https://doi.org/10.1016/j.ucl.2021.06.012
0094-0143/21/© 2021 Elsevier Inc. All rights reserved.

that give rise to the experience of orgasm, mediated through sensory fibers that course to the brain.[1] Although often perceived as one and the same, ejaculation and orgasm are 2 distinct events. Ejaculation is a peripherally mediated spinal neural response, whereas orgasm is a central "response to/perception of" the peripheral ejaculatory response. In this article the author refers primarily to ejaculation problems, recognizing that in most cases the issue involves distress about both ejaculation and orgasm.

Conceptualizing the Problem of Ejaculatory Disorders

The *problem* of ejaculatory disorders can be expressed simply: in response to penile stimulation, the time (latency) that it takes men to reach ejaculation varies, across different men (interindividually) and within the same man on different occasions (intraindividually). Interindividually means some men consistently reach ejaculation quickly, others take substantially more time, and still others require a long time, even finding it difficult to ejaculate at all (**Fig 1**). Intraindividually means latencies may vary across situations, partners, and episodes.

The sources for interindividual and intraindividual variation in ELs are different. Interindividual variation may result from various formative psychosexual experiences during critical stages of sexual development and/or from biological differences—probably genetic or epigenetic in origin—in the neurophysiological substrates that mediate

ejaculation.[1] Intraindividual variation is likely the result of contextual (psychobehavioral) factors such as levels of desire/arousal, the amount/type of stimulation, the specific type of sexual activity (intercourse, masturbation, and so forth), partner characteristics, cognitive-affective states (eg, anxiety), and other factors related to the situation, partner, or relationship.

Men with PE have very short ELs compared with other men, and they struggle to delay or control their ejaculation, as they perceive it as happening too quickly (see **Fig. 1**). Men who have DE have long latencies compared with other men, struggling to reach orgasm and sometimes giving up in frustration or when their partner is exhausted. For both disorders, men feel a lack of control over the timing of ejaculation (in either delaying or advancing it), and as a result they experience bother/distress, not only about their sense of inadequacy but also about how their condition affects their partner (**Table 1**).

DISCUSSION: PREMATURE EJACULATION
Defining Criteria, Premature Ejaculation Subtypes, and Prevalence

Defining diagnostic criteria
Contemporary diagnostic criteria for PE have incorporated 3 elements: a short EL; the lack of ability to delay ejaculation (ie, ejaculating before wanting to); and negative consequences for the man, his partner, or the relationship.[2–5] At this time, no broad consensus exists regarding

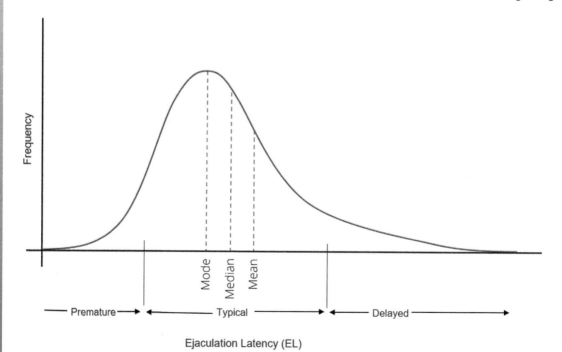

Fig. 1. Sample distribution of ejaculatory latencies, illustrating men with short, typical, and long latencies.

Table 1
Comparison and contrast of premature and delayed ejaculation

	Premature Ejaculation	Delayed Ejaculation
Ejaculatory Latency	Short, <1 or 2 min	Prolonged, >15–20 min, or giving up
Ejaculatory Control	Lack of ability to delay ejaculation	Lack of ability to hasten ejaculation
Bother/Distress	Related to self, partner, relationship	Related to self, partner, relationship
Subtypes	Lifelong, acquired, and subjective?	Lifelong and acquired

operationalizing the first criterion, that is, how to define a "short ejaculatory latency." The American Psychiatric Association's Diagnostic and Statistical Manual of Mental Disorders 5th edition (DSM-5) sets an EL threshold of 1 minute after vaginal penetration,[2] whereas the International Society of Sexual Medicine (ISSM) defines 2 types of PE (lifelong and acquired), with the distinguishing features being the time of onset within the man's sex life and the EL following heterosexual penetration. The ISSM defines *lifelong* PE as occurring before or within about 1 minute of vaginal penetration and *acquired* PE as a "clinically significant and bothersome reduction in latency, often to about 3 minutes or less."[3] In contrast, the World Health Organization's International Classification of Diseases 11th edition (ICD-11) identifies 3 forms of PE—lifelong, acquired, and subjective—but does not specify an EL for any of the subtypes..[4] Finally, in a recent reexamination of the PE diagnostic criteria, the American Urologic Association (AUA) concluded that an EL up to 2 minutes is supported by recent evidence for men with *lifelong* PE.[5–8] In addition, the AUA definition for *acquired* PE suggested that the typical EL should fall under about 2 to 3 minutes or alternatively, be reduced by about 50% relative to prior estimations.

So which, if any, EL criterion should be used? The goal of any diagnostic procedure is to reduce errors of inclusion and exclusion, that is, including men in the diagnosis who do not have the problem and excluding men from the diagnosis who do have the problem. A latency criterion is therefore relevant because it has the potential to reduce diagnostic errors. However, studies have demonstrated that (the lack of) ejaculatory control—rather than EL—plays the more central role in predicting PE status, lack of sexual satisfaction, and its associated distress/bother.[9,10] Accordingly, EL might best be viewed as a characterization of PE "risk" rather than as a precise determinant of PE or non-PE status. Specifically, an EL of less than 2 minutes captures the idea that the man ejaculates "shortly after penetration," and when used in conjunction with the other 2 criteria for PE, poor ejaculatory control and bother/distress, diagnostic errors are likely to be minimized.[5–8]

Lifelong versus acquired premature ejaculation

As noted earlier, ISSM, AUA, and ICD criteria for PE distinguish between 2 subtypes: lifelong and acquired. Lifelong PE has been present throughout the man's sexual life and typically has no clear cause (see next section). Acquired PE occurs after some period of normal ELs and results from psychological/relationship or pathophysiologic changes such as pelvic trauma, disease, or medication. Because data supporting a specific EL criterion for acquired PE are limited, thresholds have been set based on clinical expertise.[2,3,5] However, it is worth noting that recent studies suggest that the current distinction between lifelong and acquired PE may not be as robust as once presumed.[8,11,12]

Prevalence of premature ejaculation

The prevalence of *lifelong* PE in the general population of men has been estimated anywhere from 5% to 40%, depending on how PE is defined, who makes the judgment (practitioner vs patient), which populations are sampled, and whether the man seeks treatment. Estimating PE prevalence based on a single question about "ejaculating before desired" yields percentages as high as 30% to 40%,[7,8,13] but an affirmative response to this query does not categorize the man as having PE, as the man may not fulfill other criteria regarding lack of ejaculatory control and bother/distress. The true prevalence of lifelong PE is undoubtedly much lower, and recent studies on community samples that include these other 2 criteria (control and bother/distress) place it closer to 4% to 10%.[7,14] The prevalence of acquired PE has not been adequately documented at this time.

Risk Factors for and Cause of Premature Ejaculation

An integrated approach to PE encourages the practitioner to understand biological, psychological, and sociocultural factors associated with PE, particularly insofar as they affect sexual function, sexual satisfaction, and the relationship.

Biological factors

Biological factors attempt to account for consistent interindividual variations in EL. These factors may be either *physiologic* or *pathophysiologic*. Physiologic factors are inherent to the system— part of the person's hardwired neurophysiology. Pathophysiological factors are disruptions of normal biological processes, such as disease, trauma (eg, injury or surgery), and medication.

For men with *lifelong* PE, no clear *pathophysiologic* condition accounts for short ELs, although many have been suggested.[15] On the other hand, *physiologic* explanations for lifelong PE assume that interindividual ejaculatory variability results from differences in the "hard wiring" of the reflexive components of ejaculation, presumably being genetic or epigenetic in origin. Thus far, however, no clear and robust anomalies in genotype, sensorimotor response, or neurotransmitter function have been identified in men with lifelong PE or in animal models of persistent rapid ejaculators. Thus, cause-effect relationships between biological factors and *lifelong* PE remain elusive.

In contrast, men who acquire PE later in life typically suffer from some sort of precipitating or sustaining pathophysiology. Examples include lower urinary tract symptoms, endocrine problems,[3,15] and, although somewhat rare, use of medications/ drugs. Relationship factors might also play a role, but to date, documentation for such effects tends to be "case study" or anecdotal material. Men with erectile dysfunction (ED) seem to be at greater risk for PE (or vice versa), although for such men, determination of which problem—PE or ED—is primary and which is secondary, is not often clear.

Psychological factors

The term "psychological," particularly with respect to sexual dysfunction, has sometimes been misunderstood to refer to the "psychoanalytic" and "developmental/learning" approaches to sexual response, perhaps because these approaches have been associated with giants in the field—Sigmund Freud and later Masters and Johnson—who shaped much of the classic thinking about sexuality. Although these earlier interpretations have generally lost favor, to the extent that they suggested a psychosexual developmental process for PE, they remain underresearched even today.

Nevertheless, ample evidence from men's self-report suggests that their ELs are influenced by numerous contextual factors, including psychological (eg, level of emotional arousal), behavioral (eg, coital position), partner-related (eg, perceived attractiveness), and/or situational (eg, new partner or unusual place).[12,16,17] Given that men perceive such factors to affect their arousal and subsequent ELs, treatment strategies have sometimes targeted these factors as starting points for remediation. Unfortunately, well-designed studies investigating the role of psychobehavioral factors on PE are limited, a situation perhaps exacerbated by 3 decades of successful pharmacologic (selective serotonin reuptake inhibitors [SSRIs]) management of PE.

Interplay between biological and psychological factors

Biological and psychological causes do not necessarily represent mutually exclusive pathways, as it is not possible to extricate psychological processes from the biological substrates that underlie and/or mediate them.[1] Preprogrammed "hard-wired" biological systems that govern peripheral and spinal reflex processes may be differentiated from the programmable/reprogrammable "soft-wired" biological substrates that underlie psychological processes such as attention, thoughts, expectations, and feelings/anxieties that derive from past experiences and immediate context. It is not fruitful, however, to conceptualize psychological processes as somehow independent of basic biological functioning.

In summary, a man's EL *range* may be preset by biological factors, but psychological variables such as sexual desire, expectation, anxiety, attention, and arousal likely influence the intraindividual variation within that preset range. Furthermore, psychological and biological processes can exert reciprocating effects on one another: anxiety might impair sexual response, and sexual failure or impairment might lower self-confidence and increase anxiety, thereby intensifying the problem.[18–20]

Relationship and cultural factors

It has oft been stated that PE is a couple's problem. The partner of a man with PE may share in the distress, self-doubt, and sexual dissatisfaction associated with the short-lived physical/sexual intimacy common to PE,[21,22] all of which can stress the dyadic relationship. A partner having their own sexual issues (eg, sexual aversion) might also exacerbate the PE problem or interfere with treatment. In addition, culturally derived gender/sex role expectations may place further burden on the man with PE (and his partner) to follow specific sociosexual scripts that are counterproductive to ensuring mutual sexual satisfaction. Although neither relationship nor cultural factors usually account for the short ELs of PE, these factors may be highly relevant to how the couple conceptualizes the impairment and their willingness to seek and use treatment.[21]

Treating Premature Ejaculation

Although its cause is not well understood, PE is considered a manageable problem. Although the immediate goal of most treatments is to increase the man's EL, a broader and often desirable goal is to help the couple attain a more satisfying sexual relationship.

Assessment/diagnosis

Diagnosing PE typically involves 2 steps: (1) ensuring that the man truly has PE, including a medical evaluation if pathophysiologic factors are suspected for a recently acquired condition; and (2) probing biological/medical, psychological, and relationship factors that are related to the problem and/or that might enhance or interfere with treatment outcomes. Regarding the first step, men sometimes complain of ejaculating before they wish, despite having a "normal" EL. So, the EL should be relatively short (less than 1–2 min) and not fall within or near the normal range of about 6 to 10 minutes postpenetration.[8,23] In addition, the practitioner should verify that the rapid end to sexual activity results from an inability to delay ejaculation, not from loss of erection or some other reason (eg, fear of interruption). Regarding the second step, both lifelong and acquired PE should generate a brief discussion of relationship and psychological functioning that might include questions about the man's life experiences with PE, relationship quality with the partner, partner's sexual health and problems, and if relevant, cultural expectations.[21] A diagnostic interview may be supplemented with standardized assessments (**Table 2**), given as a previsit or postvisit assignment to support the PE diagnosis and assess relationship functioning.

Treatment Options Overview

Several options are available for the treatment of PE: (1) pharmacologic approaches that temporarily decrease penile sensation and/or centrally inhibit the ejaculatory response (2) surgical approaches that permanently decrease sensory input to the penis; and (3) psychobehavioral approaches that have the multiple goals, including attenuating penile input, increasing awareness of sexual arousal cues and developing control over ejaculation, establishing a positive framework for change, and encouraging patient-partner interactions that enhance sexual satisfaction. Because these treatments have been extensively reviewed elsewhere, the author provides only a broad overview that includes benefits and limitations of the various options (**Table 3**).

Pharmacologic options

Topical ointments, crèmes, gels, and sprays reduce sensory input to the penis, thus delaying/inhibiting ejaculatory response. Preparations that contain lidocaine or prilocaine or various proprietary preparations double the EL for most men with PE (eg, 2–5 min), increase the man's ejaculatory control, and improve the quality of sex life.[24] They offer an expedient and inexpensive way for increasing EL, but unless used with a condom, they may cause vaginal discomfort, hyposensitivity, or numbness.

Oral medications have varying effects on delaying ejaculation.[5,25,26] **Box 1** provides an open access link to drug doses and efficacy.[25] Several points are relevant to understanding their use in the treatment of PE.

Treatment regimens: oral medications may involve either daily dosing or "on-demand" use, that is, taking the drug several hours before anticipated sexual activity.

Neurotransmitter reuptake inhibitors (including SSRIs), known mostly for their antidepressant use, can effectively delay or inhibit ejaculation. Because neither clomipramine (a tricyclic antidepressant) nor any of the traditional SSRIs has received regulatory agency approval for PE, they must be prescribed "off-label."

Daily dosing of drugs that affect serotonergic activity, such as clomipramine, paroxetine, sertraline, fluoxetine, citalopram, and clomipramine, is effective in delaying ejaculation in most men, with paroxetine having the strongest effect (6- to 8-fold increase) (see **Box 1**). *On-demand use* of oral medications 2 to 5 hours before sexual activity imparts fewer side effects than daily dosing but is also associated with a lower efficacy. Dapoxetine, a drug developed specifically for on-demand treatment of PE (not available in the United States), is generally less effective than off-label paroxetine, delaying ejaculation by about 1 to 3 minutes.[25,27]

Other pharmacologic options are available if the aforementioned reuptake inhibitors are ineffective. Tramadol, a centrally acting synthetic opioid analgesic and weak inhibitor of reuptake of gamma aminobutyric acid, norepinephrine, and serotonin, has shown moderate success in the treatment of PE.[28] In addition, α1-adrenoceptor antagonists, widely used in the treatment of lower urinary tract symptoms, have shown some efficacy for PE (eg,[29]). However, these drugs are less optimal due to their side effects and/or lower treatment efficacy.

Treatment of PE and comorbid ED is an option for men having both problems (about one-third of men with PE). If one problem is primary over the other, that problem should be treated first. More commonly, no clear temporal order in discernible, so these men may benefit from both an SSRI and a proerectile drug such as a phosphodiesterase-5 inhibitor (PDE-5i). Because SSRIs can exacerbate an erectile problem, the addition of a PDE-5i helps the man maintain his erection and reduce performance anxiety, whereas the SSRI delays ejaculation.[30]

Table 2
Examples of useful assessment instruments for premature ejaculation and relationship functioning

Medical/Psychological Assessments

Index of Premature Ejaculation (IPE)	10-item tool assessing control over ejaculation, satisfaction with sex life, and distress in men with PE. (Althof et al., 2006, pp. 474–475, copyrighted, special access.)
Premature Ejaculation Diagnostic Tool (PEDT)	5-item tool providing diagnostic relevance to PE. Reliable, easy, fast. (Jannini et al., 2013) http://www.baus.org.uk/Resources/BAUS/Documents/PDF%20Documents/Patient%20information/PEDT.pdf
Premature Ejaculation Prevalence & Attitudes (PEPA)	Assesses basic PE parameters in 5 questions, including whether PE is considered a problem by the man and/or his partner. (Patrick et al., 2005, p. 361)
Male Sexual Health Questionnaire (MSHQ)	25-item questionnaire measuring erection, ejaculation, and satisfaction with a focus on ejaculatory function. Greater cultural sensitivity compared with some tools. (Rosen et al., 2007)

Relational Assessments

Dyadic Adjustment Scale (DAS)	A self-report measure of relationship adjustment and both partner's perception of satisfaction. (Spanier, 1989) http://trieft.org/wp-content/uploads/2010/09/DAS+1.pdf
Golombok Rust Inventory of Sexual Satisfaction (GRISS)	28-item questionnaire that assesses sexual satisfaction and dysfunction; may be used to track improvement over time as the result of medication or therapy. (Rust & Golombok, 1985) http://www.psychometrics.cam.ac.uk/productsservices/psychometric-tests/GRISS
Self-Esteem and Relationship Questionnaire (SEAR)	Short questionnaire for measuring sexual relationship, confidence, and self-esteem. (Cappelleri et al., 2004) http://www.nature.com/ijir/journal/v16/n1/fig_tab/3901095t1.html

Data from Refs.[50–56]

Surgical approaches

Although considered a last resort for men nonresponsive to pharmacologic treatment, surgical procedures include selective dorsal neurectomy and glans penis augmentation using a hyaluronic acid gel.[31] Both act by immediately and permanently reducing sensory input to the penis. Although these procedures have gained traction in Asian countries, due to possible irreversible side effects such as penile sensory loss and ED, most professional societies consider them "experimental" and do not recommend them for PE treatment.

Psychobehavioral treatment options

Psychobehavioral approaches typically combine behavioral, cognitive/affective, and relationship/couple's strategies,[21] integrated and tailored to meet the individual's or couple's needs. Any of these approaches may be combined with pharmacotherapy to optimize treatment outcomes.

Behavioral approaches date back more than half a century. Specific techniques vary but all are designed to help the man modulate levels of sexual arousal first by learning to recognize sensations associated with increasing arousal and imminent ejaculation. When these sensations are noted, men are instructed to cease penile stimulation until the sensation passes—at which point the process begins anew. The techniques are then transferred to penetrative sex with the help of the partner, where they may be supplemented with ancillary strategies that modulate the man with PE's arousal and/or enhance the partner's arousal to better synchronize sexual response.

These methods impart moderate benefits for most men with PE[32] (see **Box 2** for an open access

Table 3
Some advantages and disadvantages of various treatment options for premature ejaculation

Treatment	Advantages	Disadvantages
Pharmacologic		
Penile Topical	Robust empirical support Effective for most men Inexpensive for some options Fairly rapid effect Very targeted treatment Minimum side effects	Intrusive during sex activity Partner genital numbness during sex Required during every episode/encounter Manages, does not cure the problem Numbness may linger for a while
Oral Medications	Robust empirical support Good efficacy for most drugs Easy administration Inexpensive	Adverse effects (GI, insomnia, ED) Requires daily dosing for maximal effect On-demand requires about 2-h lead Needed for every episode/encounter Manages, does not cure the problem Not effective for some men
Surgical	Robust effect Very targeted treatment Effect is long-lasting	Potential ED, loss of penile sensation Not available in many regions of the world Expensive (generally not insured) Higher risk for complications
Psychobehavioral	No adverse effects Potential ongoing effect Can improve mutual satisfaction Address relationship fallout Increased sense of self-efficacy	Requires investment of time/effort Takes longer to achieve results Best when partner is involved Requires effort to incorporate techniques Results are less reliable/consistent May involve greater cost burden

Abbreviation: GI, gastrointestinal.

link to a summary of *behavioral* effects) unless they are suffering from anteportal ejaculation or very short ELs. Because these procedures are relatively straightforward, couples may learn them under the guidance of a nonspecialist, through tele-counseling, or even using bibliotherapy (eg,[33]).

Cognitive approaches, unlike behavioral strategies, play no direct role in lengthening EL but rather address the patient's negative fallout from sexual impairment. These interventions—usually requiring a therapist knowledgeable about sexual issues—help instill a positive attitude and support the patient's motivation for change.[18,21] Some cognitive techniques focus on identifying and countering self-defeating thoughts that may exacerbate the PE, whereas others assist men in using positive ("affirming") thoughts and in developing awareness of negative feelings/anxieties during sexual interactions, which then can be rechanneled into positive feelings/actions.[18,21]

Relationship approaches view PE as embedded in the couple's relationship and thus assume that PE may be better managed with the cooperation of the partner, not only in implementing behavioral techniques (described earlier) but also in addressing the broader impact of the PE on the couple's interactions (eg, guilt, blaming, avoidance, and so forth). They can also help the couple to better understand their respective experiences as related to the dysfunction and focus on enhancing communication, intimacy, and mutual satisfaction.[21,34]

Taking a Multimodal Approach

Both clinical experience and data suggest that combining pharmacologic and psychobehavioral approaches to PE may result in better outcomes.[35,36] Specifically, increasing EL by using a pharmacologic option may offer a renewed sense of self-efficacy for the man. At the same time, addressing sexual/relationship satisfaction may increase adherence to protocols, improve communication between partners, help the man learn techniques for controlling arousal and ejaculation, expand the sexual repertoire so both partners are satisfied, and develop positive cognitive-affective frameworks that emphasize mutual pleasuring and prepare for the possibility of relapse. The addition of psychobehavioral

---

Box 1
Quick reference link for pharmacologic efficacy in premature ejaculation treatment

Open access: https://www.ncbi.nlm.nih.gov/pmc/articles/PMC4108949/

strategies to supplement pharmacologic treatments increases ELs by an additional 1 to 3 minutes, with mutual sexual satisfaction, anxiety, and adherence to protocols also showing improvement.[32]

DISCUSSION: DELAYED EJACULATION
Defining Criteria, Delayed Ejaculation Subtypes, and Prevalence

Defining diagnostic criteria
Although there are no consensus guidelines for diagnosing DE, several common threads run through various diagnostic criteria. DSM-5[2] defines DE as a marked delay or infrequency of ejaculation occurring in about 75% to 100% of partnered sexual activity, accompanied by a desire *not* to delay the ejaculation. DSM-5 further characterizes the condition as clinically distressing, includes relevant qualifiers such as "acquired" or "lifelong," and "generalized" or "situational," and indicates the practitioner should consider 5 other factors: partner; relationship; individual vulnerability (eg, history of abuse); psychiatric comorbidity (eg, depression) and stressors; cultural/religious influences; and medical factors. The ICD-11 defines "male delayed ejaculation" as the "inability to achieve ejaculation or an excessive or increased latency of ejaculation, despite adequate sexual stimulation and the desire to ejaculate."[4] The pattern of delayed ejaculation is associated with clinically significant distress. Finally, AUA, as DSM-V, distinguishes between lifelong and acquired DE,[5] defining *lifelong* as the "consistent, bothersome inability to achieve ejaculation, or excessive latency of ejaculation, despite adequate sexual stimulation and the desire to ejaculate," and *acquired* identically except including the phrase "or *an increased latency* of ejaculation."

As with PE, the diagnostic criteria for DE suggest 3 conditions: (1) a prolonged EL or absent ejaculation; (2) the inability to ejaculate sooner despite the desire to do so; and (3) a condition that causes bother or distress. None of the definitions operationalizes a "prolonged EL," although suggestions have been offered based on data indicating a *typical* EL between 6 and 10 minutes for most men (standard deviation [SD] = ± 4 min).[8,23] Using 2 SDs greater than the mean as a criterion threshold for DE yields an EL around 18 to 20 minutes, which includes the highest 2.3% of the population. One recent study reported that men who express the "desire to ejaculate sooner during intercourse" typically had median ELs of 15 minutes, and when "an inability to ejaculate sooner" was added to this criterion, the median EL increased to 20 minutes, similar to the value based on statistical parameters noted earlier.[37] However, one problem with using a temporal criterion such as 20 minutes is that some men never reach orgasm, terminating sexual activity due to frustration, exhaustion, loss of erection, and/or partner discomfort.

Lifelong versus acquired delayed ejaculation
Practitioners may distinguish between lifelong and acquired DE. Lifelong has been present throughout the man's sexual life and has no clear cause, whereas, paralleling PE, acquired DE occurs after some period of normal ELs and results from pathophysiologic, psychological, or relationship changes. As with PE, the lack of ability to have some control over the timing of ejaculation and the related distress probably play more important roles in diagnosing a man with either lifelong or acquired DE than any specific EL threshold.

Prevalence of delayed ejaculation
DE has not attracted the same level of pharma or media attention as ED or PE. Unlike PE and ED, no pharmaceutical companies have to date vigorously studied or pursued promising biomedical treatments for DE, and no medications have received regulatory agency approval for its treatment. Except perhaps for those men/couples concerned with procreation, most men whose sexual relationships are upended by their difficulty reaching ejaculation have remained hidden from view, receiving little or no attention from the popular or medical press, or even the research community. Given this lack of visibility, together with inconsistent criteria for defining DE, the lack of expedient biomedical treatment, and the assumption that diminished ejaculatory function is a natural consequence of aging, it is not surprising that relatively little is known about DE prevalence. Nevertheless, in the past, DE had been reported at fairly low rates in the literature, typically around 3% to 5% and thus had been considered uncommon. Several recent clinical and community samples have placed the incidence substantially higher, by some estimates closer to 10% to 15% of men.[13,38,39] In one recent community sample the percentage of men indicating the "desire to ejaculate sooner" during partnered sex was around 7% to 8%, nearly identical to results from the National Health and Social Life Survey (NHSLS) in the

United States.[40] When a second condition of "lacking the ability to ejaculate sooner" was added to the criterion, the prevalence dropped to about 3% to 4%, similar to the long-assumed prevalence for this dysfunction.[37]

Risk Factors for and Cause of Delayed Ejaculation

DE may be caused by any number of factors, including an inherently higher threshold for reaching ejaculation, lack of adequate arousal, and/or lack of adequate stimulation.

Physiologic/pathophysiologic risk factors
Some men report *lifelong* difficulty reaching ejaculation. Just as men with lifelong PE, men with lifelong DE may well be biologically predisposed to having a higher threshold for orgasm—although evidence for any genetic or inherent biological abnormality is lacking. In some instances, a pathophysiologic condition may account for DE (thus acquired/secondary DE), as procedures or diseases that interfere with sympathetic or somatic innervation to the pelvic/genital region can affect ejaculatory function.[39,41] In addition, most ejaculatory problems increase with aging, so men with an inherent (biological) predisposition toward longer ELs who have functioned adequately most of their lives may begin to experience difficulty as they age. This increase may be due in part to an overall age-related decrease in general health and stamina, making intercourse more physically challenging (**Box 3**). Prolonged EL may also be due to the increased prevalence of specific diseases and/or medications that inhibit ejaculatory response (**Table 4** for such medications).[38,39]

Psychological and relationship factors
DE might be conceptualized as a problem in the stimulus → arousal pathway. That is, DE may result from (1) a lack of adequate penile stimulation, (2) lack of subjective arousal to physical and psychological stimulation, and/or (3) active interference with the arousal process.[5] Regarding the first possibility, partnered sex may not provide sufficient penile stimulation due to any number of factors, for example, an age-related decrease in penile sensitivity, or a particular masturbation style (pressure, speed, and so forth) that does not simulate partnered sex.[41] Regarding the second possibility, the man may experience insufficient *subjective sexual arousal* despite adequate physical stimulation. For example, disparity in arousal may distinguish partnered sex from masturbation, the latter sometimes involving particular sexual fantasies and erotic materials and arousal "resources" that may not be available during partnered sex.[41] Regarding the third possibility, specific thoughts

and emotions during partnered sex may *actively inhibit* or *interfere with* the arousal process in men. For example, anxiety/fear regarding adequate performance, pleasing the partner, hurting or defiling the partner, unwanted impregnation, or even semen loss (eg, Dhat syndrome, a pathologic fear that semen loss leads to loss of vitality) might inhibit arousal/ejaculation. Shame, embarrassment, and guilt surrounding the sexual act may also interfere with arousal.[5,42] Although the putative role for such factors has been based primarily on clinical experience or case reports, they highlight the need for well-designed research investigating psychological and relationship involvement in the cause or maintenance of DE.

Treating Delayed Ejaculation

A holistic approach to the treatment of DE requires exploration of physiologic, psychological, and relationship issues that might affect the man's sexual response. Although the immediate problem is that of decreasing the man's EL, a broader goal may include helping the couple achieve procreation and/or a more sexually satisfying relationship.

Assessment and diagnosis
Diagnosing DE should include 2 steps: (1) ensuring that the man meets the diagnostic criteria for DE,

---

Box 3
How physically challenging is having sex and might this account for acquired delayed ejaculation?

For a man weighing 155 pounds, intercourse (top position) burns an estimated 120 to 150 calories assuming about 30 minutes of activity. Heart rate is around 110 to 120 bpm during orgasm.

For a man weighing 180 pounds, intercourse burns an estimated 140 to 170 calories assuming about 30 minutes of activity. Heart rate may increase by another 10% to 15%.

For a man weighing 200 pounds, intercourse burns an estimated 150 to 180 calories assuming about 30 minutes of activity. Heart rate may increase by 30% over the man weighing 155 pounds, perhaps as high as 130 to 140 bpm during orgasm.

How do the aforementioned parameters compare with other physical activities? Caloric use during sex is equivalent to about 30 minutes of leisure cycling, kayaking, or brisk pace walking. Heart rate during orgasm equates with the bpm for moderately intense exercise for a 50-year-old man.

including a medical referral if pathophysiologic factors are suspected for a recently acquired condition[5] and (2) addressing specific contexts that may shed light on the cause, relationship dynamics, and consequences of the DE. Regarding the first step, the practitioner should ensure that the EL is indeed prolonged and lies substantially beyond the normal EL range for men or, alternatively, that the man terminates intercourse out of frustration or exhaustion. In addition, the practitioner should assess whether the long EL is specific to partnered sex. A brief medical history can eliminate or, alternatively, identify potential etiologies related to medication, illness, surgery, or trauma, particularly if the DE is recently acquired.[5] Regarding the second step, brief psychological and relationship histories can help reveal individual or relationship idiosyncrasies that might explain recent changes in EL, especially if normal ejaculation had been possible previously.[42] **Table 5** provides an outline of steps that might be followed in a DE evaluation; **Box 4** includes sample questions that could generate discussion and insight regarding the DE problem.

Overview of Treatment Options

Treatment options for DE are limited by the lack of accepted pharmacologic options. Treatment therefore relies more heavily on behavioral, cognitive, and relationship approaches.

Pharmacologic options

In contrast with PE, safe and effective medications that shorten the EL have remained elusive, and not for lack of testing, as many serotonergic, adrenergic, and dopaminergic agonists and antagonists have been tried.[43] Most such "experimental" drugs impart weak-to-moderate and/or inconsistent effects and many have undesirable side effects. Other agents such as testosterone have also been tested, but with minimal success (**Box 5** provides a link to an open-access article listing such agents[43]).

Psychobehavioral approaches

Psychobehavioral interventions for men with lifelong or acquired DE include a mix of behavioral, cognitive, and relational approaches and typically require a psychosexual specialist.[21]

Behavioral approaches for DE were first pioneered in the 1970s[44] and have progressed substantially since then. Some men with DE report greater satisfaction from masturbation than intercourse, perhaps because they experience difficulty ejaculating during partnered sex and/or because they rely on sexual fantasies and/or erotic material to enhance their arousal during

Table 4
Putative negative effects of various medications on erectile/arousal and ejaculatory function in men

Substance Type	Examples	Arousal and/or Erection	Orgasmic Function
Antihypertensives	α and β blockers, sympathetic inhibitors	X	X
Antidepressants	SSRIs, MAOIs, tricyclics	X	X
Antipsychotics	Phenothiazines, thioxanthenes	X	X
Antiepileptics	Gabapentin, topiramate etc.	X	X
Anxiolytics/tranquilizers	Benzodiazepines	X	
Hypnotics/sedatives	Barbiturates, alcohol	X	x
Muscle relaxants	GABA β receptor agonists	-	x
Cancer treatments	GRH agonists	X	-
Immunosuppressive	Sirolimus, everolimus	X	-
Antiandrogens	Finasteride, cyproterone acetate, etc.	X	x
Steroids	Prednisone	X	?
Analgesics	Opioids, methadone		x
Other	Antihistamines, pseudoephedrine, recreational	X	?

Abbreviations: GABA, gamma aminobutyric acid; GRH, gonadotrophin-releasing hormone.
From Rowland, David L., "Evaluation of Delayed Ejaculation" (2017). Psychology Faculty Publications. 64. https://scholar.valpo.edu/psych_fac_pub/64, with permission.

masturbation. For these men, the absence of their preferred sexual stimuli during partner sex may result in insufficient arousal to trigger ejaculation.[38,42] One long-standing approach to such situations is that of "masturbatory retraining," that is, adjusting masturbation practices so stimulation is better aligned with the experience of penetrative sex with the partner.[42,44] Adjunctive strategies may involve suspending or altering masturbatory activity during treatment (eg, permitting masturbation only with the nonpreferred hand[42]), so the man learns to redirect his arousal toward partner cues and stimulation and away from autosexual cues. The couple may also be encouraged to share fantasies, use various forms of erotica, and engage in mutual masturbation and/or body movements more consistent with what is known to trigger ejaculation. Although no large-scale studies have been conducted to support this particular approach, individual clinicians have reported positive outcomes.

Table 5
Possible steps in the evaluation of delayed ejaculation

Step	Goal	Information/Procedure Examples
Setting the tone	Establish openness and trust	Normalizing/destigmatizing the problem
Differential diagnosis	Rule out other sexual problems	Verify problem of inhibited ejaculation • Typical ejaculatory latency • Inability to affect ejaculatory latency • Significant distress
History and scope of the problem	Obtaining detailed parameters about development of the problem	Lifelong, acquired; onset, duration, situation, exacerbation, self-management, motivation for change
Medical history/examination	Pathophysiological cause	Physical examination, review of illnesses, surgeries, medications, injuries, drug use, and so forth, including general life stressors/transitions that are job-related, financial, family based, etc.
Psychosexual evaluation	Identify possible psychological and relationship predisposing factors	Current sexual practices and activities in contexts: • Predisposing religious and cultural issues, including sexual knowledge and beliefs • Masturbatory and coital activities including fantasy, use of erotic materials, and so forth. • Relationship parameters involving quality and intimacy, communication, partner attractiveness, and dysfunction
Summary of relevant factors to review with patient (and partner)	Gain patient acceptance of the problem, its cause, and encourage value/motivation for change	Verify and align clinical notes with patient and partner self-report and perceptions

From Rowland, David L., "Evaluation of Delayed Ejaculation" (2017). Psychology Faculty Publications. 64. https://scholar.valpo.edu/psych_fac_pub/64, with permission.

Box 4
Sample questions that might be asked of patients with suspected delayed ejaculation

- Has the problem been lifelong? Recent? Developed over a period of time?
- Related to any other life events? Situation specific? Illnesses? Or more generalized?
- Can the man masturbate to orgasm?
- Has there been a noticeable increase in ejaculatory latency during masturbation?
- What are the current sexual practices, in terms of coital and masturbation frequency
- Are there situations when the man is able to ejaculate with the partner (eg, masturbation, using erotic materials, specific fantasies, and so forth).

Cognitive approaches can "normalize" or help reframe the problem and thus reduce negative feelings that might inhibit sexual arousal. For example, they might help the man reduce anxiety about the problem or counter misinformation and assumptions (eg, fear about the partner dissatisfaction or disapproval) and thus help him focus more on the erotic cues from the partner/situation.[45,46]

Relationship approaches address the sexual dynamics embedded in the relationship, with strategies generally designed to enhance arousal and mitigate distress.[47] Specific approaches might include sharing sexual fantasies, having the partner assume behaviors that increase arousal, and expanding the couple's sexual repertoire to ensure mutual satisfaction. Issues having the potential to interfere with the sexual satisfaction of both partners—associated with conception/procreation, anger/resentment, and relationship control and discord—can also be explored and addressed. With the partner fully engaged and taking "co-ownership" of the problem, outcomes are likely to be more satisfying for both partners, and potential negative feelings that might arise from the partner (eg, feeling unattractive or unrousing to the man with DE) can be managed.

Integrating Treatment Options

As noted previously, combining treatment approaches may result in better outcomes for any

---

Box 5
Quick reference link for experimental drug testing effects on delayed ejaculation

https://link.springer.com/article/10.1007/s11930-020-00287-z

---

sexual problem, including DE. For example, addressing the long EL by finding ways to increase arousal and/or remove barriers to arousal *and* ensuring sexual satisfaction for both the man with DE and his partner are likely to generate better results. So, despite the lack of well-tested pharmacologic options, psychobehavioral options can (1) maximize penile sensory input; (2) use cognitive/affective strategies that enhance, or remove barriers to, arousal; and (3) encourage patient-partner interactions that ensure the mutual sexual satisfaction.

SUMMARY
A Multimodal Treatment Framework for Ejaculatory Disorders

An integrated treatment approach toward ejaculatory disorders—either PE or DE—could follow any number of paths, and practitioners will undoubtedly have their own preferences and methods. Although avoiding specific formulas, one approach might use a multisession program (perhaps 3–6 sessions) that draws from a modified PLISSIT model, a well-known model having 4 levels of intensity beginning with *Permission*, continuing with *Limited Information*, *Specific Suggestions*, and *Intensive Therapy*.[48] Although much of the progression through these sessions would focus on "content" (the information, skills, and techniques conveyed to the patient), within any treatment environment, the practitioner must also attend to "process" issues that ensure a strong working alliance with the patient/couple.[21,47] Building such rapport is particularly important when sensitive sexual issues are involved and includes expressing empathy, genuineness, and positive regard; developing the patient's motivation to change and adherence to treatment protocols; and supporting a strong sense of self-efficacy for the patient and partner.[47,49]

CLINICS CARE POINTS

Regarding Premature Ejaculation

- PE may be a lifelong condition that typically has no clear cause or pathophysiology.
- PE may be an acquired condition of recent pathophysiologic or relationship origin.
- PE is a very manageable condition.
- Patients/couples can select from a range of treatment options.
- Attention to psychological and relationship issues may improve treatment outcomes.

Regarding Delayed Ejaculation

- DE may be either lifelong or acquired; the former is poorly understood.
- Treatment options are limited as no approved pharmacologic options are available.
- Motivated patients or couples may realize significant benefit from behavioral, cognitive, and relationship strategies under the guidance of a specialist.
- These procedures help enhance arousal, remove barriers to arousal, and ensure mutual sexual satisfaction.

DISCLOSURE

The author has nothing to disclose.

REFERENCES

1. Rowland DL, Motofei IG. The aetiology of premature ejaculation and the mind-body problem: implications for practice. Int J Clin Pract 2007;61(1):77–82.
2. American Psychiatric Association. Diagnostic and statistical manual of mental disorders. 5th edition. Washington, DC: American Psychiatric Association; 2013.
3. Serefoglu EC, McMahon CG, Waldinger MD, et al. An evidence-based unified definition of lifelong and acquired premature ejaculation: report of the second international society for sexual medicine ad hoc committee for the definition of premature ejaculation. Sex Med 2014;2(2):41–59.
4. World Health Organization. ICD-11 for mortality and morbidity statistics 2020. Available at: https://icd.who.int/browse11/. Accessed January 3, 2021.
5. Disorders of Ejaculation: An AUA/SMSNA Guideline. American Urological Association. 2020. Available at: https://www.auanet.org/guidelines/disorders-of-ejaculation. Accessed January 3, 2021.
6. Janssen PKC, Waldinger MD. Men with subjective premature ejaculation have a similar lognormal IELT distribution as men in the general male population and differ mathematically from males with lifelong premature ejaculation after an IELT of 1.5 minutes (Part 2). Int J Impot Res 2019;31(5):341–7.
7. Rowland DL, Kolba TN. Understanding the effects of establishing various cutoff criteria in the definition of men with premature ejaculation. J Sex Med 2015; 12(5):1175–83.
8. Côté-Léger P, Rowland DL. Estimations of typical, ideal, premature ejaculation, and actual latencies by men and female sexual partners of men during partnered sex. J Sex Med 2020;17(8):1448–56.
9. Rowland DL, Patrick DL, Rothman M, et al. The psychological burden of premature ejaculation. J Urol 2007;177(3):1065–70.
10. Patrick DA, Rowland DL, Rothman M. Interrelationship among measures of premature ejaculation: the central role of perceived control over ejaculation. J Sex Med 2007;4(3):780–8.
11. Jern P, Gunst A, Sandqvist F, et al. Using ecological momentary assessment to investigate associations between ejaculatory latency and control in partnered and non-partnered sexual activities. J Sex Res 2011;48(4):316–24.
12. Kempeneers P, Andrianne R, Cuddy M, et al. Sexual cognitions, trait anxiety, sexual anxiety, and distress in men with different subtypes of premature ejaculation and in their partners. Sex Marital Ther 2017; 44(4):319–32.
13. Lewis RW, Fugl-Meyer KS, Corona G, et al. Definitions/epidemiology/risk factors for sexual dysfunction. J Sex Med 2010;7(4 Pt 2):1598–607.
14. Althof SE, McMahon CG, Waldinger MD, et al. An update of the international society of sexual medicine's guidelines for the diagnosis and treatment of premature ejaculation (PE). Sex Med 2014;2(2): 60–90.
15. Waldinger MD. The pathophysiology of lifelong premature ejaculation. Trans Androl Urol 2016;5(4): 424–33.
16. Althof SE, McMahon CG. Contemporary Management of Disorders of Male Orgasm and Ejaculation. Urology 2016;93:9–21.
17. Rosen RC, McMahon CG, Niederberger C, et al. Correlates to the clinical diagnosis of premature ejaculation: results from a large observational study of men and their partners. J Urol 2007;177(3):1059–64.
18. Althof SE. Psychosexual therapy for premature ejaculation. Trans Androl Urol 2016;5(4):475–81.
19. Perelman M, McMahon C, Barada J. Evaluation and treatment of ejaculatory disorders. In: Lue TF, editor. Atlas of male sexual dysfunction. Philadelphia: Current Medicine LLC; 2004. p. 127–57.
20. Rowland DL, Adamski BA, Neal CJ, et al. Self-efficacy as a relevant construct in understanding sexual response and dysfunction. J Sex Marital Ther 2015;41(1):60–71.
21. Rowland D, Cooper S. Practical tips for sexual counseling and psychotherapy in premature ejaculation. J Sex Med 2011;8(4):342–52.
22. Symonds T, Roblin D, Hart K, et al. How does premature ejaculation impact a man s life? J Sex Marital Ther 2003;29(5):361–70.
23. Waldinger M, McIntosh J, Schweitzer DH. A five-nation survey to assess the distribution of the intravaginal ejaculation time among the general male population. J Sex Med 2009;6(10):2888–95.
24. Dinsmore WW, Hackett G, Goldmeier D, et al. Topical eutectic mixture for premature ejaculation (TEMPE): a novel aerosol-delivery form of lidocaine-prilocaine for treating premature ejaculation. BJU Int 2007;99(2):369–75.

25. Cayan S, Serefoğlu EC. Advances in treating premature ejaculation. F1000 Prime Rep 2014;6:55.

26. McMahon CG, Jannini E, Waldinger M, et al. Standard operating procedures in the disorders of orgasm and ejaculation. J Sex Med 2013;10(1): 204–29.

27. Pryor JL, Althof SE, Steidle C, et al. Efficacy and tolerability of dapoxetine in treatment of premature ejaculation: an integrated analysis of two double-blind, randomised controlled trials. Lancet 2006; 368(9539):929–37.

28. Salem EA, Wilson SK, Bissada NK, et al. Tramadol HCL has promise in on-demand use to treat premature ejaculation. J Sex Med 2008;5(1):188–93.

29. Basar MM, Yilmaz E, Ferhat M, et al. Terazosin in the treatment of premature ejaculation: a short-term follow-up. Int Urol Nephrol 2005;37(4):773–7.

30. Chen J, Mabjeesh NJ, Matzkin H, et al. Efficacy of sildenafil as adjuvant therapy to selective serotonin reuptake inhibitor in alleviating premature ejaculation. Urology 2003;61(1):197–200.

31. Moon DG. Is there a place for surgical treatment of premature ejaculation? Transl Androl Urol 2016; 5(4):502–7.

32. Cooper K, Martyn-St James M, Kaltenthaler E, et al. Behavioral Therapies for Management of Premature Ejaculation: A Systematic Review. Sex Med 2015; 3(3):174–88.

33. Metz M, McCarthy B. Coping with premature ejaculation: how to overcome PE, please your partner, and have great sex. Oakland (CA): New Harbinger Publications; 2003.

34. Rosen R, Althof S. Impact of premature ejaculation: The psychological, quality of life, and sexual relationship consequences. J Sex Med 2008;5(6): 1296–307.

35. Althof S. Treatment of premature ejaculation: psychotherapy, pharmacotherapy, and combined therapy. In: Binik YM, Hall KS, editors. Principles and practice of sex therapy. 4th edition. New York: Guilford Press; 2007. p. 212–40.

36. Melnik T, Glina S, Rodrigues OM Jr. Psychological intervention for premature ejaculation. Nat Rev Urol 2009;6(9):501–8.

37. Rowland DL, Cote-Leger P. Moving Toward Empirically Based Standardization in the Diagnosis of Delayed Ejaculation. J Sex Med 2020;17(10):1896–902.

38. Rowland DL. Evaluation of Delayed Ejaculation. In: IsHak WW, editor. The Textbook of clinical sexual medicine. Cham (Switzerland): Springer; 2017. p. 241–54.

39. Butcher MJ, Serefoglu EC. Treatment of Delayed Ejaculation. In: IsHak WW, editor. The Textbook of clinical sexual medicine. Cham (Switzerland): Springer; 2017. p. 255–69.

40. Laumann EO, Paik A, Rosen RC. Sexual dysfunction in the United States: prevalence and predictors. JAMA 1999;281(6):537–44.

41. Perelman M, Rowland DL. Retarded or inhibited ejaculation (male orgasmic disorder). In: Rowland DL, Incrocci L, editors. Handbook of sexual and gender identity disorders. New York: Wiley Press; 2008. p. 100–21.

42. Perelman M. Delayed ejaculation. In: Binik YM, Hall KS, editors. Principles and practice of sex therapy. 5th edition. New York: The Guilford Press; 2014. p. 138–55.

43. Piche K, Mann U, Patel P. Treatment of Delayed Ejaculation. Curr Sex Health Rep 2020;12:251–60.

44. Masters WH, Johnson VE. Human sexual inadequacy. Boston, MA, USA: Little, Brown & Co; 1970.

45. Apfelbaum B. Retarded ejaculation, a much-misunderstood syndrome. In: Lieblum SR, Rosen RC, editors. Principles and practice of sex therapy. 2nd edition. New York: The Guilford Press; 2000. p. 205–41.

46. Rowland DL, van Diest S, Incrocci L, et al. Psychosexual factors that differentiate men with inhibited ejaculation from men with no dysfunction or another sexual dysfunction. J Sex Med 2005;2(3):383–9.

47. Rowland DL, Cooper SE. Treating men's orgasmic difficulties. In: Peterson Z, editor. The Wiley Handbook of sex therapy. West Sussex (UK): John Wiley & Sons; 2017. p. 72–97.

48. Annon JS. The PLISSIT model: A proposed conceptual scheme for the behavioral treatment of sexual problems. J Sex Educ Ther 1976;2(1):1–15.

49. Busse RT, Kratochwill TR, Elliott SN. Influences of verbal interactions during behavioral consultations on treatment outcomes. J Sch Psychol 1999;37(2): 117–43.

50. Althof S, Rosen R, Symonds T, et al. Development and validation of a new questionnaire to assess sexual satisfaction, control and distress associated with premature ejaculation. J Sex Med 2006;3(3):465–75.

51. Jannini E, McMahon C, Waldinger M, editors. Premature Ejaculation: from etiology to diagnosis and treatment. Italy: Springer-Verlag; 2013. p. 383.

52. Patrick DL, Althof SE, Pryor JL, et al. Premature ejaculation: An observational study of men and their partners. J Sex Med 2005;2(3):358–67.

53. Rosen RC, Catania JA, Althof SE, et al. Development and validation of four-item version of Male Sexual Health Questionnaire to assess ejaculatory dysfunction. Urology 2007;69(5):805–9.

54. Spanier GB. Dyadic adjustment scale manual. North Tonawanda (NY): Multi-Health Systems; 1989.

55. Rust J, Golombok S. The golombok-rust inventory of sexual satisfaction (GRISS). Br J Clin Psychol 1985; 24(1):63–4.

56. Cappelleri JC, Althof SE, Siegel RL, et al. Development and validation of the self-esteem and relationship (SEAR) questionnaire in erectile dysfunction. Int J Impot Res 2004;16(1):30–8.

Oncosexology
Sexual Issues in the Male Cancer Survivor

Carolyn A. Salter, MD, John P. Mulhall, MD, MSc, FECSM*

KEYWORDS

- Oncosexology • Cancer • Sexual dysfunction • Erectile dysfunction • Prostate cancer
- Testosterone deficiency • Peyronie's disease • Ejaculatory dysfunction

KEY POINTS

- Cancer and its associated treatments often have a negative impact on the sexual function of patients and their partners.
- Pelvic malignancies, such as prostate, bladder, or colorectal cancer, have the most significant impact on the sexual function of male cancer survivors.
- Sexual dysfunction associated with pelvic cancer treatments include erectile dysfunction, testosterone deficiency, ejaculatory dysfunction, orgasmic dysfunction, sexual incontinence, and penile shortening.

INTRODUCTION

Oncosexology is a relatively new term that refers to a multidisciplinary field addressing sexual issues in patients with cancer.[1] Physicians, nurses, psychologists, and other health care providers can all be involved in the field of oncosexology. An oncosexologist can be any of these practitioners who focus on the sexual function of patients with cancer. This discipline has developed out of a need to adequately address sexual concerns in oncology patients. Cancer remains a significant health burden in the United States, with almost 2 million new cases and more than 600,000 cancer deaths anticipated. There is a need for specialists to help cancer survivors and their partners navigate changes to sexuality related to the diagnosis and treatment of cancer.

Monitoring for patient cancer-related distress is an American College of Surgeons cancer hospital accreditation standard in the United States.[2] Although this focus on distress is warranted, the follow through for patients who express distress is suboptimal; only approximately one-third of

patients referred for distress symptoms actually obtain the desired assistance. There are many barriers to access, including time restraints, patient beliefs, logistical issues, and variability in insurance/financial issues.[2] A proposed model to address this gap in care is to identify distress and patient needs, offer support within the oncology team as appropriate, and/or refer out as needed. The oncology team should then help the patient navigate barriers to care and continue to monitor and address patient distress.[2]

The management of distress in general needs to be improved in oncology patients. Distress related to sexual issues is a particularly sensitive and important aspect of oncology-related distress. Cancer and its treatments can have direct and indirect impact on sexual function and satisfaction. Absence of sexual experience can be a source of distress. Sexual expression may also be a form of coping with distressing life circumstances and its absence can compound other forms of cancer-related distress.[3]

Historically, health care providers have not adequately discussed sexual issues with

Male Sexual and Reproductive Medicine Program, Department of Urology, Memorial Sloan Kettering Cancer Center, 16 East. 60th Street, Suite 302, New York, NY 10022, USA
* Corresponding author.
E-mail address: mulhalj1@mskcc.org

Urol Clin N Am 48 (2021) 591–602
https://doi.org/10.1016/j.ucl.2021.07.001

patients with cancer . This is of major concern, given the significant impact of cancer and cancer treatments on sexual functioning. It is estimated that 40% to 100% of patients with cancer experience perturbations in sexual functioning. Patients with pelvic cancers tend to have greater risks with respect to sexual dysfunctions.[4] Despite this, many patients with cancer are not counseled on sexual side effects. A study of nearly 500 patients with colorectal cancer (CRC) found that only 16% of patients said that their medical team discussed sexual concerns with them.[5] Among patients with prostate cancer (PCA), few report being counseled on penile length loss, Peyronie disease (PD), and/or anejaculation after prostate cancer treatment such as radical prostatectomy (RP).[6]

Self-identified oncosexologists tend to be more engaged and inquisitive regarding a patient's experience of sexual distress during or after treatment. However, even among these providers, up to 10% may not address sexual issues with patients. A survey of self-reported oncosexology providers who attended a "Cancer, Sexuality and Fertility" meeting demonstrated that only 90% endorsed discussing sexuality with patients. Almost 7% of these practitioners noted they felt uncomfortable discussing sexual concerns with patients, and most had no experience discussing sexuality with adolescent patients.[4]

Fortunately, research has shown that training practitioners can improve their handling of oncosexology issues. A review of these interventions evaluated 7 studies that aimed to improve sexual health knowledge of providers and increase their comfort level with these discussions. Interventions included either face-to-face workshops or lectures or online video-based training. End-points were assessed anywhere from 3 weeks to 16 months after the interventions and included self-reported questionnaires that ranged from sexual health knowledge and attitudes to frequency discussing the topic, and provider comfort level. Many studies showed that with training of health care providers, there may be a durable improvement in their knowledge and comfort level regarding sexual concerns. This has the end result of an increase in the frequency with which providers discuss sex with patients.[7] Increasing these conversations is vital, as it has been shown to improve sexual function in patients with cancer . Of patients with hematologic cancer status-post stem cell transplantation, those who had been counseled on sexual side effects had fewer sexual problems at 3 years after treatment (r = −0.43, P = .02).[8]

These data demonstrate a clear need to expand the field of oncosexology and better counsel patients with cancer on the sexual impact of their disease and treatments. Sexual functioning should be discussed to assess baseline symptoms and in the context of the impact of various treatment options.[3] This article discusses sexual issues in male patients with cancer , with a specific focus on men with prostate malignancies, as these men are at high risk for sexual dysfunction (**Box 1**). Readers interested in oncosexology in women are referred to the Mindy Goldman and Mary Kathryn Abel's article, "Oncology Survivorship and Sexual Wellness for Women," elsewhere in this issue.

IMPACT OF CANCER DIAGNOSIS ON SEXUAL FUNCTION

Any cancer diagnosis can affect patients' sexual function, and cancer treatments often compound this issue. A survey of 2500 patients with cancer demonstrated that 44% of patients endorsed sexual symptoms. More than half of patients answered that they had unmet informational needs. Of these patients seeking information, 50% sought information of the impact of cancer on their spouse or their relationship. Patients with sexual side effects were 2 times more likely to have questions on the impact of cancer on their relationship (odds ratio [OR] 2.05, 95% confidence interval [CI] 1.54–2.72).[9] Clearly, sexual side effects of cancer and its treatments are common and leads to patient concern about their relationships.

The impact of PCA on sexual function can be profound. Analysis of almost 60,000 patients with PCA in the United Kingdom showed that 81% of these men had sexual issues related to their cancer and treatment. Surprisingly, 55.8% of them had not received any treatment for these sexual issues.[10] Clearly there is a high burden of unmet needs in this population.

Couples-based intervention may be particularly helpful for men and their partners who are struggling with cancer-related sexual issues. A randomized trial in 189 post-RP patients with PCA and their female partners compared "usual care" (ie, printed education materials and standard medical care) to peer support or nurse support (ie, phone calls for support or counseling from either peers or nurses, respectively, as well as written and audiovisual materials) over a 5-year span. There was clear benefit to both experimental arms compared with control for men adhering to erectile dysfunction (ED) treatment. At time points of 2, 3, 4, and 5 years post-RP, the men in the treatment

Box 1
Sexual conditions associated with prostate cancer treatment

Erectile dysfunction

Orgasmic dysfunction

  Anorgasmia

  Dysorgasmia

  Delayed orgasm

  Change in orgasm intensity

Ejaculatory dysfunction

  Anejaculation

  Decreased volume

  Premature ejaculation

Sexual incontinence

  Arousal incontinence

  Climacturia

Low libido

Loss of penile length

Peyronie's disease

arms reported higher overall use of ED treatments, to include phosphodiesterase 5 inhibitors (PDE5i), intracavernosal injections (ICI), or vacuum erection devices (VED) ($P<.05$ for both groups compared with control).[11] At 2 years, 61% of the usual care group used ED treatments compared with 89% in peer and 88% in nurse support groups; at 3 years, this was 55% in usual care versus 80% in peer support and 81% in nurse support. This trend continued at 4 years, with 47% of usual care and 87% and 79% of peer and nurse support, respectively, using ED treatments. Similar results were seen at year 5, with 54% of usual care, 87% of peer support, and 80% of nurse support patients using ED treatments.[11] Interestingly, although the support groups used more ED treatment, there was no difference in sexual satisfaction and function, as measured by the International Index of Erectile Function (IIEF), among the 3 groups.[11]

IMPACT OF MALE SEXUAL DYSFUNCTION ON PARTNERS

Sexual well-being in patients with cancer is often overlooked; the sexual well-being of partners of patients with cancer is similarly poorly understood and often neglected. The unmet needs and stressors facing the partners of patients with cancer can have a negative effect on both members of the dyad.[12] A survey of 113 female partners of patients with PCA noted key themes of coping with changes to their relationship and the emotional distress of dealing with their partners' illness. Women had a range of responses, from complaining of inconvenience due to changes in sex life to lamenting the complete loss of their sexual relationship.[13] The impact on partners is further demonstrated with quantitative data. Eighty-eight pairs of patients with PCA and their partners were surveyed at 6 and 12 months after PCA diagnosis. At 6 months, 51% of partners noted a very or somewhat negative impact on their sexual relationship, and this increased to 71% at 12 months. The overall relationship suffered as well, with 10% of partners noting a very or somewhat negative impact at 6 months, which increased to 14% at 12 months postdiagnosis.[14]

The impact on partners is less well studied in gay or bisexual men. A review of PCA in this population noted unique challenges. A firmer erection is needed for insertive anal intercourse, and thus the sexual role of the patient may be changed. Fewer than half of insertive partners are able to always remain insertive postoperatively. Similarly, due to discomfort or lack of pleasure postoperatively, receptive partners may also change their sexual roles. As not all gay or bisexual men are versatile (acting as insertive and receptive partner), this can impact the couples' sexual relationship.[15] Clearly, patients and their partners (regardless of sexual orientation) need resources to help mitigate this decline in their sexual and overall relationship.

PELVIC MALIGNANCIES

Pelvic malignancies, such as PCA, CRC, or bladder cancer (BCA), arguably have the most significant impact on sexual function and have been the best studied with respect to oncosexology. Although this article focuses on PCA, some general guidance on management of other pelvic malignancies can be derived from these data.

ERECTILE DYSFUNCTION

ED is multifactorial in patients with cancer . Psychological issues, such as anxiety, depression, or relationship stressors can contribute to ED in all male patients with cancer .[6] Although clearly all patients with cancer are at increased risk, arguably no oncology patients are more at risk for ED than men with PCA.

The rate of ED after an RP is difficult to compare given that many studies do not mention how ED was defined or the timepoint it was defined. Patient populations also vary between studies. The published literature thus has a broad range of 6% to 68%.[16] From a purely function perspective, erectile function (EF) recovery can be conceptualized as the ability to achieve and maintain an erection that allows for satisfying sexual activity. Using this definition, rates of satisfactory EF at 12 months post-RP can be anywhere from 25% to 77%.[16] The International Consultation for Sexual Medicine (ICSM) recommends that researchers use validated instruments[16] for future studies to allow for comparisons between series and to provide patients with more realistic expectations.

ED is also common in men after a radical cystoprostatectomy (CP), with ED rates as high as 94% in the literature and up to half of patients being sexually inactive postoperatively.[3] Likewise, ED is high in patients with CRC. Unsurprisingly, this is higher in patients with rectal compared with colon cancer. Eighty-six percent of all patients with rectal cancer endorse sexual dysfunction compared with 39% of patients with colon cancer .[3]

Factors predicting EF recovery include younger age, bilateral nerve-sparing surgery, and better preoperative EF.[16] A common practice in men after RP or radiation therapy (RT) for PCA is a program referred to as penile rehabilitation. Penile rehabilitation is nonspecific, but is broadly intended to enhance recovery of penile erections after cancer treatment. Penile rehabilitation protocols vary widely, but typically include routine or even daily dosing of PDE5i, which can be given in a low dose daily and/or on demand dosing to enhance erections. Rehab ICI or VED is used by many.[6]

Existing data on penile rehabilitation comes from varied sources using different protocols and outcome measures and is hence difficult to compare. The ICSM is unable to recommend a specific rehabilitation protocol as optimal after PCA treatment.[6] Furthermore, the American Urological Association (AUA) guidelines on ED concluded, based on a review of all randomized placebo-controlled studies of PDE5I for rehabilitation after RP, that there is no evidence that PDE5I-based penile rehabilitation protocol leads to improved recovery of spontaneous erection function.[17]

PDE5I-based penile rehabilitation remains generally safe, and it is our practice that men take a low-dose PDE5i daily, with at least 1 full dose each week to try to achieve an erection. If men are unable to achieve an erection satisfactory for penetration with the full dose PDE5i by 6 weeks postoperatively, then they remain on the low dose daily and perform ICI at least once a week to induce an erection.

Ejaculatory Dysfunction

Although ED is arguably the most common sexual change in male patients with cancer , there are numerous other changes that can occur in these men. This includes ejaculatory dysfunction, which comprises anejaculation, change in ejaculate volume, and premature ejaculation.

Anejaculation refers to the absence of antegrade ejaculate efflux at the time of orgasm. This can be due to failure of emission, where ejaculate is not released, or retrograde ejaculation, where the ejaculate travels backwards into the bladder due to bladder neck dysfunction. Anejaculation is universal after RP, as surgery involves removal of the organs responsible for production of more than 95% of the content of semen. This should be discussed with all patients preoperatively, as natural conception is no longer be possible.[6] Aside from effects on fertility, anejaculation can have a significant impact on men, as it can affect body image and feelings of masculinity. There is also thought that the absence of ejaculate may reduce orgasmic intensity.[6]

Anejaculation can also occur with prostate RT but to a lesser degree. This has been noted in 11% of men undergoing prostate external beam RT (EBRT)[18] and approximately 19% of men undergoing brachytherapy. Of those men who maintained ejaculation, almost all (85%) reported reduced ejaculate volume. Interestingly, the addition of androgen deprivation therapy (ADT) did not affect ejaculatory function ($P > .05$).[19] Another study evaluated 364 men who had RT, including EBRT, and brachytherapy ± ADT. Men were followed for a mean of 6.0 ± 4.5 years. Anejaculation was seen in 16% of men at 1 year, 69% at 3 years, and 89% at 5 years. At their last visit, 72% of men reported anejaculation. Variables associated with greater risk for anejaculation included age older than 65 years (OR 2.8; 95% CI 1.8–4.2; $P < .01$), baseline prostate volume <40 g (OR 1.8; 95% CI 1.3–6.1; $P < .01$), use of ADT (OR 2.2; 95% CI 1.9–9.8; $P < .01$) and a total RT dose of greater than 100 Gy (OR 1.6; 95% CI 1.4–7.2; $P < .05$).[20]

Premature ejaculation (PE) is common in patients with cancer, although there is no specific organic mechanism through which cancer or its treatments leads to PE. In general, the rates of PE are difficult to establish, given various definitions used. This can range in the literature from 3% when using a strict definition of chronic and consistent intravaginal ejaculatory latency time of less than 1 minute coupled with absence of sense of control and personal bother to 78% in men reporting any history of ejaculating before they wished to do so.[21] The data are limited when specifically evaluating men with cancer. An assessment was conducted in 1202 men newly diagnosed with PCA who were referred to urology for treatment discussion. PE was diagnosed by physicians using the PE Diagnostic Tool, which is based on Diagnostic and Statistical Manual of Mental Disorders, Fourth Edition, Text Revision (DSM-IV-TR) criteria for PE and hence lack a robust time-based criterion. The rates were high at 63.7% for PE and 66.2% for ED (as measured by the IIEF-5).[22] Predictors of PE included IIEF-5 scores (β 0.58 [0.03], P = .007), which suggests that these 2 disorders are associated.[22] These data support the notion that acquired PE is strongly linked to ED; the estimated prevalence for clinical PE may be artificially elevated in this study, as the DSM-IV-TR definition is outdated and does not include essential time-based criteria.

Orgasmic Dysfunction

Many men after PCA treatment notice some form of orgasmic dysfunction, such as change in orgasm intensity, inability to reach orgasm (anorgasmia), delayed orgasm, or pain with orgasm (dysorgasmia). Changes in orgasm intensity may be psychological or physical and related to changes in pelvic floor muscle contraction and/or ejaculation; data on this topic are sparse.[6] Dysorgasmia is poorly understood. The etiology is proposed to be from spasms of pelvic floor musculature or issues at the vesicourethral anastomosis. Many patients experience a reduction in symptoms after treatment with an alpha blocker such as tamsulosin.[6]

In a series of more than 250 men post-RP, 5% had complete anorgasmia, whereas 57% had delayed orgasm; 60% noted a decrease in orgasm intensity, and 10% had dysorgasmia.[23] Orgasmic dysfunction has also been studied in men post-RT for PCA. A survey of more than 100 men status-post EBRT ± ADT noted common orgasmic changes in these men; 15% reported dysorgasmia, 24% had anorgasmia, 40% reported delayed ejaculation, and 44% reported decreased orgasmic intensity.[18] In men status-post brachytherapy ± ADT, 30% had dysorgasmia and 10% anorgasmia. Interestingly, ADT did not increase the risk of orgasmic dysfunction in these men (P>.05).[19]

Sexual Incontinence

Sexual incontinence is composed of arousal incontinence (ie, urine leakage with foreplay or arousal) and climacturia (ie, orgasm-associated incontinence). These conditions are not as well studied as other sexual changes in patients with PCA, but they are known to occur after RP and to a lesser extent RT.[18,23] The RP literature is more robust, with multiple studies describing sexual incontinence postoperatively.

With regard to climacturia, the rate ranges from 20% to 93% based on the definition used.[23–29] For example, Choi and colleagues[25] report the lowest end of the spectrum at 20% of men post-RP, but they used a definition of 3 or more episodes of climacturia. Conversely, Barnas and colleagues[29] reported a 93% rate of climacturia, as defined by ≥1 episode. However, this study design was a retrospective survey with a 68% response rate, which could have introduced bias and thus contributed to these higher rates.

Data on arousal incontinence (AI) is limited, but this entity has been described in 38% of post-RP men without diurnal incontinence and in 82% of men undergoing a sling or artificial sphincter placement for stress urinary incontinence post-RP.[30,31] A larger series of prostatectomy patients noted 49% of men endorsed experiencing AI after their surgery.[32]

In a series of more than 250 sexually active men post-RP, 38% endorsed sexual incontinence when surveyed between 3 to 36 months postoperative; 29% of men reported AI and 27% had climacturia (there was overlap between these groups). On multivariate analysis of predictors of sexual incontinence, the only significant factor was more severe stress urinary incontinence (SUI) as measured by the International Consultation on Incontinence Questionnaire (OR 1.17; 95% CI 1.10–1.25; P<.0001).[23]

When specifically evaluating AI, more severe SUI was still a predictor. A total of 226 men post-RP were queried on AI. At a mean of 18.3 ± 5.5 months after surgery, 49% of men endorsed experiencing AI at some point during their recovery. On multivariate analysis of predictors of AI, worsening SUI, as measured by increasing pads per day (OR 1.55; 95% CI 1.12–2.13; P = .01) and the absence of hypertension (hypertension OR 0.44; 95% CI 0.25–0.80; P = .01), was associated with AI.[32]

The available evidence suggests against a close link between climacturia and SUI. A study evaluating predictors of climacturia showed that none of the factors analyzed, such as age, time since surgery, urinary flow rate, stress incontinence (as defined as >1 pad per day), or urinary symptoms as measured by the International Prostate Symptom Score, were associated with climacuturia.[26] There are some data to suggest a link between functional urethral length and climacturia. A small functional urodynamics study showed men with climacturia post-RP had shorter functional urethral length at 20.3 ± 4.03 mm compared with controls at 35.2 ± 4.81 mm (P = .02).[33]

Strategies to manage sexual incontinence include limiting fluid intake, urinating before sexual activity, and/or using condoms.[34] We have also recommended use of a variable tension penile loop worn at the base of the penis, as this has been shown to eliminate climacturia in almost half of patients and improved symptoms in the remaining paitients.[35] This band may be less useful in patients with AI, as it can be more difficult to predict arousal.

Peyronie Disease

One of the most underrecognized sexual change associated with PCA treatment is PD. PD is characterized by penile deformity, such as curvature, waisting, or indentation, and can be associated with penile pain. In a group of more than 250 men post-RP, 10% noted a new penile curvature postoperatively.[23] A larger series evaluated more than 1000 men post-RP at a mean time of 13.9 ± 0.7 months after surgery and found that 15.9% had new-onset PD postoperatively. On multivariate analysis for incident PD in these men, younger age (per 5 years) and white race (compared with nonwhite) were both associated with higher risk (OR 1.28; 95% CI 1.24–1.32 and OR 4.08; 95% CI 1.73–9.58, respectively).[36] Although the data are even more limited with RT, a series of more than 100 men status-post RT ± ADT noted that 12% endorsed new penile curvature and 6% had penile pain.[18] More research is needed to fully elucidate the rates of PD in patients with PCA after RT and RP.

Penile Shortening

Penile length loss is common after PCA treatment and has been linked to treatment regret.[37] Proposed etiologies include sympathetic hyperinnervation or structural changes, such as fibrosis or collagenization from cavernous nerve injury or cavernosal hypoxia.[38] Men post-RP have been noted to endorse subjective length loss, but there are limited data on objective measurements. With regard to subjective report, a series of more than 250 men post-RP showed that almost half (47%) reported >1 cm length loss.[23] On multivariate analysis, risks of self-reported penile shortening included ED (Erectile Hardness Score < 3 with OR 1.81; 95% CI 1.07–3.10) and increasing body mass index (BMI) calculated by self-reported height and weight (OR 1.10; 95% CI 1.02–1.19; P = .01). The only protective factor was unilateral

or bilateral nerve-sparing surgery (OR 0.32; 95% CI 0.16–0.95; P = .0005) compared with bilateral non–nerve-sparing.[23]

Although subjective length loss is common, objective data indicate that penile length loss is less common than self-report would indicate. This could, however, be in part due to differing measuring techniques. The most common way to measure stretched flaccid length it to place axial traction on the penis and measure from coronal sulcus to penopubic junction.[39] This can underestimate penile length by up to 23% depending on the amount of traction and whether the suprapubic fat pad is compressed or not.[39]

One study used a single evaluator and measured stretched flaccid length from pubic bone to coronal sulcus preoperatively and then at 2 and 6 months post-RP.[40] EF was measured via the IIEF erectile function domain (EFD). Men were recommended for a penile rehabilitation protocol of a low dose of sildenafil nightly and a full dose twice a week to induce an erection. The men were separated based on PDE5i compliance into a group who "always" took the PDE5i compared with those in all other frequencies of compliance, from never to frequently. At 6 months, fewer of the compliant patients had length loss at 25% compared with the men with less frequent PDE5i use at 52% (P = .03).[40] The PDE5i-compliant patients had no penile length loss at 6 months (difference of +1 ± 6.7 mm, P = .37), whereas the noncompliant group experienced length loss (−4.4 ± 16.6 mm, P<.002).[40] On multivariate analysis of stretched flaccid penile length loss, both "always" using PDE5i and EFD score at 6 months were associated with less length loss (β = −0.54, P = .002 and β = −0.35, P = .05, respectively).[40]

Although less well described, there are also data indicating penile length loss after radical CP for BCA. A series of 151 men post-CP evaluated EF via the IIEF-5 and asked subjective questions on perceived penile length. At a median follow-up of 28 months, these men had severe ED with a mean IIEF-5 of 3. More than half reported penile length loss, and of those, 55% reported a loss of greater than 1 inch.[41] On multivariate analysis of predictors of length loss, severe ED (defined as IIEF-5 score 1–7) and higher BMI were associated with length loss (OR 3.712; 95% CI 1.43–9.64; P = .0071 and OR 1.198; 95% CI 1.38–10.53; P = .006, respectively).[41]

Surgery is not the only cause of penile length loss in patients with cancer . A survey of more than 100 men who had EBRT ± ADT 3 months to 5 years prior inquired about subjective length loss; 44% endorsed penile length loss of >1 cm.[18] Factors analyzed included not receiving ADT, the duration of ADT, cancer tumor stage, BMI, Charlson comorbidity index, and ED (as measured by an erectile hardness scale score of 1 or 2) On logistic regression analysis, none of the factor analyses predicted length loss.[18] A series of 47 men had 9 months of ADT and 70 Gr of RT. Flaccid length was measured at baseline and then every 3 months for 18 months. Flaccid penile length decreased from 14.20 ± 1.10 cm at baseline to 8.60 ± 1.06 cm at 18 months (P<.001).[42] These studies are limited in that there are no data on RT alone.

A large series of almost 950 men treated with RT for biochemical recurrence after PCA treatment had an overall subjective rate of penile shortening of 2.63%. Interestingly, length loss was reported by no patients in the RT alone group compared with 2.67% in the RT plus ADT group (P = .016).[43] This suggests that ADT as opposed to RT is what leads to penile length loss in these men. This is supported by a study of men who received ADT as primary continuous therapy for PCA. Thirty-nine men had stretched flaccid length measured at baseline and then every 3 months for 24 months. Results showed a steady decline in penile length that stabilized by 15 months after initiation of ADT. The mean length went from 10.76 ± 1.92 cm pre-ADT to 8.05 cm ± 1.36 after 24 months of treatment (P<.001).[44]

Although penile length loss is clearly common after PCA treatment, there are data to suggest that this can be reduced. As mentioned previously, daily PDE5i use was associated with preserved length in RP patients compared with those with less frequent use.[40] VEDs have also been investigated for penile length preservation. A review article summarized that penile shortening and loss of girth was reported in 45% to 71% of men post-RP who did not use a VED compared with 3.5% to 27% of men who used VED (no P-value provided).[45] Existing data are hampered by the absence of randomization, blinding, and control interventions, so these conclusions should be interpreted with caution; better designed studies are required.

TESTICULAR CANCER

Patients with testicular cancer (TCA) can experience significant changes in their sexual health, from erectile and ejaculatory dysfunction to testosterone deficiency (TD). These changes can be psychologically devastating, as most patients with TCA are young and may not be in stable supportive relationships.

Ejaculatory Dysfunction

Ejaculatory dysfunction is common in men with TCA after retroperitoneal lymph node dissection (RPLND) due to damage to lumbar sympathetic nerves. Up to 50% of patients with TCA have ejaculatory dysfunction.[3] With newer nerve-sparing techniques (when possible from an oncologic perspective), there is less risk of anejaculation in these men.[46] Both a modified unilateral template or a nerve-sparing technique have been shown to preserve antegrade ejaculation in many men. For primary RPLND, the rates of preserved ejaculation range from 75% to 100% and 25% to 100% for post-chemo RPLND.[46] Given that many men with TCA are young, the risk of anejaculation and its implications on fertility should be discussed before RPLND.

Testosterone Deficiency

Men with TCA are at risk for TD; this may be the result of treatments but could also be attributable to testicular dysgenesis syndrome. Testicular dysgenesis is a putative syndrome that involves endocrine disruption during fetal development, leading to a constellation of symptoms to include hypospadias, cryptorchidism, infertility, and TCA.[47] The fact that many men with TCA have pre-existing TD and/or impaired spermatogenesis in non–cancer-containing testicle supports this notion.[47] One series showed that 5% of patients with TCA had TD before orchiectomy, increasing to 16% when assessed at 1-month post-orchiectomy.[48] This suggests that these men are predisposed to TD, and that further loss of testicular tissue exacerbates the issue.

Treatment for TCA clearly compounds the risk of TD. For example, data on men with TCA has shown that chemotherapy has a clear dose-response relationship with TD due to the gonadotoxicty.[49] Retroperitoneal radiation for metastatic disease can also lead to TD due to scatter to the testes.[50] An abdominal radiation dose of 30 Gy is associated with a 0.09 to 0.32 Gy to the testes, which leads to a slightly increased risk of TD due to Leydig cell damage.[50]

In an elegant meta-analysis, rates of TD were assessed in standard chemotherapy, nonconventional chemotherapy (essentially high-dose) and RT as compared with orchiectomy alone.[49] The lowest risk of TD was with RT (OR 1.6; 95% CI 1.0–2.4; P = .03). This was followed by conventional chemotherapy regimens, which had an OR of 1.8 (95% CI 1.3–2.5; P = .0007). The highest risk of TD was with nonconventional chemotherapy (OR 3.1; 95% CI 2.0–4.8; P<.001).[49]

Low Libido

Libido, or sex drive, is another form of sexual dysfunction that is multifactorial and can have organic as well as psychological components. Although this can happen to any patient with cancer, the effects are often more noticeable in younger patients (such as men with TCA), as these patients often have a higher pre-illness libido.

One study evaluated 129 consecutive patients with TCA 3 to 5 years after treatment compared with 916 age-matched controls. Sexual dysfunction was self-reported using epidemiologic study questions. After controlling for comorbidities, patients with TCA were more likely to have low libido (OR 6.7; 95% CI 2.1–21) compared with controls.[51]

Another study followed patients longitudinally. They used a Dutch questionnaire on sexual function and administered it to patients with TCA post-orchiectomy but preradiation, and then again 3 and 6 months after radiation[52]; 23% of the patients reported a decrease in sexual interest. Many men endorsed body image issues due to testicular loss, and in 13% of men, this led to concern about having sexual relations with their partners.[52]

TD is thought to be an etiology of impairment of sexual desire. Testosterone has a clear link to libido, and thus this can be affected with systemic illness, CT, or abdominal/pelvic RT, as these can all lead to TD. The general link between TD and libido was evaluated in a study of 400 healthy men aged 20 to 50 years. These men all received 16 weeks of ADT and either testosterone gel in concentrations of 1.25 g, 2.5 g, 5g, or 10g daily or a placebo gel. Results showed a stepwise decrease in libido as testosterone replacement decreased. This demonstrates how sex drive is intricately linked to testosterone levels.[53]

However, low libido is multifactorial and there are additional factors at play, especially in patients with cancer . In the aforementioned study of patients with TCA versus controls, TD, as defined by a luteinizing hormone (LH) level greater than 10 IU/L or testosterone less than 10 nmol/L (288 ng/dL) was not associated with low libido (OR 1.2; 95% CI 0.11–14).[51] Another study evaluated men with bilateral orchiectomies who were on intramuscular testosterone every 3 weeks. They were evaluated with laboratory tests and questionnaires 1 day after injection, mid-cycle, and just before injection.[54] With respect to libido, men were asked to grade it from a scale of 1 to 10 with 1 being absent and 10 being very strong. Three of 7 patients reported low libido before injection; however, their testosterone levels were no different from men who did not complain of low libido.[54] This demonstrates the multifactorial nature of this condition and suggests that some men may be more sensitive to changes in testosterone and its impact on libido.

Erectile Dysfunction

Patients with TCA are at risk for ED given the frequency of TD in this population. In general, there is a clear link between TD and ED. In the aforementioned study with young men receiving ADT and then testosterone gel versus placebo, results show a link between ED and testosterone, but only at subphysiologic levels of testosterone. A decline in EF was only seen in the men on placebo or on the lowest testosterone dose of 1.25 g daily, but the men on 2.5 to 10 g daily did not experience a change in their erections ($P<.05$).[53] Normal EF is testosterone-dependent, but only at lower levels. Hence, men undergoing cancer treatment may be at higher risk for hormone-deficiency–related ED because many cancer treatments may lead to TD.

Patients with TCA can also be at risk for ED independent of their testosterone levels. In the aforementioned study on patients with TCA versus controls, the patient with cancer had higher rates of ED (OR 3.8; 95% CI 1.4–10).[51] However, ED was not associated with TD (OR 1.1; 95% CI 0.26–4.5).[51]

HEMATOLOGIC MALIGNANCIES

Patients with hematologic malignancies, especially those undergoing stem cell transplantation (SCT), are at high risk for sexual dysfunction. These patients require high-dose chemotherapy, usually involving alkylating agents, which are highly gonadotoxic. Total body irradiation (TBI) can also damage the testes and penis, thus further contributing to sexual dysfunction.[55] Patients with an allogeneic SCT will typically require immunosuppressants, which can further worsen hormonal status and sexual function.[55] This section focuses on TD, ED, and low libido in these men.

Testosterone Deficiency

The etiology of TD in men undergoing SCT is multifactorial and can include chemotherapy, TBI, and chronic corticosteroids.[55] In a series of 16 men status-post SCT, 88% had elevated follicle-stimulating hormone and 47% elevated LH; 38% of these men had low testosterone.[56] The impact of these specific hormonal perturbations on sexual function remains ambiguous.

Erectile Dysfunction and Low Libido

ED in patients with hematological malignancy may be multifactorial, related to TD, autonomic neuropathy from chemotherapy, TBI, and/or psychogenic causes.[3,55] A case-control series of men undergoing SCT evaluated patients pretransplantation, 6 months after, and 1, 2, 3, and 5 years post-SCT and compared their results at 5 years with age-matched controls (eg, siblings or friends of the patients or community-based volunteers).[57] One hundred percent of controls had been sexually active in the past month compared with 82% of patients ($P = .04$). Sexual function was assessed via the Sexual Function Questionnaire, and the sexual function mean score was slightly lower in patients (3.2 ± 1.0) compared with controls (3.7 ± 0.6); $P = .01$.[57] Forty-six percent of male patients had at least 1 sexual complaint compared with 21% in male controls ($P = .05$). Delayed ejaculation was the most common sexual complaint (27% of men), but ED was also common, with problems achieving erection in 23% and problems maintaining erection in 23%. These rates were lower in controls, with only 3% having delayed ejaculation, 6% had difficulty achieving erection, and 9% had difficulty maintaining an erection.[57]

In the aforementioned study of hormone changes after SCT, TD was a significant predictor of low libido ($P = .008$).[56] A decrease in sex drive and sexual activity is common after SCT. Of 34 men after SCT for leukemia, 56% noted a decreased interest in sex, 59% decreased sexual pleasure, and 62% had decline in sexual activity based on answers to study-specific, single-item questions.[58] When followed longitudinally, it is clear that these problems persist for years after SCT. At 5 years post-SCT, 23% of men noted low libido. Of men who were not sexually active, low libido was one of the most common reasons cited for lack of sexual activity.[57]

Although not evaluating ED or libido per se, a longitudinal study evaluated sexual activity in patients post-SCT, which can be considered a surrogate for sexual dysfunction. Patients were interviewed pretransplantation and then 6 months and 1 and 3 years afterward. Pretransplant men were most concerned with lack of sexual interest (46%), but this shifted to concern regarding body appearance in 61% of men at 3 years.[8] Of 90 men who were sexually active pretransplant, only 18 were active at 1 and 3 years after treatment.[8]

RECOMMENDATIONS

The aforementioned data demonstrate the breadth and prevalence of aspects of sexual dysfunction seen in male patients with cancer. A diagnosis of cancer itself can lead to various sexual side effects. This is further compounded by various treatments, such as chemotherapy, radiation, surgery, and ADT. We recommend a discussion of sexual functioning be initiated by providers early on in the process, typically following the initial cancer diagnosis. The impact of all oncologic treatment modalities on sexual functioning also should be discussed. Patient and partner goals need to be addressed, as this may impact treatment decisions. Throughout the treatment and recovery process, men should be routinely queried about the presence of sexual dysfunction and have a thorough discussion of their treatment options.

With regard to radical pelvic surgery or radiation, we recommend all men with any possible interest in future sexual function undergo a penile rehabilitation program. As mentioned previously, at our institution, this involves a low-dose PDE5i daily with 1 full treatment dose at least once a week. Any patient who is not able to achieve a penetration-hardness erection by 6 weeks is taught to perform ICI weekly in lieu of the test dose.

Any patient undergoing chemotherapy or TBI needs to be counseled on the risk of TD. They should be regularly screened for symptoms. If there is clinical concern for TD based on signs or symptoms, they should have 2 early morning testosterone labs as per the AUA guidelines.[59] If their testosterone is low in the context of signs and symptoms, testosterone therapy should be offered.

SUMMARY

In summation, the emerging field of oncosexology focuses on the sexual consequences of cancer and its treatments. As many patients are not being appropriately counseled on sexual consequences, it is imperative that health care practitioners provide adequate information on the sexual dysfunction associated with cancer treatment. Although pelvic cancer, especially genitourinary malignancy, has higher risk of sexual dysfunction, these changes can occur in all patients with cancer. The etiology is often multifactorial, with psychological and organic components at play. TD from chronic illness, CT, RT, or ADT can contribute to ED, low libido, and ejaculatory and orgasmic dysfunction. Pelvic surgery or RT can remove or damage the ejaculatory apparatus, as well as the cavernous nerves responsible for normal EF. With appropriate treatment and counseling, oncosexologists can help patients to navigate these sexual changes.

CLINICS CARE POINTS

- Health care providers need to discuss sexual issues with patients with cancer, including potential adverse effects of all treatment options.
- Many patients with cancer endorse sexual dysfunction and associated unmet informational and/or treatment needs.
- Pelvic malignancies, such as prostate, bladder, or colorectal cancer, have high rates of sexual dysfunction.
- Sexual dysfunction in male patients with cancer include ED, ejaculatory dysfunction, orgasmic dysfunction, PD, low libido, TD, and penile shortening.
- Penile rehabilitation is recommended after pelvic cancer treatment; however, there are no data to suggest the superiority of one rehabilitation protocol over another.

DISCLOSURE

The authors have nothing to disclose.

REFERENCES

1. Enzlin PAIDC. The emerging field of 'oncosexology': recognising the importance of addressing sexuality in oncology. Belgium J Med Oncol 2011;5:44–9.
2. Allen JO, Zebrack B, Wittman D, et al. Expanding the NCCN guidelines for distress management: a model of barriers to the use of coping resources. J Community Support Oncol 2014;12:271–7.
3. Sadovsky R, Basson R, Krychman M, et al. Cancer and sexual problems. J Sex Med 2010;7:349–73.
4. Almont T, Farsi F, Krakowski I, et al. Sexual health in cancer: the results of a survey exploring practices, attitudes, knowledge, communication, and professional interactions in oncology healthcare providers. Support Care Cancer 2019;27:887–94.
5. Almont T, Bouhnik AD, Ben Charif A, et al. Sexual health problems and discussion in colorectal cancer patients two years after diagnosis: a national cross-sectional study. J Sex Med 2019;16:96–110.
6. Salonia A, Adaikan G, Buvat J, et al. Sexual rehabilitation after treatment for prostate cancer-part 2: recommendations from the Fourth International Consultation for Sexual Medicine (ICSM 2015). J Sex Med 2017;14:297–315.
7. Albers LF, Palacios LAG, Pelger RCM, et al. Can the provision of sexual healthcare for oncology patients be improved? A literature review of educational interventions for healthcare professionals. J Cancer Surviv 2020;14:858–66.
8. Humphreys CT, Tallman B, Altmaier EM, et al. Sexual functioning in patients undergoing bone marrow transplantation: a longitudinal study. Bone Marrow Transplant 2007;39:491–6.
9. Bernat JK, Wittman DA, Hawley ST, et al. Symptom burden and information needs in prostate cancer survivors: a case for tailored long-term survivorship care. BJU Int 2016;118:372–8.
10. Downing A, Wright P, Hounsome L, et al. Quality of life in men living with advanced and localised prostate cancer in the UK: a population-based study. Lancet Oncol 2019;20:436–47.
11. Chambers SK, Occhipinti S, Stiller A, et al. Five-year outcomes from a randomised controlled trial of a couples-based intervention for men with localised prostate cancer. Psychooncology 2019;28:775–83.
12. Loeb S, Salter CA, Nelson CJ, et al. A call to arms: increasing our understanding of the impact of prostate cancer on the sexual health of partners. J Sex Med 2020;17:361–3.
13. Tanner T, Galbraith M, Hays L. From a woman's perspective: life as a partner of a prostate cancer survivor. J Midwifery Womens Health 2011;56:154–60.
14. Ramsey SD, Zeliadt SB, Blough DK, et al. Impact of prostate cancer on sexual relationships: a longitudinal perspective on intimate partners' experiences. J Sex Med 2013;10:3135–43.
15. McInnis MK, Pukall CF. Sex after prostate cancer in gay and bisexual men: a review of the literature. Sex Med Rev 2020;8:466–72.
16. Salonia A, Adaikan G, Buvat J, et al. Sexual rehabilitation after treatment for prostate cancer-part 1: recommendations from the Fourth International Consultation for Sexual Medicine (ICSM 2015). J Sex Med 2017;14:285–96.
17. Burnett AL, Nehra A, Breau RH, et al. Erectile dysfunction: AUA Guideline. J Urol 2018;200:633–41.
18. Frey A, Pedersen C, Lindberg H, et al. Prevalence and predicting factors for commonly neglected sexual side effects to external-beam radiation therapy for prostate cancer. J Sex Med 2017;14:558–65.
19. Huyghe E, Delannes M, Wagner F, et al. Ejaculatory function after permanent 125I prostate brachytherapy for localized prostate cancer. Int J Radiat Oncol Biol Phys 2009;74:126–32.
20. Sullivan JF, Stember DS, Deveci S, et al. Ejaculation profiles of men following radiation therapy for prostate cancer. J Sex Med 2013;10:1410–6.
21. Serefoglu EC, McMahon CG, Waldinger MD, et al. An evidence-based unified definition of lifelong and acquired premature ejaculation: report of the

second international society for sexual medicine ad hoc committee for the definition of premature ejaculation. Sex Med 2014;2:41–59.

22. Lin CY, Burri A, Pakpour AH. Premature ejaculation and erectile dysfunction in Iranian prostate cancer patients. Asian Pac J Cancer Prev 2016;17:1961–6.

23. Frey A, Sonksen J, Jakobsen H, et al. Prevalence and predicting factors for commonly neglected sexual side effects to radical prostatectomies: results from a cross-sectional questionnaire-based study. J Sex Med 2014;11:2318–26.

24. O'Neil BB, Presson A, Gannon J, et al. Climacturia after definitive treatment of prostate cancer. J Urol 2014;191:159–63.

25. Choi JM, Nelson CJ, Stasi J, et al. Orgasm associated incontinence (climacturia) following radical pelvic surgery: rates of occurrence and predictors. J Urol 2007;177:2223–6.

26. Lee J, Hersey K, Lee CT, et al. Climacturia following radical prostatectomy: prevalence and risk factors. J Urol 2006;176:2562–5 [discussion: 65].

27. Koeman M, van Driel MF, Schultz WC, et al. Orgasm after radical prostatectomy. Br J Urol 1996;77:861–4.

28. Nilsson AE, Carlsson S, Johansson E, et al. Orgasm-associated urinary incontinence and sexual life after radical prostatectomy. J Sex Med 2011;8:2632–9.

29. Barnas JL, Pierpaoli S, Ladd P, et al. The prevalence and nature of orgasmic dysfunction after radical prostatectomy. BJU Int 2004;94:603–5.

30. Guay A, Seftel AD. Sexual foreplay incontinence in men with erectile dysfunction after radical prostatectomy: a clinical observation. Int J Impot Res 2008;20:199–201.

31. Jain R, Mitchell S, Laze J, et al. The effect of surgical intervention for stress urinary incontinence (UI) on post-prostatectomy UI during sexual activity. BJU Int 2012;109:1208–12.

32. Bach PV, Salter CA, Katz D, et al. Arousal incontinence in men following radical prostatectomy: prevalence, impact and predictors. J Sex Med 2019;16:1947–52.

33. Manassero F, Di Paola G, Paperini D, et al. Orgasm-associated incontinence (climacturia) after bladder neck-sparing radical prostatectomy: clinical and video-urodynamic evaluation. J Sex Med 2012;9:2150–6.

34. Mendez MH, Sexton SJ, Lentz AC. Contemporary review of male and female climacturia and urinary leakage during sexual activities. Sex Med Rev 2018;6:16–28.

35. Mehta A, Deveci S, Mulhall JP. Efficacy of a penile variable tension loop for improving climacturia after radical prostatectomy. BJU Int 2013;111:500–4.

36. Tal R, Heck M, Teloken P, et al. Peyronie's disease following radical prostatectomy: incidence and predictors. J Sex Med 2010;7:1254–61.

37. Nguyen PL, Alibhai SM, Basaria S, et al. Adverse effects of androgen deprivation therapy and strategies to mitigate them. Eur Urol 2015;67:825–36.

38. Mulhall JP. Penile length changes after radical prostatectomy. BJU Int 2005;96:472–4.

39. Shindel LLAA. Penile length and its preservation in men after radical prostatectomy. Curr Sex Health Rep 2019;11:3890398.

40. Berookhim BM, Nelson CJ, Kunzel B, et al. Prospective analysis of penile length changes after radical prostatectomy. BJU Int 2014;113:E131–6.

41. Loh-Doyle JC, Han J, Ghodoussipour S. Factors associated with patient-reported penile length loss after radical cystoprostatectomy in male patients with bladder cancer. J Sex Med 2020;17:957–63.

42. Haliloglu A, Baltaci S, Yaman O. Penile length changes in men treated with androgen suppression plus radiation therapy for local or locally advanced prostate cancer. J Urol 2007;177:128–30.

43. Parekh A, Chen MH, Hoffman KE, et al. Reduced penile size and treatment regret in men with recurrent prostate cancer after surgery, radiotherapy plus androgen deprivation, or radiotherapy alone. Urology 2013;81:130–4.

44. Park KK, Lee SH, Chung BH. The effects of long-term androgen deprivation therapy on penile length in patients with prostate cancer: a single-center, prospective, open-label, observational study. J Sex Med 2011;8:3214–9.

45. Pahlajani G, Raina R, Jones S, et al. Vacuum erection devices revisited: its emerging role in the treatment of erectile dysfunction and early penile rehabilitation following prostate cancer therapy. J Sex Med 2012;9:1182–9.

46. Masterson TA, Cary C, Rice KR, et al. The evolution and technique of nerve-sparing retroperitoneal lymphadenectomy. Urol Clin North Am 2015;42:311–20.

47. Wohlfahrt-Veje C, Main KM, Skakkebaek NE. Testicular dysgenesis syndrome: foetal origin of adult reproductive problems. Clin Endocrinol (Oxf) 2009;71:459–65.

48. Wiechno PJ, Kowalska M, Kucharz J, et al. Dynamics of hormonal disorders following unilateral orchiectomy for a testicular tumor. Med Oncol 2017;34:84.

49. Bandak M, Jorgensen N, Juul A, et al. Testosterone deficiency in testicular cancer survivors - a systematic review and meta-analysis. Andrology 2016;4:382–8.

50. La Vignera S, Cannarella R, Duca Y, et al. Hypogonadism and sexual dysfunction in testicular tumor survivors: a systematic review. Front Endocrinol (Lausanne) 2019;10:264.

51. Eberhard J, Stahl O, Cohn-Cedermark G, et al. Sexual function in men treated for testicular cancer. J Sex Med 2009;6:1979–89.

52. Wortel RC, Ghidey Alemayehu W, Incrocci L. Orchiectomy and radiotherapy for stage I-II testicular seminoma: a prospective evaluation of short-term effects on body image and sexual function. J Sex Med 2015;12:210–8.

53. Finkelstein JS, Yu EW, Burnett-Bowie SA. Gonadal steroids and body composition, strength, and sexual function in men. N Engl J Med 2013;369:2457.

54. van Basten JP, van Driel MF, Jonker-Pool G, et al. Sexual functioning in testosterone-supplemented patients treated for bilateral testicular cancer. Br J Urol 1997;79:461–7.

55. Yi JC, Syrjala KL. Sexuality after hematopoietic stem cell transplantation. Cancer J 2009;15:57–64.

56. Schimmer AD, Ali V, Stewart AK, et al. Male sexual function after autologous blood or marrow transplantation. Biol Blood Marrow Transplant 2001;7:279–83.

57. Syrjala KL, Kurland BF, Abrams JR, et al. Sexual function changes during the 5 years after high-dose treatment and hematopoietic cell transplantation for malignancy, with case-matched controls at 5 years. Blood 2008;111:989–96.

58. Claessens JJ, Beerendonk CC, Schattenberg AV. Quality of life, reproduction and sexuality after stem cell transplantation with partially T-cell-depleted grafts and after conditioning with a regimen including total body irradiation. Bone Marrow Transplant 2006;37:831–6.

59. Mulhall JP, Trost LW, Brannigan RE, et al. Evaluation and management of testosterone deficiency: AUA Guideline. J Urol 2018;200:423–32.

Energy-Based Therapies for Erectile Dysfunction
Current and Future Directions

Raghav Pai, BS[a], Jesse Ory, MD[a], Carlos Delgado, BS[b],
Ranjith Ramasamy, MD[a],*

KEYWORDS

- Low-intensity shock wave therapy • Radial shock wave therapy • Restorative therapy
- Erectile dysfunction

KEY POINTS

- A growing body of data supports shock wave therapy as a safe and effective treatment modality for erectile dysfunction (ED), particularly in men who are responders to phosphodiesterase-5 inhibitor (PDE5i) therapy.
- There are important distinctions regarding energy source and transfer that must be carefully considered when interpreting existing data and applying them to practice.
- Published studies on shock wave treatment for ED are limited by short follow-up durations, lack of heterogeneity in patient selection, and variability in shock wave treatment protocol.

INTRODUCTION

Erectile dysfunction (ED) is defined as the consistent or recurrent inability of a man to attain and/or maintain a penile erection sufficient for sexual activity and is a common condition worldwide.[1] ED has been shown to be associated with a variety of comorbidities that affect both patients' physical and mental health, including cardiovascular disease, anxiety, and depression.[2] The prevalence of ED is expected to increase throughout the world, with some estimates predicting that 322 million men will be affected globally by 2025, a 111% increase from 1995.[3] Although there are many therapeutic options available for men with ED, management has changed little since the approval of phosphodiesterase-5 inhibitors (PDE5i) in 1998.[4] Approximately, 30% of men do not respond to PDE5i therapy and many others find that these medications cause undesirable side effects.[5] As a result, PDE5is have been

reported to have discontinuation rates of approximately 4% per month and almost 50% after 1 year.[6] In the setting of PDE5i failure, the next steps in management typically involve more invasive therapy, including injections of erectogenic medications and penile prosthesis. Therefore, there is a clear need for new, noninvasive treatment options for men with ED.

Energy-based therapies have been proposed as a novel, nonsurgical, restorative treatment option for ED. A variety of energy sources have been used, most prominently shock waves. Shock waves are a form of acoustic energy that can be targeted and focused on highly specific anatomic regions.[7] Shock waves are known to have mechanically disruptive effects, impacts on tissue regeneration, and anti-inflammatory properties. These properties have made shock wave energy of interest for several medical applications.[8] Examples of use include the management of

Conflict of Interest: The authors have no conflict of interests to disclose.
Funding sources: None.
[a] Department of Urology, Miller School of Medicine, University of Miami, Miami, FL 33136, USA;
[b] Technologico de Monterrey, School of Medicine and Health Science, Avenue Morones Prieto 3000, Monterrey, Nuevo León 64710, Mexico
* Corresponding author.
E-mail address: ramasamy@miami.edu

Urol Clin N Am 48 (2021) 603–610
https://doi.org/10.1016/j.ucl.2021.06.013

nephrolithiasis, in calcific coronary plaque modification, and musculoskeletal regeneration.[9–11]

Shock wave therapy for use in ED typically uses either low-intensity extracorporeal shock wave therapy (Li-ESWT) or radial shock wave therapy. Li-ESWT is similar to extracorporeal shock wave therapy (ESWT) that is used in other medical applications, except that it works at a lower energy level and the shock waves are spread over a larger focal volume.[12] Radial shock waves, however, are pressure waves that use maximum pressures that are approximately 100 times lower and pulse durations that are about 1000 times longer than Li-ESWT.[13,14] **Fig. 1** demonstrates the differences in the waveforms between Li-ESWT and radial shock wave therapy. Because of differences between these types of shock waves, radial shock wave therapy is classified as an FDA Class I device and does not require medical supervision, whereas Li-ESWT is a class II device, requiring medical supervision. As there is little to no peer-reviewed published literature regarding the efficacy of radial shock waves in the treatment of ED, this technology will not be considered in this article.

The mechanism by which Li-ESWT may improve erectile function remains unclear but is thought to stem at least in part from stimulation of mechano-sensors throughout the endothelium in the penile vasculature. This stimulation in turn induces neo-angiogenic processes allowing for greater blood flow throughout the corpus cavernosum.[15] In addition to neoangiogenesis, rat models of ED have shown that Li-ESWT may induce migration of progenitor cells that can improve microcirculation and contribute to nerve regeneration.[16] Li-ESWT has also been thought to contribute to the overall decline in cell stress responses and inflammation in penile tissue, which can further contribute to increased blood flow and smooth muscle relaxation.[15] In fact, Lue et al. used a rat model of pelvic neurovascular injuries to demonstrate that Li-ESWT can induce endogenous progenitor cell recruitment and subsequent Schwann cell activation allowing for angiogenesis along with tissue and nerve regeneration.[17] Similar findings have been demonstrated in many other animal models of ED and there have been numerous proposed specific cellular pathways implicated.[18] This is of particular interest as Li-ESWT for the management of ED is generally regarded as safe, with few to no reported adverse effects.[19]

Since Li-ESWT was introduced in 2010, there have been numerous randomized controlled trials (RCTs), as well as meta-analyses evaluating, and in most cases supporting, the efficacy of Li-ESWT.[20–23] Despite this, multiple sexual health organizations and guidelines remain restrictive in their endorsement of this technology, recommending use only in the setting of an institutional review board (IRB)-approved clinical trial.[24–26] Nevertheless, interest in this technology for ED remains quite high.[27,28] In this article, we critically analyze the literature to determine which men are most likely to benefit from Li-ESWT for ED and to delineate data necessary to establish whether or not Li-ESWT will be a new standard of care in ED management.[29] Most studies of Li-EWT have been conducted on men with vasculogenic ED. Moreover, few if any studies have evaluated the efficacy of Li-ESWT in men with ED related to radical pelvic surgery, neurogenic ED, and diabetes.

LITERATURE REVIEW
Phosphodiesterase-5 Inhibitor Responders

Many RCTs investigating the use of Li-ESWT in ED treatment have focused on efficacy in men who are responders to PDE5i therapy. This is an important group to study as it represents the majority of patients with ED and Li-ESWT has the potential to reduce or even eliminate reliance on medication. This is of particular import for men with contraindications to PDE5i use, such as those taking nitrates for angina, and those who have moderate to severe side effects.[30]

The first peer-reviewed published investigation of Li-ESWT for ED was a prospective cohort study by Vardi and colleagues in 20 PDE5i responsive men with vasculogenic ED with International Index of Erectile Function Erectile Function Domain (IIEF-EF) scores between 5 and 19 as well as abnormal nocturnal penile tumescence parameters. All participants underwent a 4-week PDE5i washout period. The participants were administered LI-ESWT to the penile shaft and crura at 5 different sites for 2 sessions a week for 3 weeks with a total of 1500 shocks per treatment. This protocol was repeated after a 3-week period of no treatment. This pilot study was quite successful, with a significant increase in mean IIEF-EF scores from 13.5 ± 4.1 to 20.9 ± 5.8 at 1-month follow-up. Improvements in mean IIEF-EF score remained unchanged at 6-month follow-up, with half of the participants no longer requiring PDE5i therapy.[20]

These promising results led to further study by this same group. In 2012, the first randomized, double-blind, sham-controlled trial of Li-ESWT was reported. In this study, 67 men with ED who were PDE5i responders were randomized to receive Li-ESWT therapy or sham therapy after a 4-week PDE5i washout period. The Li-ESWT cohort received 2 treatment sessions per week for 3 weeks, which were repeated after a 3-week

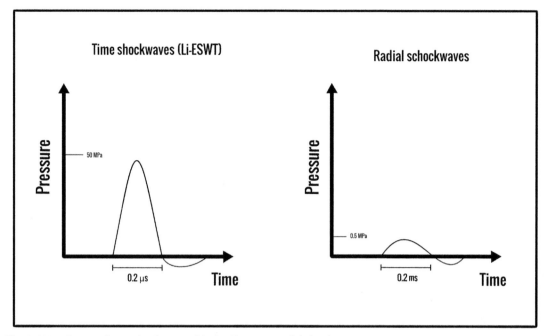

Fig. 1. Waveforms of true shockwaves (Li-ESWT) versus radial shockwaves.

period of no treatment. The participants received 1500 shocks in each treatment session. The authors measured erectile function before the first treatment as well as 1 month after the final treatment. Both cohorts had similar baseline measures of erectile function with a mean IIEF-EF score of 11.5 ± 0.86 and 12.6 ± 0.75 in the sham and treatment group, respectively. There was a significant improvement in erectile function in the treatment group at 1-month follow-up, with a mean IIEF-EF increase of 6.7 ± 0.9 versus 3.0 ± 1.4 in the Li-ESWT and placebo cohorts, respectively. Importantly, more than 40% of the men in the treatment group were newly able to achieve erections hard enough for penetration in the treatment group compared with none in the placebo.[31]

Numerous subsequent studies on Li-ESWT for ED have yielded similar results. In a recent meta-analysis conducted by Sokolakis and colleagues, 6 of the 13 RCTSs on Li-ESWT for ED were focused on men who were PDE5i responders and all of these studies demonstrated a positive effect of Li-ESWT on ED compared with placebo.[22] These results are encouraging but substantial limitations remain to be addressed. The follow-up durations in the RCTs that have been conducted have been quite short, with 4 of the 6 RCTs focusing on PDE5i responders in the aforementioned meta-analysis having follow-up durations of under 6 weeks.[21] This is important as studies evaluating the efficacy of Li-ESWT in

patients with even mild forms of ED have shown that the benefits of treatment are not durable at 2 years in at least a quarter of patients.[32] Therefore, it is essential that additional RCTs with longer follow-up durations be conducted to understand how the extent to which patients may experience durable benefit from this therapy.

Phosphodiesterase-5 Inhibitor Nonresponders

PDE5i nonresponders represent a unique group that could significantly benefit from Li-ESWT.[33] Men who fail PDE5i often must turn to more invasive treatment options, including intracorporal injections or surgery for placement of an inflatable penile prosthesis. Unfortunately, studies reporting the efficacy of Li-ESWT in PDE5i nonresponders are scant and until recently have been limited to prospective single-arm cohort studies. Both of the most recent meta-analyses by Dong and colleagues and Sokolakis and colleagues included only one RCT by Kitrey and colleagues that focused on PDE5i nonresponders.[21,22,34] Since these two meta-analyses were published, a more recent randomized, double-blind, sham-controlled trial was conducted in 2020 in which 76 patients with vascular ED who were nonresponders to PDE5i therapy were assigned to either Li-ESWT or a sham probe. The participants had a baseline median IIEF-EF score of 12 (IQR 8–17) and 13 (IQR 8–17) in the treatment and placebo group, respectively, as well a median baseline Erection Hardness Score (EHS) score of 2 (IQR 1–3) in both groups. At the 3-month follow-up, the median change in IIEF-EF from baseline in the Li-ESWT and sham group was 3.5 (IQR 0–10) and −0.5 (IQR -11 to 1) respectively. At 6 months, 52.5% of participants in the treatment group had an EHS of greater than 2, which is consistent with erections sufficient for penetration, compared with 27.8% in the sham group.[35] Overall, this study showed how Li-ESWT can provide a modest improvement in erectile function in specific groups of patients who are nonresponders to PDE5i therapy. Nevertheless, similar to the majority of RCTs studying Li-ESWT in PDE5i responders, this study was limited by its short follow-up duration of only 6 months. In addition, this study did not reach a clinically significant endpoint which is defined as the minimally clinically important difference in IIEF-EF scores, which varies with a baseline level of erectile function, and is defined as 2, 5, and 7 in those with mild, moderate, and severe ED, respectively.[36] In addition, other than the study by Kitrey and colleagues described below, this is the only sham-controlled RCT evaluating the use of Li-ESWT in PDE5i nonresponders.[30,34]

Li-ESWT was shown to convert men from PDE5i nonresponders to PDE5i responders in one sham-controlled RCT. Kitrey and colleagues conducted a prospective, randomized, double-blind placebo-controlled study in 58 patients with vasculogenic ED who stopped using PDE5i therapy because of a lack of efficacy. Participants had a median IIEF-EF score of 7 and 8 in the treatment and placebo group, respectively, and all participants had an EHS of 2 or less with PDE5i therapy. At 1-month follow-up, 54.1% of participants in the treatment group were able to achieve an erection hard enough for vaginal penetration with PDE5i therapy compared with 0% in the placebo group.[34] A therapy that may allow men to become PDE5i responders may of great utility as an alternative to proceeding to invasive treatments. Although these results are intriguing, data from longer duration studies with a large sample size are necessary before Li-ESWT can be recommended to men who are PDE5i nonresponders.

Erectile Dysfunction in Diabetic Men

In 2019, Spivak and colleagues identified and analyzed 5 double-blind, sham-controlled trials that did not exclude men with diabetes. The study extracted data on 109 men with diabetes who underwent Li-ESWT. Of these, 61 men were PDE5i responders and 48 were nonresponders. Li-ESWT was effective in both groups of diabetic patients, with a mean change in IIEF-EF scores between the treatment and placebo groups of 6.4 (1.6 ± 3.4 vs 8.0 ± 5.5), 4.8 (3.6 ± 5.2 vs 8.4 ± 5.0), and 5.4 (5.4 ± 0.5 vs 5.9 ± 5.1) at 1, 6, and 12 months after the last shock wave treatments, respectively. Among PDE5i nonresponders, 55% were responsive to PDE5i after Li-ESWT corresponding to a change in mean IIEF-EF at 1 month follow-up from −0.5 ± 2.0 to 5.4 ± 5.9 in the placebo and experimental group in this cohort, respectively. As would be expected, PDE5i responders had better outcomes than the PDE5i nonresponders.[37] Although this study speaks to the efficacy of Li-ESWT in this population, dedicated RCTs for diabetic men need to be conducted to better determine the extent to which this therapy may be beneficial in this population. Furthermore, men should be further classified by the extent and control of their diabetes to better elucidate which diabetic men may most benefit from Li-ESWT.

Erectile Dysfunction in Men after Pelvic Surgery

There are certain patient populations for whom Li-ESWT trials have failed to find any efficacy. This has held especially true in men who have undergone radical prostatectomy or radical cystoprostatectomy. Radical pelvic surgery was an exclusion criterion for most RCT evaluating Li-ESWT for ED. Baccaglini and colleagues led the first RCT of Li-ESWT for ED related to nerve-sparing radical prostatectomy. The study enrolled 92 men who were randomly assigned to either receive a PDE5i or combination therapy with Li-ESWT and PDE5i postoperatively following removal of the transurethral catheter. All men received 5 mg/d of tadalafil postoperatively and the Li-ESWT cohort received one session of Li-ESWT per week with 2400 shocks per session for a total of 8 weeks. At 8-week follow-up, the men in the combination therapy cohort were found to have an improvement in median IIEF-EF score compared with the PDE5i only cohort with a median IIEF-EF score of 12 (IQR 9.3–15.8) and 10.0 (IQR 7.0–11.0), respectively. However, despite statistical significance, the study did not reach the primary clinical endpoint defined as a ≥4-point difference in mean IIEF-EF scores between the arms.[38] A similar study by Zewin and colleagues evaluated the role of Li-ESWT for ED in male patients who underwent nerve-sparing cystoprostatectomy. The study included 128 patients who were randomized to Li-ESWT, PDE5i, or control arm. All men had received surgery within 5 years of the date the study was conducted. The participants in the Li-ESWT cohort received 12 sessions of Li-ESWT with a total of 1500 shocks per treatment session. Patients in the Li-ESWT and control arms did not use adjunctive PDE5i. Potency recovery rates, defined as ≥5 point increase in IIEF-EF score and/or erection sufficient for vaginal penetration, at 9-month follow-up were 76.2%, 79.1%, and 60.5% in the Li-ESWT, PDE5i, and control arms, respectively. The researchers did not find a statistically significant difference in erectile function between these groups at any follow-up periods.[39] Furthermore, potency recovery rates in this study were likely higher than other nerve-sparing cystectomy series because of the young age of the patients (53 ± 6 years) and because all surgeries were carried out by a single expert surgeon. Overall, existing data suggest that although Li-ESWT may be safe in postpelvic surgery patients, it is unlikely to be effective as a monotherapy.

Erectile Dysfunction in Men after Renal Transplant

ED is prevalent in over half of sexually active male renal transplant patients.[40] ED in renal transplant patients is often multifactorial, involving vascular, neurogenic, and pharmacologic causes.

Furthermore, there is some concern that PDE5i may alter serum levels of immunosuppressive drugs.[41] In the only sham-controlled RCT in this population, Yamacake and colleagues recruited 20 patients with a minimum interval of 6 months postrenal transplant who were equally randomized among a Li-ESWT and placebo group. All participants were required to discontinue PDE5i use at least a month before treatment and throughout the study period. The Li-ESWT cohort received 2 treatment sessions per week for 3 weeks with a total of 2000 shocks per session. The 2 cohorts had similar baseline IIEF-EF scores of 10.9 ± 5.1 and 14.9 ± 3.0 and the mean change in IIEF-EF scores at 4 month follow-up were 6.3 and 1.6 for the Li-ESWT and placebo cohorts, respectively.[41] Although small, this study suggests that renal transplant patients with ED may benefit from Li-ESWT.

Optimal Low-Intensity Extracorporeal Shock Wave Therapy Protocols

The studies that have evaluated the efficacy of Li-ESWT in ED treatment have had significant heterogeneity in their treatment protocols. Unfortunately, the number of trials investigating unique treatment protocols has also been quite limited. The recent

---

Table 1
Summary of the limitations of current RCTs evaluating Li-ESWT in ED treatment

Limitation	Description
Professional urologic and sexual health associations have advised restricting Li-ESWT use in ED to clinical trials.	Lack of unequivocal evidence and long-term follow-up duration have led to skepticism about the true efficacy of Li-ESWT in ED.
Most RCTs evaluating Li-ESWT in ED have limited follow-up durations.	The most recent meta-analyses of RCTs report follow-up durations between 1 mo and 1 y. Prospective cohort studies that have been conducted with lengthier follow-up durations report diminished efficacy after 1 y.
Many of the RCTs evaluating Li-ESWT in ED are not adequately powered or are missing power calculations altogether.	Approximately, half of the RCTs included in the most recent meta-analyses are missing power calculations. Limited sample sizes and lack of appropriate power calculations lead to uncertainty of the trial's statistical accuracy.
Treatment protocols that have been used in the RCTs evaluating Li-ESWT in ED have not been consistent.	RCTs have used varying treatment durations, number of shocks, and types of shockwave lithotripters. This leads to ambiguity as to the most efficacious protocol in ED treatment.
There are certain patient populations in which Li-ESWT in ED has not been shown to be effective or there is limited data.	The RCTs that have been conducted on men who have underwent pelvic surgery have not shown Li-ESWT to be effective. Limited data exist in diabetic men.

meta-analysis by Sokolakis and colleagues identified only 3 RCTs that compared two different Li-ESWT protocols.[22] In one of these RCTs, Katz and colleagues compared a protocol involving 5 daily sessions of 720 shocks to 6 daily sessions of 600 shocks for a period of 2 weeks. Men who were taking a PDE5i were assigned a 4-week washout period before starting the study and remained free of PDE5i use throughout the study. Although both protocols involved a total of 3600 shocks throughout the course of the study, the first protocol failed to show any difference in IIEF scores at 6 months while the second protocol showed a significant increase of 4.2 points in mean IIEF scores.[29] This indicated that the intense daily application of shocks failed to produce the same results as distributing fewer shocks over a longer period. Kalyvianakis and colleagues also led an RCT involving 42 PDE5i responders in which they tried to compare the efficacy of Li-ESWT in patients who received either 6 (Group A) or 12 (Group B) treatment sessions within a 6-week period. Men who were taking PDE5is underwent a 4-week washout period and remained free of PDE5i use throughout the study. All participants received 5000 shocks per treatment session. Furthermore, those who completed 6-month follow-up were offered 6 additional sessions. The researchers found that when examining the impact of the total number of sessions received, 62%, 74%, and 83% of patients achieved an MCID in IIEF-EF score compared with baseline after 6, 12, and 18 sessions, respectively.[42] As a whole, this study demonstrated that the total number of Li-ESWT sessions has a significant impact on the efficacy of treatment. It also demonstrated that there may be a benefit in retreating patients at specific intervals. Although the current literature gives us some understanding of how to optimize treatment protocols, a larger number of RCTs and meta-analyses comparing protocols must be conducted. This will allow for less heterogeneity and the identification of specific protocols that can best benefit patients.

SUMMARY

Numerous RCTs have demonstrated the efficacy of Li-ESWT in ED treatment. Furthermore, the safety of Li-ESWT has been well-established with none of the RCTs included in recent meta-analyses reporting any significant adverse effects.[21,22] Both urologists and patients have also expressed great interest in this novel therapy.[27,43] Nevertheless, RCTs that have been conducted have not used consistent treatment protocols and additional studies are required to determine

which treatment protocols (in terms of number of shocks, location of shocks, intervals between treatment, and frequency of treatment sessions) are optimal. It is conceivable that patient factors may modulate treatment response and that there may not be an optimal "one-size-fits-all" approach.

Currently, most of the successful studies on Li-ESWT in ED treatment have been on men with vasculogenic ED, particularly those who are still responsive to PDE5i. Li-ESWT appears to lack efficacy in men who have undergone pelvic surgery. Other populations, including diabetic men and men who have had a renal transplant, have been incompletely evaluated as to the efficacy of Li-ESWT for ED. Therefore, additional studies in carefully categorized populations are necessary to properly evaluate what populations may best benefit from Li-ESWT.

It is also crucial to assess the long-term efficacy of Li-ESWT to determine how it may best be incorporated into ED treatment. The short follow-up duration of most current RCTs, as well as the small number of men recruited, creates a disadvantage in determining who would best benefit from Li-ESWT and how it can be optimally incorporated into treatment plans.

Overall, despite the growing evidence of efficacy, these limitations have led major urologic and sexual health societies to restrict Li-ESWT as an experimental treatment.[24,26] **Table 1** summarizes the limitations of the RCTs evaluating the use of Li-ESWT in ED treatment. Appropriately powered RCTs with longer follow-up durations, homogenous treatment protocols, and diverse patient populations are required to determine the role of Li-ESWT in ED management. Until such data become available, clinicians should use Li-ESWT only in the context of appropriate patient counseling and safety protocols.

CLINICS CARE POINTS

- Li-ESWT is a noninvasive restorative treatment option for ED with minimal adverse effects.

- Numerous small RCTs have demonstrated the efficacy and safety of Li-ESWT for the management of ED.

- The bulk of data on Li-ESWT for ED has been focused on short-term efficacy in PDE5i responders, a population in which there is evidence for substantial efficacy.

- There are few RCTs on the use of Li-ESWT for ED treatment in PDE5i nonresponders and nonvascular ED.
- Limitations in existing clinical trials of Li-ESWT for ED include short follow-up durations, small sample sizes, and variability in treatment protocols.
- Future studies to expand the prime-time use of Li-ESWT in ED will need to focus on conducting additional RCTs with more diverse patient populations, longer follow-up durations, and larger sample sizes.

REFERENCES

1. Raheem OA, Natale C, Dick B, et al. Novel treatments of erectile dysfunction: review of the current literature. Sex Med Rev 2020;9(1).
2. Christensen BS, Grønbæk M, Osler M, et al. Associations between physical and mental health problems and sexual dysfunctions in sexually active danes. J Sex Med 2011;8(7):1890–902.
3. Goldstein I, Goren A, Li VW, et al. Epidemiology update of erectile dysfunction in eight countries with high burden. Sex Med Rev 2020;8(1):48–58.
4. Moon DG. Evolution of phosphodiesterase-5 inhibitors. World J Mens Health 2015;33(3):123–4.
5. Giuliano F, Joussain C, Denys P. Safety and efficacy of intracavernosal injections of abobotulinumtoxinA (Dysport(®)) as add on therapy to phosphdiesterase type 5 inhibitors or prostaglandin E1 for erectile dysfunction-case studies. Toxins (Basel) 2019;11(5).
6. Corona G, Rastrelli G, Burri A, et al. First-generation phosphodiesterase type 5 inhibitors dropout: a comprehensive review and meta-analysis. Andrology 2016;4(6):1002–9.
7. Gruenwald I, Appel B, Kitrey ND, et al. Shockwave treatment of erectile dysfunction. Ther Adv Urol 2013;5(2):95–9.
8. Kamel FH, Basha M, Alsharidah A, et al. Efficacy of extracorporeal shockwave therapy on cervical myofascial pain following neck dissection surgery: a randomized controlled trial. Ann Rehabil Med 2020; 44(5):393–401.
9. Cao L, Wang YQ, Yu T, et al. The effectiveness and safety of extracorporeal shock wave lithotripsy for the management of kidney stones: A protocol of systematic review and meta-analysis. Medicine (Baltimore) 2020;99(38):e21910.
10. Karimi Galougahi K, Patel S, Shlofmitz RA, et al. Calcific Plaque Modification by Acoustic Shock Waves: Intravascular Lithotripsy in Coronary Interventions. Circ Cardiovasc Interv 2020;14(1): e009354. https://doi.org/10.1161/CIRCINTERVENTIONS.120.009354.
11. Simplicio CL, Purita J, Murrell W, et al. Extracorporeal shock wave therapy mechanisms in musculoskeletal regenerative medicine. J Clin Orthop Trauma 2020;11(Suppl 3):S309–18.
12. Zou Z-J, Tang L-Y, Liu Z-H, et al. Short-term efficacy and safety of low-intensity extracorporeal shock wave therapy in erectile dysfunction: a systematic review and meta-analysis. Int Braz J Urol 2017; 43(5):805–21.
13. McClure SR, Sonea IM, Evans RB, et al. Evaluation of analgesia resulting from extracorporeal shock wave therapy and radial pressure wave therapy in the limbs of horses and sheep. Am J Vet Res 2005;66(10):1702–8.
14. Katz JE, Clavijo RI, Rizk P, et al. The basic physics of waves, soundwaves, and shockwaves for erectile dysfunction. Sex Med Rev 2020;8(1):100–5.
15. Sokolakis I, Dimitriadis F, Teo P, et al. The basic science behind low-intensity extracorporeal shockwave therapy for erectile dysfunction: a systematic scoping review of pre-clinical studies. J Sex Med 2019;16(2):168–94.
16. Lin G, Reed-Maldonado AB, Wang B, et al. In situ activation of penile progenitor cells with low-intensity extracorporeal shockwave therapy. J Sex Med 2017;14(4):493–501.
17. Li H, Matheu MP, Sun F, et al. Low-energy shock wave therapy ameliorates erectile dysfunction in a pelvic neurovascular injuries rat model. J Sex Med 2016;13(1):22–32.
18. Liu T, Shindel AW, Lin G, et al. Cellular signaling pathways modulated by low-intensity extracorporeal shock wave therapy. Int J Impot Res 2019;31(3): 170–6.
19. Chung E, Cartmill R. Evaluation of clinical efficacy, safety and patient satisfaction rate after low-intensity extracorporeal shockwave therapy for the treatment of male erectile dysfunction: an Australian first open-label single-arm prospective clinical trial. BJU Int 2015;115(Suppl 5):46–9.
20. Vardi Y, Appel B, Jacob G, et al. Can low-intensity extracorporeal shockwave therapy improve erectile function? A 6-month follow-up pilot study in patients with organic erectile dysfunction. Eur Urol 2010; 58(2):243–8.
21. Dong L, Chang D, Zhang X, et al. Effect of low-intensity extracorporeal shock wave on the treatment of erectile dysfunction: a systematic review and meta-analysis. Am J Mens Health 2019;13(2). 1557988319846749.
22. Sokolakis I, Hatzichristodoulou G. Clinical studies on low intensity extracorporeal shockwave therapy for erectile dysfunction: a systematic review and meta-analysis of randomised controlled trials. Int J Impot Res 2019;31(3):177–94.
23. Clavijo RI, Kohn TP, Kohn JR, et al. Effects of low-intensity extracorporeal shockwave therapy on

erectile dysfunction: a systematic review and meta-analysis. J Sex Med 2017;14(1):27–35.

24. Hatzimouratidis K, Giuliano F, Moncada I, et al. EAU guidelines on erectile dysfunction, premature ejaculation, penile curvature and priapism 2019.

25. Burnett AL, Nehra A, Breau RH, et al. Erectile dysfunction: AUA guideline. J Urol 2018;200(3):633–41.

26. POSITION STATEMENT: ED Restorative (Regenerative) Therapies (shock waves, autologous platelet rich plasma, and stem cells). Sexual Medicine Society of North America. Available at: https://www.smsna.org/V1/images/SMSNA_Position_Statement_RE_Restorative_Therapies.pdf. Accessed December 22, 2020.

27. Capogrosso P, Di Mauro M, Fode M, et al. Low-intensity extracorporeal shockwave therapy among urologist practitioners: how the opinion of urologists changed between 2016 and 2019. Int J Impot Res 2020.

28. Towe M, El-Khatib F, Osman M, et al. "Doc, if it were you, what would you do?": a survey of Men's Health specialists' personal preferences regarding treatment modalities. Int J Impot Res 2020.

29. Katz JE, Molina ML, Clavijo R, et al. A phase 2 randomized trial to evaluate different dose regimens of low-intensity extracorporeal shockwave therapy for erectile dysfunction: clinical trial update. Eur Urol Focus 2018;4(3):336–7.

30. Schoofs E, Fode M, Capogrosso P, et al, for the European Association of Urology Young Academic Urologists Men's Health G. Current guideline recommendations and analysis of evidence quality on low-intensity shockwave therapy for erectile dysfunction. Int J Impot Res 2019;31(3):209–17.

31. Vardi Y, Appel B, Kilchevsky A, et al. Does low intensity extracorporeal shock wave therapy have a physiological effect on erectile function? Short-term results of a randomized, double-blind, sham controlled study. J Urol 2012;187(5):1769–75.

32. Kitrey ND, Vardi Y, Appel B, et al. Low intensity shock wave treatment for erectile dysfunction-how long does the effect last? J Urol 2018;200(1):167–70.

33. Patel P, Fode M, Lue T, et al. Should low-intensity extracorporeal shockwave therapy be the first-line erectile dysfunction treatment for nonresponders to phosphodiesterase type 5 inhibition? Eur Urol Focus 2019;5(4):526–8.

34. Kitrey Noam D, Gruenwald I, Appel B, et al. Penile low intensity shock wave treatment is able to shift PDE5i nonresponders to responders: a double-blind, sham controlled study. J Urol 2016;195(5):1550–5.

35. Vinay J, Moreno D, Rajmil O, et al. Penile low intensity shock wave treatment for PDE5I refractory erectile dysfunction: a randomized double-blind sham-controlled clinical trial. World J Urol 2020;39:2217–22. https://doi.org/10.1007/s00345-020-03373-y.

36. Rosen RC, Allen KR, Ni X, et al. Minimal clinically important differences in the erectile function domain of the International Index of Erectile Function scale. Eur Urol 2011;60(5):1010–6.

37. Spivak L, Shultz T, Appel B, et al. Low-Intensity Extracorporeal Shockwave Therapy for Erectile Dysfunction in Diabetic Patients. Sex Med Rev 2019. https://doi.org/10.1016/j.sxmr.2019.06.007. S2050-0521(19)30072-1.

38. Baccaglini W, Pazeto CL, Corrêa Barros EA, et al. The role of the low-intensity extracorporeal shockwave therapy on penile rehabilitation after radical prostatectomy: a randomized clinical trial. J Sex Med 2020;17(4):688–94.

39. Zewin TS, El-Assmy A, Harraz AM, et al. Efficacy and safety of low-intensity shock wave therapy in penile rehabilitation post nerve-sparing radical cystoprostatectomy: a randomized controlled trial. Int Urol Nephrol 2018;50(11):2007–14.

40. Malavaud B, Rostaing L, Rischmann P, et al. High prevalence of erectile dysfunction after renal transplantation. Transplantation 2000;69(10):2121–4.

41. Yamaçake KGR, Carneiro F, Cury J, et al. Low-intensity shockwave therapy for erectile dysfunction in kidney transplant recipients. A prospective, randomized, double blinded, sham-controlled study with evaluation by penile Doppler ultrasonography. Int J Impot Res 2019;31(3):195–203.

42. Kalyvianakis D, Memmos E, Mykoniatis I, et al. Low-intensity shockwave therapy for erectile dysfunction: a randomized clinical trial comparing 2 treatment protocols and the impact of repeating treatment. J Sex Med 2018;15(3):334–45.

43. Patel P, Huang C, Molina M, et al. Clinical trial update on shockwave therapy and future of erectile function restoration. Int J Impot Res 2019;31(3):206–8.

Stem Cell and Gene-Based Therapy for Erectile Dysfunction
Current Status and Future Needs

Ethan L. Matz, MD, Ryan P. Terlecki, MD*

KEYWORDS

- Mesenchymal stem cells • Gene therapy • Erectile dysfunction • Nitric oxide

KEY POINTS

- Stem cell therapy for erectile dysfunction has been effective in improving intracorporal pressure in animal models; small human trials have pointed toward efficacy.
- Gene therapy for erectile dysfunction aims to increase high expression efficacy for upstream genes in the erectogenic pathway and has promising results in models.
- Stem cell and gene therapy for erectile dysfunction are currently appropriate only within the context of clinical trial and should be used with caution.

INTRODUCTION

The high prevalence of erectile dysfunction (ED) and the associated detriment to quality of life for affected men and their partners underscores the need for effective therapy for this troubling condition.[1] Contemporary algorithms for ED management rely on the on-demand use of self-administered medications or surgical placement of a prosthetic device to offset the disease process and allow for sexual activity.[2] Although the introduction of effective oral and injectable agents for ED were revolutionary breakthroughs, no contemporary treatment options have been shown to restore the natural erectile physiology. Additionally, medications may be contraindicated, intolerable, unaffordable, or ineffective in many instances. Mechanical replacement of function, either through external or internal devices, has proven effective for many men, but remains generally less satisfactory than native function and carries associated risk.[3]

Given the large number of factors deemed contributory to development of ED, behavioral modifications (eg, weight loss, exercise, tobacco cessation) and optimization of conditions such as diabetes, hypertension, hypogonadism, and vascular disease are indicated.[4] Even when patients are compliant and successful with such measures, improvements in erectile function tend to be modest and frequently insufficient to meet the needs of most patients.

The desire for restorative, rather than palliative, management strategies for ED has stimulated interest in gene- and cell-based therapies. Herein, we present a brief overview of the relevant physiology and pathophysiology for these targeted therapies, describe the existing data to support these novel therapeutics, and highlight areas for future research. Therapies such low intensity shock wave therapy and platelet-rich plasma (PRP) are also advertised as regenerative therapies for ED.[5–7] Readers interested in energy-based therapies for ED are Raghav Pai and colleagues' article, "Energy-based Therapies for Erectile Dysfunction: Current and Future Directions," in this issue. We do not address PRP in detail in this report because, to our knowledge at the time of this writing, there is a paucity of published peer-reviewed data on this technology for management of ED.

Department of Urology, Wake Forest School of Medicine, Medical Center Boulevard, Winston-Salem, NC 27157, USA
* Corresponding author.
E-mail address: rterlecki@wakehealth.edu

Urol Clin N Am 48 (2021) 611–619
https://doi.org/10.1016/j.ucl.2021.06.014
0094-0143/21/© 2021 Elsevier Inc. All rights reserved.

INSIGHT FROM PHYSIOLOGY

This article is not designed to provide an exhaustive overview of the complex cascade involved in the male erection. However, several steps are relevant to past and current research aimed at identification and further development of restorative therapy. Because the etiology of ED (in the absence of pure psychogenic dysfunction) can involve hormonal, neuronal, or vascular pathology, the targets of investigative research vary.[8]

In the cavernous arteries and spongy tissues of the penile corpora cavernosa, neuronal nitric oxide synthase (nNOS) and endothelial nitric oxide synthase (eNOS) produce nitric oxide, which leads to the production of cyclic guanosine monophosphate (cGMP). The downstream effects of cGMP are mediated by a number of cellular pathways, many of which involve calcium, and result in smooth muscle relaxation, corporal dilation, and subsequent venous occlusion, which ultimately produces an erection.[9] Penile flaccidity returns as cGMP is hydrolyzed by phosphodiesterase type 5 (PDE-5).

Penile innervation is principally supplied by the cavernous nerve originating from the pelvic ganglia and containing both sympathetic and parasympathetic fibers.[10] During pelvic surgery (eg, radical prostatectomy), mechanical or thermal nerve injury may produce changes at the peripheral nerve cell body and target organ, resulting in ED.[11] Fortunately, the peripheral nervous system has a higher recovery potential relative to the central nervous system, and neurotrophins have been shown to result in erectile functional recovery in animal models.[12]

A patient's hormonal balance is also relevant to erectile function. In addition to the physical development of the penis and influence on libido, androgens are also essential to maintaining erectile physiology with an influence on the endothelium as well as the smooth muscle and fibroelastic properties of the corpora cavernosa.[13] Animal studies have demonstrated that decreases in testosterone levels result in changes to adrenergic and nonadrenergic receptor density and responsiveness, as well as alterations in nNOS activity.[14,15] Clinical studies have shown the association between testosterone replacement and improved frequency and rigidity of erections.[16] The conversion of testosterone to estradiol also has complex ramifications to erectile function; research on human tissue has shown that estrogen receptors are abundantly located throughout the corpora and around the neurovascular bundle.[17] Negative feedback mediated by estradiol receptors at the level of the brain and pituitary can result in indirect effects by lowering testosterone. However, direct effects are also possible, because exogenous estrogen has also been shown to lower smooth muscle within the corpora, with a corresponding increase in connective tissue.[18] Of note, estradiol levels were notably higher among men with ED attributed to venous leak, with authors speculating that this process was mediated by an influence on venous tone.[19]

The ultimate goal of any restorative ED therapy is to recreate the neurovascular milieu that permits spontaneous erectile responses. Development of a one-size-fits-all solution is complicated by the variety of etiologies. Thus, it is advantageous to study restorative therapies across a variety of models as vascular end-organ damage is distinct from what occurs after neurogenic injury (eg, after prostatectomy).

Numerous small animal (mostly rodent) models have been developed for studying pathophysiology and treatment response in ED. An early model described by Lue and colleagues[20] was based on ligation of the bilateral internal iliac arteries and could be considered a proxy for severe vascular disease. A cavernous nerve crush injury has been used within a rodent model of ED related to prior pelvic surgery; this approach may be used with or without concomitant internal pudendal bundle ligation.[21] Leuprolide acetate and orchiectomy have both been used to model the human condition of ED related to low serum testosterone levels.[22] A rodent model of ED related to diabetes may be achieved by using either streptozocin injection (models type 1 diabetes) or a high-fat diet in rats with or without propensity to develop abnormalities of glucose metabolism (models type 2 diabetes).[23,24] Another simple model for ED involves the use of aged rats that are otherwise healthy.[25,26]

MESENCHYMAL STEM CELLS

Mesenchymal stem cells (MSC) are a pluripotent adult stem cell population capable of both self-renewal and differentiation into multiple cell lines.[27] There are a variety of sources of MSC. Bone marrow–derived stem cells (BMSC), adipose-derived stem cells (ASC), amniotic fluid stem cells (AFSC), placental stem cells (PSC), and urine-derived stem cells have all been used in animal and human trials for management of ED and/or impaired penile hemodynamics.

The minimally immunogenic state of MSCs makes them an attractive therapeutic option. MSCs express low amounts of MHC class 1 and no MHC class 2 in their undifferentiated state.[28,29] Thus, autologous or allogenic MSC preparations seem practical. Banas and colleagues examined the immunogenic characteristics of amnion-derived multipotent progenitor cells.[30] A low level of MHC 1 were seen and no MHC 2 antigens were detected. Additionally, these cells lacked costimulatory molecules B7-1 and B7-2. Cultured peripheral blood mononuclear cells did not react to these AMPs and actually had an immunomodulatory effect when prompted. Of note, MSC cell types seem to differ slightly in their immunogenic profiles. For example, BMSC seem to be more immunomodulatory than PSC.[31]

The mechanism(s) of MSC-induced functional recovery is/are not well-elucidated. Traditionally, 2 schools of thought existed regarding the therapeutic ability of these cells. These schools include cellular differentiation and direct integration into the target tissue and paracrine effects of the delivered MSC producing a more favorable cellular milieu. The total paracrine effect of the MSCs is not well-known, although the composition of the media produced by the cell has been reported.[32] It is likely that MSC functionality is related to paracrine immunomodulation rather than the direct action of the cells or integration of the cells into the existing matrix.[33,34] Cytokine and growth factor release seems to be the most likely fundamental therapeutic mechanism of stem cells in tissue.

Evidence in support of this hypothesis stems from animal studies indicating that intracavernous injection of conditioned media from PSC induces erectile functional recovery in the form of increased intracorporal pressure/mean arterial pressure ratio at a level just below that of the cellular-based product.[32] Improvement from conditioned media (CM) produced from PSC (acellular) and directly from PSC administration (cellular) resulted in functional recovery to 57.1% and 66.6% of AMC groups, respectively.

Multiple cell-labeling experiments have attempted to track the fate of injected stem cells.[35] Fandel and colleagues labeled ASCs with 5-ethynyl-2-deoxyuridine before intracavernosal injection.[36] They produced ED in their model by crushing the cavernous nerve bilaterally. Histology demonstrated a higher concentration of cells in the major pelvic ganglion and cavernous nerve at the site of injury. Under a dual labeling system described by Dou and colleagues,[37] real-time in vivo imaging demonstrated cell migration to the area of injury at the pelvic crush sites and near immediate washout from the corpora. The proposed mechanism for this migration is still debated; however, Fandel and colleagues[36] postulated that stromal cell-derived factor 1 attracted the ASCs to the site of cavernous nerve injury.

Bone marrow was the first reported source of MSC.[38] In 2010, Kendirci and associates[39] performed intracavernosal injections of BMSC activated by antibodies against p75 nerve growth factor receptor and noted improved erectile function in a rat model. Although both activated and unactivated cells seemed to produce a restorative effect, this effect was more pronounced with activated cells. Another study with BMSCs evaluated the outcomes of injecting cells both intracavernosally and intraperitoneally.[40] Both approaches resulted in some degree of erectile functional recovery. Intracavernosal injection, however, was far superior to intraperitoneal injection with return of function equal to 90% to 100% of sham controls. Although efficacious, bone marrow aspiration to procure stem cells is invasive and tends to provide a low cellular yield.[40,41]

Surgically extracted fat may be used to procure ASC. Adipose tissue is ubiquitous and morally acceptable; although its procurement is not without risk, lipoaspiration is generally better tolerated than other means of MSC procurement.[42] Xu and colleagues[43] used ASC to produce microtissues that were injected into rat corpora, with a comparison arm involving injection of free ASC. Both the microtissues and free ASC resulted in erectile functional recovery, with the microtissues producing a significantly better response. Fandel and colleagues[36] described an animal model where ASC were injected intracavernosally in animals undergoing sham surgery and in another arm with bilateral cavernous nerve injury. Significantly more labeled ASC were seen at the major pelvic ganglion and animals with intracavernosal injection of ASC saw a significantly better recovery of erectile function as measured by intracorporal pressure at 7 and 28 days.

MSC from amniotic and placental sources have also shown promise.[31,44] Extraction of MSC from the mature placenta has become the method of choice as amniocentesis has fallen out of favor. Amniotic fluid cells, not from mature placenta, have been shown to produce erectile functional recovery versus control (saline injected animals), as recorded by maximum intracorporal pressure/mean arterial pressure (0.52, 0.26; $P<.05$) in an animal pelvic neurovascular injury model.[45] Gu and colleagues[46] subsequently evaluated PSC, extracted from mature placenta, also demonstrating functional recovery significantly better than controls (60% improved at the 12 week time point as compared with AMC) as demonstrated by intracorporal pressure/mean arterial pressure. Improved penile hemodynamic response in both of these studies was observed at 12 weeks after injection, implying a durable effect.

Urine-derived stem cells, procured from voided urine samples, are attractive given the ease of procurement, ability to forego enzymatic digestion, and a lower cost profile.[47–49] Animal data suggest that urine-derived stem cells may afford some functional recovery in vitro, but in vivo results from animal model studies are lacking.[50]

A diverse mixture of secreted growth factors, cytokines, and chemokines is present within the CM across MSC subtypes.[41] This "secretome" is of interest as a potential therapeutic modality. Lee and colleagues[51] found that the application of CM from human embryonic stem cells accelerated wound healing. Likewise, Kim and colleagues[52] saw similar changes with increased collagen type 1 deposition using CM from ASC. CM from PSC were examined in vitro and in an animal model to determine cytokine make-up and changes in erectile function.[32] Intracavernosal injection of PSC, CM of PSC, serum-free media, and phosphate-buffered saline, with serum-free media and phosphate-buffered saline acting as controls, was performed in an animal model of neurovascular ED and the intracorporal pressure/mean arterial pressure was recorded at 6 weeks. There was an improvement in the intracorporal pressure/mean arterial pressure by 57.1% and 66.6% in CM of PSC and PSC, respectively.

Despite promising data from animal models, human studies of MSC for the management of ED are scant. The vast majority of published studies are fraught with experimental flaws, low numbers of participants, and absence of control groups. Bahk and colleagues[53] injected umbilical MSC intracavernosally across 7 had patients with ED and diabetes. All 7 patients absence of erections, despite medications, for at least 6 months and received intracavernosal injections of 1.5×10^7 human umbilical cord blood stem cells. When coupled with PDE-5 inhibitors, there was rigidity sufficient for penetration in 2 patients. There were improvements in reported outcomes (International Index of Erectile Function [IIEF-5], Sexual encounter profile, Global Assessment Questionnaire, and erection diary) for up to 11 months in 1 patient.

Yiou and colleagues[54] performed intracavernosal injection of BMSC in 12 men with medication-refractory ED after radical prostatectomy at increasing doses (2×10^7, 2×10^8, 1×10^9, and 2×10^9). Erectile function was assessed with IIEF-15, erection hardness scale, and color duplex Doppler ultrasound examination. At 6 months, there were significant improvement in intercourse satisfaction and erectile function components of the IIEF and improvements of the erection hardness scale (2.6 ± 1.1 and 1.3 ± 0.8,

respectively; $P = .008$). Outcomes seemed to be somewhat dose dependent.

Haahr and colleagues[55] performed a single intracavernosal injection of ASC into 17 men after radical prostatectomy to examine safety. The amount of ASC was proportional to the amount of lipoaspirant with a mean of 1.4×10^5 per gram of fat, correlating with 8.4 to 37.2 million ASC injected. Five patients reported adverse events related to the lipoaspiration or injection that were all minor and included pain at the procedural sites or penile hematoma. Eight of the 17 men treated recovered their erectile function to a level that permitted penetrative sex.

Finally, Levy and coworkers[56] recruited men with ED for at least 6 months with an IIEF of less than 21. All participants refrained from using PDE-5 inhibitors at the time of study and underwent a 4-week washout if used previously. All 8 men previously required injectable medication for erection. One milliliter of PSC diluted in 2 mL of isotonic saline was prepared, and a single injection of 1.5 mL was injected into the base of each corpus cavernosum. The exact number of cells was unknown owing to the proprietary formulation. Evaluation was performed at 6 weeks, 3 months, and 6 months. At follow-up, 3 men were able to achieve erections without additional medications, 4 required low-dose PDE-5 inhibitors, and 1 required additional injectable therapy.

GENE THERAPY

Gene therapy aims to transform the function of existing cell populations. Despite initial interest, the field has been slow to develop secondary to safety concerns related to gene therapy-related deaths in the late 1990s and early 2000s.[57] Unlike approaches to malignancies and systemic inflammatory diseases, where the goal of genetic therapy is high expression efficiency leading to a robust systemic impact, strategies targeting ED aim for minimal cellular perturbation with minimal systemic effects. Gene therapy may be administered with vectors or without (sometimes known as naked DNA).[57] The vector is the package in which the gene is placed, and these vectors are usually viral.[58] The optimal technique for gene transfer, particularly to the penis, remains unclear; however, the benign nature of ED and the local smooth muscle targets allow for plasmid-free, naked DNA, transfer.

The most prominent gene therapy candidate for treatment of ED is the calcium sensitive potassium channels (Maxi-K), a regulator of intracellular calcium.[59] Results from the first human trial of gene transfer of Maxi-K channels were published in

2006.[60] In this study, a single dose of *h*Maxi-K (human) was injected into the corpora of a small group of men who were monitored for 24 weeks. Three men were treated at each of 3 dosages of 500, 1000, and 5000 μg, and 2 men treated at 7500 μg. No adverse events were reported and no plasmids (evidence of residual genetic material) were detected in the semen of the treated men. There was a trend toward improved erectile function on the IIEF that was maintained at 24 weeks at the 2 higher dosages (5000 μg and 7500 μg). Despite apparent safety and possible efficacy, no subsequent studies have been published on this treatment modality.

The investigation of gene therapy to stimulate alternative molecular signaling pathways has included study of nitric oxide synthase (NOS), which is known to be germane to erectile function in men.[9] After intracorporal injection of an adenoviral vector containing the gene for eNOS, aged rats demonstrated increased levels of eNOS, cGMP, and a higher intracorporal pressure as compared with vehicle alone.[61] Another study placed adenoviral vectors containing the eNOS gene into MSC before also performing intracavernosal injection among aged rats.[62] Treated animals manifested increased levels of eNOS protein, NOS activity, and cGMP. Viral vector-based gene therapy specific to nNOS and inducible NOS may improve erectile function in animal models.[63,64] Penile nNOS was transfected into 5-month and 24-month aged rats. intracorporal pressure was increased in aged rats compared with controls when electroporated penile nNOS was transfected into these animals.[63]

Growth factors such as vascular endothelial growth factor (VEGF), neurotrophin-3, glial cell-derived neurotrophic factor (GDNF), and brain-derived neurotrophic factor have been postulated to enhance erectile function. In a diabetic rat model, Bennett and colleagues[65] examined herpes simplex virus (HSV)–mediated neurotrophin-3 transmission. Injection of HSV-NT3 was compared with injection of the β-galactosidase (Lac-z) gene, acting as a control, inserted into HSV. The researchers noted significantly higher density of NOS-stained neurons and higher intracorporal pressure levels in the neurotrophin-3 group as compared with the Lac-z group.

GDNF is part of the transforming growth factor-β family and has a role in the maintenance of autonomic axons.[66] These neurons are found within the penis and GDNF has a role in their survival and regeneration.[67] Two studies by Kato and colleagues[68,69] examined HSV delivery of GDNF and neurturin (NTN) in an animal model of cavernous nerve injury. intracorporal pressure and histology were evaluated at 2 and 4 weeks after the injection of HSV-GDNF and HSV-NTN around the site of injury. At 4 weeks, the intracorporal pressure was significantly improved (approximately twice as high as control) in groups treated with GDNF and NTN when compared with HSV transfected with green fluorescent protein and lacZ. The HSV-NTN groups were shown to have significantly higher levels of fluorogold positive neurons in the major pelvic ganglion than the control groups.

Studies involving animal models have shown that administration of VEGF after arterial injury better facilitates recovery of erectile function, with increased levels of neuronal nitric oxide among treated participants.[70] Animals treated with VEGF, bovine serum albumin, and phosphate-buffered saline at concentrations of 2 and 4 μg were examined at different times. At 6 weeks, there was a significant improvement in erectile function as noted by increased intracorporal pressure/mean arterial pressure.

Choe and colleagues[71] examined sonic hedgehog (SHH), a known regulator of penile smooth muscle. Their laboratory designed a nanofiber hydrogel capable of injection into the cavernosa aimed at extended release after cavernous nerve injury in an animal model. Rats were injected with SHH concentrations of 6.25 μg per rat (1×) or 2× (n = 5). SHH suppressed apoptosis and preserved smooth muscle by 48% while delivering the SHH to the cavernous nerve and cavernosa in combination preserved smooth muscle at 100%.

Although not gene therapy, injection of MSC or platelet-based therapies have been promoted with hopes of increasing the presence of VEGF and possibly improving the density of healthy vascular channels, but washout remains a major concern and the evidence of benefit is lacking. There are minimal human data examining PRP for ED. One small study addressed the safety profile of using PRP for multiple genitourinary conditions.[72]

CONCERNS AND LIMITATIONS

Ethical concerns exist in regard to stem cell and gene therapies. The appealing nature of autologous restorative therapy across the spectrum of disease, coupled with the slow regulatory process, may tempt providers and patients to pursue or offer therapies with poorly understood benefits and risks.[73] Direct-to-consumer marketing in men's health is increasing, evidenced by the ability to obtain prescription medications without ever meeting a provider.[74] Predatory practices by clinics targeting men with ED have been investigated repeatedly and reported in popular news outlets.[75] This multibillion dollar per year industry in the United States has led to unevidenced, expensive, and potentially dangerous interventions.[76] The Sexual Medicine Society of North America has warned against the inappropriate use of cell-based and gene therapies. Although the Sexual Medicine Society of North America recognizes the merits of research and "strongly supports the development of novel erectogenic therapies," they also assert that these novel therapeutics should be considered experimental and administration conducted only under research protocols in compliance with institutional review board approval."[77]

It is important to consider the placebo effect, the phenomenon of improvement in symptoms based on patient belief and desire for a positive outcome. The placebo effect is particularly strong with respect to issues in sexuality; participants in the placebo arm of studies on erectogenic therapy often have statistically meaningful improvements in their self-evaluated erectile function.[78] Younger patients, those with milder ED, and men with substantial psychological dimensions to their ED may be particularly susceptible to this and more hence more likely to fall prey to therapies of unclear verified benefit.[79,80] The possibility of a strong placebo effect must be considered in any study involving a novel therapeutic in a small subset of men with no placebo group (eg, as in most of the human studies of gene and stem cell therapy to date).

FUTURE DIRECTIONS

The future direction of cellular therapies must be large-scale human studies. There are very few, if any, large, randomized, placebo-controlled studies in the field of novel therapeutics for ED. Thus, coordinated multicenter studies of adequate power are required. Efforts must establish safety and efficacy, as well as optimal dosing and delivery. Despite the number of animal studies suggesting benefit, more translation to human trials is essential. Comparisons between cellular and cell-free (eg, CM) therapies should continue as the latter may obviate some cost and ethical concerns if deemed satisfactory.

SUMMARY

Stem cell and gene therapy represent a promising area of study relative to developing truly restorative options for erectile function. The data from animal studies are impressive, but larger human trials are necessary. Given existing fears, it seems important that the future of valuable research isn't jeopardized by opportunists. Both studies and clinical interventions should be conducted ethically, with appropriate patient counseling and fully informed consent.

CLINICS CARE POINTS

- Stem cell and gene therapy for Erectile dysfunction is only currently appropriate within the context of clinical trial.
- Patients asking about stem cell and gene therapy for ED should be informed of the current SMSNA position statement.
- Sexual health and urologic providers can consider participating in well run clinical trials if/when they become approved.

DISCLOSURE

R.P. Terlecki: Consultant/Advisory Board/Grant support for Boston Scientific; Grant support for Department of Defense. E.L. Matz: nothing to disclose.

REFERENCES

1. Araujo A, Mohr B, McKinlay J. Changes in sexual function in middle-aged and older men: longitudinal data from the Massachusetts Male Aging Study. J Am Geriatr Soc 2004;52(9):1502–9.
2. Burnett A, Nehra A, Breau R, et al. Erectile dysfunction: AUA guideline. 2018.
3. Bettocchi C, Palumbo F, Spilotros M, et al. Patient and partner satisfaction after AMS inflatable penile prosthesis implant. J Sex Med 2010;7(1 PART 1): 304–9.
4. Wing RR, Rosen RC, Fava JL, et al. Effects of weight loss intervention on erectile function in older men with type 2 diabetes in the Look AHEAD Trial. J Sex Med 2010;7(1 PART 1):156–65.
5. Li H, Matheu MP, Sun F, et al. Low-energy Shock Wave Therapy Ameliorates Erectile Dysfunction in a Pelvic Neurovascular Injuries Rat Model. J Sex Med 2016;13(1):22–32.
6. Man L, Li G. Low-intensity extracorporeal shock wave therapy for erectile dysfunction: a systematic review and meta-analysis. Urology 2018;119:97–103.
7. Qiu X, Lin G, Xin Z, et al. Effects of low-energy shockwave therapy on the erectile function and tissue of a diabetic rat models. J Sex Med 2009; 6(SUPPL. 6):1–9.
8. Lue TF. Physiology of penile erection and pathophysiology of erectile dysfunction. In: Alan W Partin. Campbell- Philadelphia, PA:Elsevier; Walsh Urology. 26th edition. 2016. p. 612–42.

9. Lue TF. Erectile Dysfunction. N Engl J Med 2000; 342(24):1802–13.

10. Jung J, Jo HW, Kwon H, et al. Clinical neuroanatomy and neurotransmitter-mediated regulation of penile erection. Int Neurourol J 2014;18(2):58–62.

11. Burnett AL. Erectile function outcomes in the current era of anatomic nerve-sparing radical prostatectomy. Rev Urol 2006;8(2):47–53.

12. Chen KC, Minor TX, Rahman NU, et al. The additive erectile recovery effect of brain-derived neurotrophic factor combined with vascular endothelial growth factor in a rat model of neurogenic impotence. BJU Int 2005;95(7):1077–80.

13. Isidori AM, Buvat J, Corona G, et al. A critical analysis of the role of testosterone in erectile function: from pathophysiology to treatment - A systematic review. Eur Urol 2014;65(1):99–112.

14. Reilly C, Stopper V, Mills T. Androgens modulate the alpha-adrenergic responsiveness of vascular smooth muscle in the corpus cavernosum. J Androl 1997;18(1):26–31.

15. Lugg J, Ng C, Rajfer J, et al. Cavernosal nerve stimulation in the rat reverses castration-induced decrease in penile NOS activity. Am J Physiol Endocrinol Metab 1996;271(2 34–2).

16. Chiang HS, Cho SL, Lin YC, et al. Testosterone gel monotherapy improves sexual function of hypogonadal men mainly through restoring erection: evaluation by IIEF score. Urology 2009;73(4):762–6.

17. Dietrich W, Haitel A, Huber JC, et al. Expression of Estrogen Receptors in Human Corpus Cavernosum and Male Urethra. J Histochem Cytochem 2004; 52(3):355–60.

18. Srilatha B, Adaikan PG. Estrogen and phytoestrogen predispose to erectile dysfunction: do ER-α and ER-β in the cavernosum play a role? Urology 2004; 63(2):382–6.

19. Mancini A, Milardi D, Bianchi A, et al. Increased estradiol levels in venous occlusive disorder: a possible functional mechanism of venous leakage. Int J Impot Res 2005;17(3):239–42.

20. El-Sakka a, Yen TS, Lin CS, et al. Traumatic arteriogenic erectile dysfunction: a rat model. Int J Impot Res 2001;13(3):162–71.

21. Bochinski D, Lin GT, Nunes L, et al. The effect of neural embryonic stem cell therapy in a rat model of cavernosal nerve injury. BJU Int 2004;94(6):904–9.

22. Traish AM, Munarriz R, O'Connell L, et al. Effects of medical or surgical castration on erectile function in an animal model. J Androl 2003;24(3):381–7.

23. Castela Â, Costa C. Molecular mechanisms associated with diabetic endothelial-erectile dysfunction. Nat Rev Urol 2016;13(5):266–74.

24. Chiou W-F, Liu H-K, Juan C-W. Abnormal protein expression in the corpus cavernosum impairs erectile function in type 2 diabetes. BJU Int 2010;105(5): 674–80.

25. Lin JSN, Tsai YS, Lin YM, et al. Age-associated changes in collagen content and its subtypes within rat corpora cavernosa with computerized histomorphometric analysis. Urology 2001;57(4):837–42.

26. Davila HH, Rajfer J, Gonzalez-Cadavid NF. Corporal veno-occlusive dysfunction in aging rats: evaluation by cavernosometry and cavernosography. Urology 2004;64(6):1261–6.

27. Park JS, Suryaprakash S, Lao Y-H, et al. Engineering mesenchymal stem cells for regenerative medicine and drug delivery. Methods 2015;84:3–16.

28. Le Blanc K, Tammik C, Rosendahl K, et al. HLA expression and immunologic properties of differentiated and undifferentiated mesenchymal stem cells. Exp Hematol 2003;31(10):890–6.

29. Mangir N, Akbal C, Tarcan T, et al. Mesenchymal stem cell therapy in treatment of erectile dysfunction: autologous or allogeneic cell sources? Int J Urol 2014;21(12):1280–5.

30. Banas RA, Trumpower C, Bentlejewski C, et al. Immunogenicity and immunomodulatory effects of amnion-derived multipotent progenitor cells. Hum Immunol 2008;69(6):321–8.

31. Fazekasova H, Lechler R, Langford K, et al. Placenta-derived MSCs are partially immunogenic and less immunomodulatory than bone marrow-derived MSCs. J Tissue Eng Regen Med 2011;5: 684–92.

32. Matz EL, Thakker PU, Gu X, et al. Administration of secretome from human placental stem cell-conditioned media improves recovery of erectile function in the pelvic neurovascular injury model. J Tissue Eng Regen Med 2020;1–9. https://doi.org/ 10.1002/term.3105.

33. Peak TC, Anaissie J, Hellstrom WJG. Current Perspectives on Stem Cell Therapy for Erectile Dysfunction. Sex Med Rev 2016;4(3):247–56.

34. Lin C-S. Advances in stem cell therapy for the lower urinary tract. World J Stem Cells 2010;2(1):1–4.

35. Lin C-S, Xin Z-C, Wang Z, et al. Stem cell therapy for erectile dysfunction: a critical review. Stem Cells Dev 2012;21(3):343–51.

36. Fandel TM, Albersen M, Lin G, et al. Recruitment of intracavernously injected adipose-derived stem cells to the major pelvic ganglion improves erectile function in a rat model of cavernous nerve injury. Eur Urol 2012;61(1):201–10.

37. Dou L, Matz EL, Gu X, et al. Non-invasive cell tracking with brighter and red-transferred Luciferase for potential application in stem cell therapy. Cell Transplant 2019;28(12):1542–51.

38. Oliveira MS, Barreto-Filho JB. Placental-derived stem cells: culture, differentiation and challenges. World J Stem Cells 2015;7(4):769–75.

39. Kendirci M, Trost L, Bakondi B, et al. Transplantation of nonhematopoietic adult bone marrow stem/progenitor cells isolated by p75 nerve growth factor

receptor into the penis rescues erectile function in a rat model of cavernous nerve injury. J Urol 2010; 184(4):1560–6.

40. Ryu JK, Kim DH, Song KM, et al. Intracavernous delivery of clonal mesenchymal stem cells restores erectile function in a mouse model of cavernous nerve injury. J Sex Med 2014;11(2):411–23.

41. Jayaraman P, Nathan P, Vasanthan P, et al. Stem cells conditioned medium: a new approach to skin wound healing management. Cell Biol Int 2013; 37(10):1122–8.

42. Albersen M, Fandel TM, Lin G, et al. Injections of adipose tissue-derived stem cells and stem cell lysate improve recovery of erectile function in a rat model of cavernous nerve injury. J Sex Med 2010;7(10): 3331–40.

43. Xu Y, Guan R, Lei H, et al. Therapeutic potential of adipose-derived stem cells-based micro-tissues in a rat model of postprostatectomy erectile dysfunction. J Sex Med 2014;11(10):2439–48.

44. Yuan W, Zong C, Huang Y, et al. Biological, immunological and regenerative characteristics of placenta-derived mesenchymal stem cell isolated using a time-gradient attachment method. Stem Cell Res 2012;9(2):110–23.

45. Gu X, Shi H, Matz E, et al. Long-term therapeutic effect of cell therapy on improvement in erectile function in a rat model with pelvic neurovascular injury. BJU Int 2019;124(1):145–54.

46. Gu X, Thakker PU, Matz EL, et al. Dynamic Changes in Erectile Function and Histological Architecture After Intracorporal Injection of Human Placental Stem Cells in a Pelvic Neurovascular Injury Rat Model. J Sex Med 2020;17(3):400–11.

47. Bharadwaj S, Liu G, Shi Y, et al. Characterization of Urine-Derived Stem Cells Obtained from Upper Urinary Tract for Use in Cell-Based Urological Tissue Engineering. Tissue Eng A 2011;17(15–16): 2123–32.

48. Wu S, Wang Z, Bharadwaj S, et al. Implantation of autologous urine derived stem cells expressing vascular endothelial growth factor for potential use in genitourinary reconstruction. J Urol 2011;186(2): 640–7.

49. Liu G, Wang X, Sun X, et al. The effect of urine-derived stem cells expressing VEGF loaded in collagen hydrogels on myogenesis and innervation following after subcutaneous implantation in nude mice. Biomaterials 2013;34(34):8617–29.

50. Wu S, Liu Y, Bharadwaj S, et al. Human urine-derived stem cells seeded in a modified 3D porous small intestinal submucosa scaffold for urethral tissue engineering. Biomaterials 2011;32(5):1317–26.

51. Lee MJ, Kim J, Chung H-M, et al. Enhancement of wound healing by secretory factors of endothelial precursor cells derived from human embryonic stem cells. Cytotherapy 2011;13(2):165–78.

52. Kim W-S, Park B-S, Sung J-H, et al. Wound healing effect of adipose-derived stem cells: a critical role of secretory factors on human dermal fibroblasts. J Dermatol Sci 2007;48(1):15–24.

53. Bahk JY, Jung JH, Han H, et al. Treatment of diabetic impotence with umbilical cord blood stem cell intra-cavernosal transplant: preliminary report of 7 cases. Exp Clin Transplant 2010;8(2):150–60.

54. Yiou R, Hamidou L, Birebent B, et al. Safety of intra-cavernous bone marrow-mononuclear cells for post-radical prostatectomy erectile dysfunction: an open dose-escalation pilot study. Eur Urol 2016;69(6): 988–91.

55. Haahr MK, Jensen CH, Toyserkani NM, et al. Safety and potential effect of a single intracavernous injection of autologous adipose-derived regenerative cells in patients with erectile dysfunction following radical prostatectomy: an open-label phase I clinical trial. EBioMedicine 2016;5:204–10.

56. Levy JA, Marchand M, Iorio L, et al. Determining the feasibility of managing erectile dysfunction in humans with placental-derived stem cells. J Am Osteopath Assoc 2016;116(1):e1–5.

57. Melman A, Davies KP. Gene therapy in the management of erectile dysfunction (ED): past, present, and future. ScientificWorldJournal 2009;9:846–54.

58. Melman A, Rojas L, Christ G. Gene transfer for erectile dysfunction: will this novel therapy be accepted by urologists? Curr Opin Urol 2009;19(6):595–600.

59. Christ G, Spray D, Brinkt P. Characterization of K currents in cultured human corporal smooth muscle cells. J Androl 1993;14(5):319–28.

60. Melman A, Bar-Chama N, McCullough A, et al. hMaxi-K gene transfer in males with erectile dysfunction: results of the first human trial. Hum Gene Ther 2006;17(12):1165–76.

61. Champion HC, Bivalacqua TJ, D'Souza FM, et al. Gene transfer of endothelial nitric oxide synthase to the lung of the mouse in vivo. Circ Res 1999;84(12):1422–32.

62. Bivalacqua TJ, Deng W, Kendirci M, et al. Mesenchymal stem cells alone or ex vivo gene modified with endothelial nitric oxide synthase reverse age-associated erectile dysfunction. Am J Physiol Heart Circ Physiol 2007;292(3):1278–90.

63. Magee TR, Ferrini M, Garban HJ, et al. Gene therapy of erectile dysfunction in the rat with penile neuronal nitric oxide synthase. Biol Reprod 2002;67(3):1033–41.

64. Garbán H, Marquez D, Magee T, et al. Cloning of rat and human inducible penile nitric oxide synthase. Application for gene therapy of erectile dysfunction. Biol Reprod 1997;56(4):954–63.

65. Bennett N, Kim J, Wolfe D, et al. Improvement in erectile dysfunction after neurotrophic factor gene therapy in diabetic rats. J Urol 2005;173(5):1820–4.

66. Markus A, Patel TD, Snider WD. Neurotrophic factors and axonal growth. Curr Opin Neurobiol 2002; 3:523–31.

67. Palma CA, Keast JR. Structural effects and potential changes in growth factor signalling in penis-projecting autonomic neurons after axotomy. BMC Neurosci 2006;7:1–12.

68. Kato R, Wolfe D, Coyle CH, et al. Herpes simplex virus vector-mediated delivery of neurturin rescues erectile dysfunction of cavernous nerve injury. Gene Ther 2009;16(1):26–33.

69. Kato R, Wolfe D, Coyle CH, et al. Herpes simplex virus vector-mediated delivery of glial cell line-derived neurotrophic factor rescues erectile dysfunction following cavernous nerve injury. Gene Ther 2007; 14(18):1344–52.

70. Lee M-C, El-Sakka AI, Graziottin TM, et al. The effect of vascular endothelial growth factor on a rat model of traumatic arteriogenic erectile dysfunction. J Urol 2002;167(2 Pt 1):761–7.

71. Choe S, Kalmanek E, Bond C, et al. Optimization of Sonic hedgehog delivery to the penis from selfas-sembling nanofiber hydrogels to preserve penile morphology after cavernous nerve injury. Nanomedicine 2019. https://doi.org/10.1016/j.nano.2019. 102033.

72. Matz EL, Pearlman AM, Terlecki RP. Safety and feasibility of platelet rich fibrin matrix injections for treatment of common urologic conditions. Investig Clin Urol 2018;59:61–5.

73. Cui T, Kovell R, Brooks D, et al. A Urologist's Guide to Ingredients Found in Top-Selling Nutraceuticals for Men's Sexual Health. J Sex Med 2015;12(11): 2105–17.

74. Shahinyan RH, Amighi A, Carey AN, et al. Direct-to-consumer internet prescription platforms overlook crucial pathology found during traditional office evaluation of young men with erectile dysfunction. Urology 2020. https://doi.org/10.1016/j.urology. 2020.03.067.

75. Houman JJ, Eleswarapu SV, Mills JN. Current and future trends in men's health clinics. Transl Androl Urol 2020;9(I):S116–22.

76. Krader CG. Marketing used by men's health clinics is cause for concern. Urol Times 2020.

77. America SMS of N. POSITION STATEMENT : ED Restorative (Regenerative) Therapies (Shock Waves , Autologous Platelet Rich Plasma , and Stem Cells).; 2020.

78. Chen KK, Hsieh JT, Huang ST, et al. ASSESS-3*: a randomised, double-blind, flexible-dose clinical trial of the efficacy and safety of oral sildenafil in the treatment of men with erectile dysfunction in Taiwan. Int J Impot Res 2001;13(4):221–9.

79. Mulhall JP, Carlsson M, Stecher V, et al. Predictors of Erectile Function Normalization in Men With Erectile Dysfunction Treated With Placebo. J Sex Med 2018;15(6):866–72.

80. Stridh A, Pontén M, Arver S, et al. Placebo responses among men with erectile dysfunction enrolled in phosphodiesterase 5 inhibitor trials: a systematic review and meta-analysis. JAMA Netw Open 2020;3(3):e201423.

UNITED STATES POSTAL SERVICE

Statement of Ownership, Management, and Circulation
(All Periodicals Publications Except Requester Publications)

1. Publication Title	2. Publication Number	3. Filing Date
UROLOGIC CLINICS OF NORTH AMERICA	000 – 711	9/18/2021

4. Issue Frequency	5. Number of Issues Published Annually	6. Annual Subscription Price
FEB, MAY, AUG, NOV	4	$395.00

7. Complete Mailing Address of Known Office of Publication *(Not printer)* *(Street, city, county, state, and ZIP+4®)*
ELSEVIER INC.
230 Park Avenue, Suite 800
New York, NY 10169

Contact Person
Malathi Samayan

Telephone *(Include area code)*
91-44-4299-4507

8. Complete Mailing Address of Headquarters or General Business Office of Publisher *(Not printer)*
ELSEVIER INC.
230 Park Avenue, Suite 800
New York, NY 10169

9. Full Names and Complete Mailing Addresses of Publisher, Editor, and Managing Editor *(Do not leave blank)*

Publisher *(Name and complete mailing address)*
Dolores Meloni, ELSEVIER INC.
1600 JOHN F KENNEDY BLVD. SUITE 1800
PHILADELPHIA, PA 19103-2899

Editor *(Name and complete mailing address)*
KERRY HOLLAND, ELSEVIER INC.
1600 JOHN F KENNEDY BLVD. SUITE 1800
PHILADELPHIA, PA 19103-2899

Managing Editor *(Name and complete mailing address)*
PATRICK MANLEY, ELSEVIER INC.
1600 JOHN F KENNEDY BLVD. SUITE 1800
PHILADELPHIA, PA 19103-2899

10. Owner *(Do not leave blank. If the publication is owned by a corporation, give the name and address of the corporation immediately followed by the names and addresses of all stockholders owning or holding 1 percent or more of the total amount of stock. If not owned by a corporation, give the names and addresses of the individual owners. If owned by a partnership or other unincorporated firm, give its name and address as well as those of each individual owner. If the publication is published by a nonprofit organization, give its name and address.)*

Full Name	Complete Mailing Address
WHOLLY OWNED SUBSIDIARY OF REED/ELSEVIER, US HOLDINGS	1600 JOHN F KENNEDY BLVD. SUITE 1800 PHILADELPHIA, PA 19103-2899

11. Known Bondholders, Mortgagees, and Other Security Holders Owning or Holding 1 Percent or More of Total Amount of Bonds, Mortgages, or Other Securities. If none, check box ☐ None

Full Name	Complete Mailing Address
N/A	

12. Tax Status *(For completion by nonprofit organizations authorized to mail at nonprofit rates) (Check one)*
The purpose, function, and nonprofit status of this organization and the exempt status for federal income tax purposes:
☒ Has Not Changed During Preceding 12 Months
☐ Has Changed During Preceding 12 Months *(Publisher must submit explanation of change with this statement)*

PS Form **3526**, July 2014 *(Page 1 of 4) (see instructions page 4))* PSN: 7530-01-000-9931 **PRIVACY NOTICE:** See our privacy policy on www.usps.com.

---

13. Publication Title	14. Issue Date for Circulation Data Below
UROLOGIC CLINICS OF NORTH AMERICA	MAY 2021

15. Extent and Nature of Circulation

		Average No. Copies Each Issue During Preceding 12 Months	No. Copies of Single Issue Published Nearest to Filing Date
a. Total Number of Copies *(Net press run)*		310	259
b. Paid Circulation *(By Mail and Outside the Mail)*	(1) Mailed Outside-County Paid Subscriptions Stated on PS Form 3541 *(Include paid distribution above nominal rate, advertiser's proof copies, and exchange copies)*	147	117
	(2) Mailed In-County Paid Subscriptions Stated on PS Form 3541 *(Include paid distribution above nominal rate, advertiser's proof copies, and exchange copies)*	0	0
	(3) Paid Distribution Outside the Mails Including Sales Through Dealers and Carriers, Street Vendors, Counter Sales, and Other Paid Distribution Outside USPS®	113	80
	(4) Paid Distribution by Other Classes of Mail Through the USPS *(e.g. First-Class Mail®)*	0	0
c. Total Paid Distribution *(Sum of 15b (1), (2), (3), and (4))*		260	197
d. Free or Nominal Rate Distribution *(By Mail and Outside the Mail)*	(1) Free or Nominal Rate Outside-County Copies included on PS Form 3541	34	46
	(2) Free or Nominal Rate In-County Copies Included on PS Form 3541	0	0
	(3) Free or Nominal Rate Copies Mailed at Other Classes Through the USPS *(e.g. First-Class Mail)*	0	0
	(4) Free or Nominal Rate Distribution Outside the Mail *(Carriers or other means)*	0	0
e. Total Free or Nominal Rate Distribution *(Sum of 15d (1), (2), (3) and (4))*		34	46
f. Total Distribution *(Sum of 15c and 15e)*		294	243
g. Copies not Distributed *(See Instructions to Publishers #4 (page #3))*		16	16
h. Total *(Sum of 15f and g)*		310	259
i. Percent Paid *(15c divided by 15f times 100)*		88.43%	81.06%

*If you are claiming electronic copies, go to line 16 on page 3. If you are not claiming electronic copies, skip to line 17 on page 3.

16. Electronic Copy Circulation

	Average No. Copies Each Issue During Preceding 12 Months	No. Copies of Single Issue Published Nearest to Filing Date
a. Paid Electronic Copies	▲	
b. Total Paid Print Copies (Line 15c) + Paid Electronic Copies (Line 16a)	▲	
c. Total Print Distribution (Line 15f) + Paid Electronic Copies (Line 16a)	▲	
d. Percent Paid (Both Print & Electronic Copies) (16b divided by 16c × 100)	▲	

☒ I certify that 50% of all my distributed copies (electronic and print) are paid above a nominal price.

17. Publication of Statement of Ownership
☒ If the publication is a general publication, publication of this statement is required. Will be printed in the NOVEMBER 2021 issue of this publication. ☐ Publication not required.

18. Signature and Title of Editor, Publisher, Business Manager, or Owner

Malathi Samayan - Distribution Controller

Malathi Samayan Date 9/18/2021

I certify that all information furnished on this form is true and complete. I understand that anyone who furnishes false or misleading information on this form or who omits material or information requested on the form may be subject to criminal sanctions (including fines and imprisonment) and/or civil sanctions (including civil penalties).

PS Form **3526**, July 2014 *(Page 3 of 4)* **PRIVACY NOTICE:** See our privacy policy on www.usps.com.

Printed and bound by CPI Group (UK) Ltd, Croydon, CR0 4YY

08/05/2025

01864697-0009